Integrated Care

Creating Effective Mental and Primary Health Care Teams

Integrated Care

Creating Effective Mental and Primary Health Care Teams

Anna Ratzliff
Jürgen Unützer
Wayne Katon
Kari A. Stephens
University of Washington School of Medicine, Seattle, Washington, USA

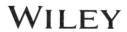

Library of Congress Cataloging-in-Publication Data

Ratzliff, Anna, 1972–, author.
 Integrated care : creating effective mental and primary health care teams / Anna Ratzliff, Jürgen Unützer, Wayne Katon, Kari A. Stephens.
  p. ; cm.
 Includes bibliographical references and index.
 ISBN 978-1-118-90002-4 (pbk.), 978-1-118-90004-8 (e-PDF), and 978-1-118-90003-1 (e-Pub)
 I. Jürgen Unützer, author. II. Katon, Wayne, author. III. Stephens, Kari Astley, author. IV. Title.
 [DNLM: 1. Mental Health Services. 2. Primary Health Care—methods. 3. Delivery of Health Care, Integrated—methods. 4. Evidence-Based Medicine—methods. 5. Mental Disorders—drug therapy. 6. Patient Care Team. WM 30.1]
 RA418
 362.1—dc23
                                        2015036828

Cover design by Wiley
Cover image: ©iStock.com/Jeja

Printed in the United States of America
FIRST EDITION

PB Printing 10 9 8 7 6 5 4 3 2 1

Contents

We dedicate this book to the memory of Wayne Katon, our friend, colleague and mentor. Wayne's research and clinical work for more than three decades helped establish the evidence-base for collaborative care and his ongoing mentorship gave us the practice experience and support to write this book.

—Anna Ratzliff, Jürgen Unützer, Kari A. Stephens

Preface Using Collaborative Care to Create Effective Mental and Primary Health Care Teams

Anna Ratzliff, Wayne Katon, and Jürgen Unützer

What is Collaborative Care?

Collaborative Care is more than just bringing a mental health provider to a primary care setting. In Collaborative Care, a team of providers, including the patient's primary care provider, a behavioral health provider or care manager, and a psychiatric consultant, work together to provide evidence-based mental health care to populations of patients. To provide Collaborative Care, a group of providers must function as a team and share a workflow to provide evidence-based mental health.

Evidence-Based Care: A large body of evidence shows that Collaborative Care improves mental health outcomes in primary care settings. This approach has been recommended as a best practice by the Surgeon General's Report on Mental Health and the President's New Freedom Commission on Mental Health.

Not Care as Usual: Before starting a Collaborative Care program, a team must develop a clear sense of what kind of care will be provided and how success will be measured.

What makes Collaborative Care effective? The principles of Collaborative Care

Although programs may vary in how their team works together, expert consensus suggests that to be effective Collaborative Care addresses the following five principles.

Patient-Centered Team Care: A team of providers effectively work together to provide patient-centered care using a shared care plan.

Population-Based Care: Tracking all patients receiving care proactively through a registry so no patients "fall through the cracks."

Measurement-Based Treatment to Target: Systematic use of clinical outcome measures to support treatment and treatment adjustments.

Evidence-Based Care: Delivery of evidence-based psychosocial and pharmacological treatments.

Accountable Care: The team and the health care organization are responsible for individual patients and patient populations reaching treatment targets and conduct ongoing quality improvement.

How can this book support the work of a Collaborative Care team?

This book is designed to help teams work together to assess for and treat patients with common mental health disorders in a primary care setting. Although many of the evidence-based treatments used to treat common mental health disorders are discussed in subsequent chapters, this book is not meant to be a comprehensive guide on how to deliver all aspects of care. This book models how the tasks required to successfully assess and treat patients for common mental health disorders can be shared by a team using Collaborative Care. Additionally, this book:

- Helps teams develop integrated workflows and facilitate effective communication about common clinical problems that the team will encounter.
- Can be shared by the whole team so that each team member may better understand the work of the other team members.
- Focuses on adult populations. Although there are Collaborative Care models for pediatric populations, the majority of conditions and treatments reviewed here are for adult populations.
- Provides a quick overview of each team member's role in assessment and treatment in each chapters' "working as a team" boxes.
- Offers quick access to answers to the following common questions when sharing a clinical workflow:
  - What is my role in the care of this patient?
  - How will the other team members work with the patient?
  - How can we share care more effectively?

This book is designed for a Collaborative Care team that is already working together. If you have not yet started working as a team, a more formal team building process will be an important first step to form a Collaborative Care Team. We encourage you consider looking at the following resources:

UWAIMS Center: http://aims.uw.edu/

Qualis Safety-Net Medical Home Initiative: http://www.safetynetmedicalhome.org/change-concepts

SAMSHA/HRSA: http://www.integration.samhsa.gov/workforce/teammembers

How would this patient be treated in the clinic system you work in?

This book will help your team provide a structured, team approach, providing effective care for the common mental health disorders encountered in primary care settings. As an introduction to this book we want you to consider the following patient and the care the patient would receive in your clinic setting.

Case

Mr A, 31-year-old male, presents to his primary care doctor asking for "sleeping pills." His PCP takes a history and finds out he has not been sleeping well for the last month, he has been struggling to get work and missed a few days, he has difficulty concentrating and his wife is frustrated because he has "just checked out." His PCP suspects he may be experiencing depression.

- How much of this patient's care would you be able to provide in your primary care setting?
- Which providers would work with this patient? Would you work as a team?
- How would you make a diagnosis?
- Do you have a system to make sure he would not "fall through the cracks" if he missed a follow-up appointment?
- How would you track his response to treatment?
- Do you have experience with the evidence-based treatments you might need to treat him to achieve remission?
- What tools and resources would you use to help you treat him?
- Do you have a system in place to monitor the quality of care delivered at your clinic?

Now consider how the Principles of Collaborative Care can influence Mr. A's treatment:

Case example:
- **Patient centered team care:** Mr. A's PCP introduces him to Collaborative Care and the idea that a team of providers will work with him to provide care for his depression right in the primary care clinic. That very first day he meets his Care Manager (a licensed behavioral health professional), starts a mental health assessment and is offered information about depression treatment options. His Care Manager also recognizes how much Mr. A's sleep disturbance is bothering him, so she discusses sleep hygiene with him on that first visit.

(Continued)

- **Population-based care:** The Care Manager enters Mr. A into the clinic patient registry. This is an important step because Mr A missed his follow-up visit due to oversleeping. His Care Manager is able to engage Mr A over the phone to return for follow-up care at the next available appointment. This approach allows the team to track all the current patients being followed for depression in the clinic and make sure no patients "fall through the cracks."
- **Measurement-based treatment to target:** At every visit, Mr A's team makes sure he completes a depression measure (in this case the Patient Health Questionaire-9) to assess the severity of his symptoms. Mr A is started on antidepressant medication but needs several adjustments before this medication is effective. Using measurement to assess depression helps the team make decisions about when to intensify treatment.
- **Evidence-based care:** After the initial assessment, Mr A's Care Manager discusses his case with the psychiatric consultant by presenting his case over the telephone. Although the psychiatric consultant does not meet Mr A, the psychiatric consultant is able to provide guidance about evidence-based medication treatment and brief behavioral interventions validated for use in primary care to treat depression. The psychiatric consultant is also available to provide guidance to the PCP about intensification of medication treatment for Mr A's depression.
- **Accountable care:** On the patient level, the whole team is committed to adjusting Mr A's treatment until his depression symptoms are significantly improved. At an organizational level, the team that takes care of Mr A engages in regular quality improvement efforts. For example, when they examine their data on follow-up visits, the team realizes that many patients miss their early follow-up visits. The clinic begins a program to track follow-up visits and make outreach phone calls for missed appointments. These quality improvement efforts provide the accountability the clinical team needs to systemically improve outcomes.

Mr A's depression goes into remission, and he is able to continue working and improve his relationship with his wife. By using Collaborative Care, Mr. A's team is able to deliver high-quality care that improves outcomes, is associated with high patient satisfaction, and contains cost.

Book structure

Each of the clinical chapters in this book follows a format designed to make it easy for the clinical team to work together to assess and treat patients. Readers performing any of the roles on a Collaborative Care team can read this book and learn practical skills from its case examples. Each chapter will start with a general overview of the condition in the **Clinical Impact** section. Team assessment is often a new skill for providers who have generally completed this step on their own. The **Assessment** section breaks the patient assessment process down into two phases. Finally, the **Treatment** section breaks down treatment into the three phases.

The **Working as a Team** sections provide a sample case and an outline of how a team can share the assessment and treatment responsibilities. More detailed resources on the evidence-based treatment for common psychiatric disorders exist, and this book is no replacement. Rather our chapters outline principles unique to a Collaborative Care team approach to assessment and treatment in a primary care setting. Special attention is devoted to highlighting how the principles of Collaborative Care may be incorporated into the treatment process. Additional information about effective treatment strategies for the Collaborative Care team is reviewed in two chapters: Chapter 10, "Evidence-Based Psychopharmacology for the Collaborative Care Team," and Chapter 11, "Evidence-Based Behavioral Interventions for the Collaborative Care Team."

Toolkit inventory checklist

Team members working together to provide Collaborative Care as a team is often a new way of working. The following checklist can be helpful in assessing if your team has all the tools and skills needed to begin working as a Collaborative Care team. This list is not comprehensive, but gives a categorical list of basic tools, procedures, and protocols needed across the team to be effective.

Collaborative Care toolkit inventory

Principles	Toolkit inventory	Yes?	For more information
Patient-Centered Team Care	Introducing the Integrated Care Team Approach	☐	Chapter 1
	Team Communication Strategies	☐	Chapter 1
	Psychoeducation	☐	Chapter 1, Diagnosis Specific Chapters
	Team Goal Setting	☐	Chapter 1, Chapter 10

(Continued)

(*Continued*)

Principles	Toolkit inventory	Yes?	For more information
Population-Based Care	Effective Engagement	☐	Chapter 10
	Registry Tracking	☐	Chapter 1, Appendix
	Caseload Management	☐	Chapter 1
Tracking and Treatment to Target	Use of Behavioral Health Measures	☐	Chapter 1, Diagnosis Specific Chapters, Appendix
	Measurement Based Practice	☐	Chapter 1, Diagnosis Specific Chapters
	Stepped Care Approach	☐	Chapter 1, Diagnosis Specific Chapters
Evidence-Based Practices	Differential Diagnosis Techniques	☐	Chapter 1, Diagnosis Specific Chapters
	Evidence-Based Behavioral Interventions	☐	Diagnosis Specific Chapters, Chapter 10
	Evidence-Based Psychopharmacology	☐	Diagnosis Specific Chapters, Chapter 11
	Suicidal and Homicidal Protocols	☐	Online Materials
	Crisis Management	☐	Chapter 9, Online Materials
Accountable Practice	Quality Improvement Goals	☐	Chapter 1
	Quality Improvement Approach	☐	Chapter 1

Acknowledgments

"We thank the many patients and providers who have worked with us to learn how to deliver more effective mental health care in primary care settings and inspire us to continuously to improve the care we deliver.

"We also would like to thank the AIMS Center staff with special appreciation to Lindsay Baldwin, Melissa Farnum, Alan Godjics, Andrea Panniero and Rebecca Sladek for their support in this effort."

Integrated Care

Creating Effective Mental and Primary Health Care Teams

Chapter 1 Working as a Team to Provide Collaborative Care

Anna Ratzliff, Joseph Cerimele, Wayne Katon, and Jürgen Unützer

Effective integration of mental and primary health care requires the effective sharing of tasks among members of a Collaborative Care team that works together with the patient as the center of the team's efforts. This chapter reviews typical team-member roles, a model of a shared clinical workflow, and core Collaborative Care skills and tools.

Collaborative Care team roles

Focusing on the function, rather than title or previous role, of team members ensures that all the critical tasks of a Collaborative Care program are delivered to provide effective patient care. A formal team-building process can facilitate Collaborative Care implementation. Common roles on a Collaborative Care team include (Figure 1.1):

- Patient
  - The most important person on the team!
  - Works with the primary care provider (PCP) and the behavioral health provider (BHP)/care manager (CM).
  - Reports changes in health, symptoms, and functioning.
  - Sets goals for treatment with the team.
  - Tracks clinical progress using patient-reported outcome measures.
  - Asks questions and discusses concerns about care.
  - Understands treatment plan, including goals of behavioral interventions and names/doses of medications.

Integrated Care: Creating Effective Mental and Primary Health Care Teams, First Edition.
Anna Ratzliff, Jürgen Unützer, Wayne Katon, and Kari A. Stephens.
© 2016 John Wiley & Sons, Inc. Published 2016 by John Wiley & Sons, Inc.

- Primary care provider (PCP)
  - Clinician degrees may include MD, DO (doctor of osteopathic medicine), ARNP (advanced registered nurse practitioner), and NP (nurse practitioner).
  - Oversees all aspects of patient's care.
  - Introduces Collaborative Care team, often with "warm handoff."
  - Diagnoses common mental disorders.
  - Prescribes medications to treat psychiatric illnesses as appropriate.
  - Adjusts treatment in consultation with BHP/care manager, psychiatric consultant, and other behavioral health providers.
- Behavioral health provider (BHP)
  - Clinician degrees may include MSW, LCSW, RN, MA, PhD, and PsyD.
  - Works closely with PCP and helps manage a caseload of patients in primary care (care manager).
  - Facilitates patient engagement and education.
  - Performs structured initial and follow-up assessments.
  - Systematically tracks treatment response using behavioral health measures.
  - Provides brief, evidence-based behavioral interventions or refers to other BHP for these services.
  - Supports medication management by PCPs.
    - Helps patient identify where to get medications.
    - Encourages and supports medication adherence.
    - Brings concerns about medications or side effects to PCP, and schedules PCP visit to adjust treatments as appropriate.
  - Reviews challenging patients in systematic, weekly case review with the psychiatric consultant.
  - Facilitates referrals to other services (e.g., substance abuse treatment, specialty care, and community resources) as needed.
  - Prepares patient for relapse prevention.
- Psychiatric consultant (PC)
  - Psychiatrist or other expert in psychiatry and psychopharmacology.
  - Supports PCPs and BHPs, providing regular (weekly) and as-needed consultation on a caseload of patients followed in primary care.
  - Focuses on patients who are not improving and who need treatment adjustment or intensification.
  - Available to provide in-person or telemedical consultation or, for complex or persistently ill patients, referral.
  - Provides education and training for primary care providers and BHPs as appropriate.

- Other behavioral health providers
  - These may include chemical dependency counselors or other licensed behavioral health professionals.
  - Deliver specialized evidence-based counseling/psychotherapy (individual or group).
  - Support behavioral health interventions focused on health behaviors.
  - Provide chemical dependency counseling/treatment.
  - Facilitate other mental health or substance abuse services.
- Other partners important to include in team building
  - CEO, administrators, medical directors, clinic managers.
  - Medical and mental health leaders/champions.
  - Receptionists/front desk staff, medical assistants.

Collaborative Care shared workflow

A typical course of Collaborative Care will involve contributions from the entire team over a relatively short period of time. Figure 1.2 shows a typical course of Collaborative Care for a common mental health disorder, such as depression. Patients will be identified, assessed, and treated, and complete an episode of care, including relapse prevention.

Figure 1.3 shows common tasks accomplished as part of Collaborative Care. Some clinics may add additional tasks to meet the needs of specific populations or to target specific health problems. For each task, a team will need to decide how, when, where, and by whom the task will be completed as part of a shared workflow. A shared clinical flowchart can be useful to illustrate the process of care when a patient comes to the clinic. Handoffs and communication among team members require special attention. Every clinic's flowchart will be unique.

Core Collaborative Care skills and tools

Skills training (summarized below) will need to be completed before launching a Collaborative Care program.

Introducing the Collaborative Care team approach to the patient

It is important to introduce the patient to the concept of team-based care and to explain how a team of providers will work together to deliver care in the familiar primary care setting. One of the best ways to do this is to have the PCP introduce the patient to the BHP in person, providing a "warm handoff."

Collaborative Care Team Structure

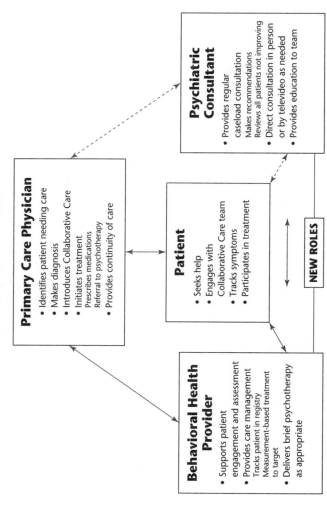

Figure 1.1 Model integrated behavioral health team: There are two new roles added to the primary care setting, a behavioral health provider and a psychiatric consultant. The solid arrows indicate regular communication and the dashed arrows represent as-needed communication.

	Initial Assessment	Initial Treatment	Follow-Up Treatment			Completion and Relapse Prevention
Time In Treatment	Week 1	Week 1	Weeks 2–Week 16			Week 16 and Beyond
PCP	X	X	X		X	X
BHP	X	X	X X X X X X X X X			X
Psychiatric Consultant		X	X	X	X	X

Figure 1.2 Typical timeline of treatment in Collaborative Care.

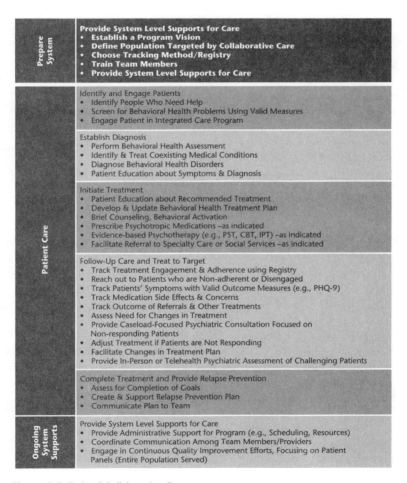

Prepare System

Provide System Level Supports for Care
- **Establish a Program Vision**
- **Define Population Targeted by Collaborative Care**
- **Choose Tracking Method/Registry**
- **Train Team Members**
- **Provide System Level Supports for Care**

Patient Care

Identify and Engage Patients
- Identify People Who Need Help
- Screen for Behavioral Health Problems Using Valid Measures
- Engage Patient in Integrated Care Program

Establish Diagnosis
- Perform Behavioral Health Assessment
- Identify & Treat Coexisting Medical Conditions
- Diagnose Behavioral Health Disorders
- Patient Education about Symptoms & Diagnosis

Initiate Treatment
- Patient Education about Recommended Treatment
- Develop & Update Behavioral Health Treatment Plan
- Brief Counseling, Behavioral Activation
- Prescribe Psychotropic Medications –as indicated
- Evidence-based Psychotherapy (e.g., PST, CBT, IPT) –as indicated
- Facilitate Referral to Specialty Care or Social Services –as indicated

Follow-Up Care and Treat to Target
- Track Treatment Engagement & Adherence using Registry
- Reach out to Patients who are Non-adherent or Disengaged
- Track Patients' Symptoms with Valid Outcome Measures (e.g., PHQ-9)
- Track Medication Side Effects & Concerns
- Track Outcome of Referrals & Other Treatments
- Assess Need for Changes in Treatment
- Provide Caseload-Focused Psychiatric Consultation Focused on Non-responding Patients
- Adjust Treatment if Patients are Not Responding
- Facilitate Changes in Treatment Plan
- Provide In-Person or Telehealth Psychiatric Assessment of Challenging Patients

Complete Treatment and Provide Relapse Prevention
- Assess for Completion of Goals
- Create & Support Relapse Prevention Plan
- Communicate Plan to Team

Ongoing System Supports

Provide System Level Supports for Care
- Provide Administrative Support for Program (e.g., Scheduling, Resources)
- Coordinate Communication Among Team Members/Providers
- Engage in Continuous Quality Improvement Efforts, Focusing on Patient Panels (Entire Population Served)

Figure 1.3 Tasks of Collaborative Care.

Another communication strategy is to use a flyer to introduce the care team and each team member's role.

Key information to be shared with the patient:
- The patient is an important member of the team.
- All team members will share one treatment plan to support patient-centered goals.
- The PCP will oversee all aspects of patient care at the clinic.
- The care manager works closely with the patient and the PCP to implement a treatment plan, including keeping track of treatment progress and providing counseling.
- The psychiatric consultant does not see all patients in person but provides valuable expertise to guide treatment for all patients.

Team functioning

Sharing care is often a new skill for care-team members. Effective communication is fundamental to providing high-quality shared care. One of the major challenges to team function around behavioral health is that providers have often trained in "cultures" with different orientations. This culture clash can make it difficult to plan and implement truly integrated behavioral health plans, unless effective team building occurs.

Key strategies to strengthen team functioning include:

Sharing goals: Describe a clear set of behavioral health goals at the organization level. At the patient level, the goal is to have one treatment plan that is shared by all team members. This will often require practical troubleshooting in how to document and share information in electronic medical record systems.

Building mutual trust: Consider opportunities to foster mutual trust and skill building among the care team. Sharing patient success stories and challenges at provider meetings can strengthen team members' commitment to sharing care.

Clarifying roles and workflow: Taking time to establish clear roles and shared workflows is important to support effective teamwork. Workflows should be regularly reviewed as a team to identify areas in which additional problem solving is needed.

Strengthening communication strategies: Agree on communication strategies, including in-person communication, tasking or electronic communication, or using the electronic medical record. Consider daily or weekly huddles to facilitate rapid team communication around challenging patients and organizing team priorities.

Accountable practice

The core concept of accountable clinical care is identifying goals, defining ways to measure those goals, and then regularly reviewing progress toward goals. Accountable practice is key for effective Collaborative Care at the patient and population levels. Common targets for behavioral health teams include access to care, number of patients served, patient satisfaction, patient-reported outcomes using standard measurements (such as the Patient Health Questionnaire, or PHQ-9, for depression), and costs. Many teams find using familiar quality-improvement strategies, such as a Plan-Do-Study-Act (PDSA) cycle, helpful in supporting accountable practice.

Key strategies for accountable care include:

Identify goals: All team members should have a clear understanding of both patient- and program-level goals.

Define measurements: Identify key measurements and strategies to obtain data on these measures in your organization.

Review progress: Regular review of data can help all team members identify areas for improvement. If real-time data on key measures are available, any member of the behavioral health team can examine current data on both process and outcome data to assess progress toward shared goals. This allows teams to nimbly respond to unmet goals.

Registry

A registry is a list of all the patients currently being cared for by a provider or clinic, and is used to keep track of a defined population of patients. Registries allow teams to track patient progress and to reach out to patients who have been identified in the registry as needing help but may have "fallen through the cracks." This concept may be familiar to primary care practitioners, as many clinics keep registries for other chronic medical conditions, such as diabetes. Using a registry, or having the ability to proactively engage patients in care when they have been "lost to follow-up," is especially important with mental health disorders such as depression and anxiety, as symptoms of these disorders often include isolation and low motivation. (See online materials for more information on registries.)

Key strategies for effective registry use:

- Typically, each patient is assigned to a specific behavioral health care manager. Date of enrollment, dates of follow-up contacts, and scores on outcome measures (such as the PHQ-9) are examples of information commonly included in a registry.

- More sophisticated registries have such capabilities as reporting percent improvement for a patient, percentage of the entire patient panel population improved, or reminders for key clinical processes.

Collaborative Care assessment

This information is not meant to replace detailed resources on patient assessment; rather, this book outlines principles for how a team can share assessment of patients in primary care. Special attention is devoted to highlighting how Collaborative Care principles may be incorporated into the assessment process.

Identify chief complaint, associated somatic and psychological symptoms, functional impairment, and safety concerns

Clinicians will identify patients either when they present with symptoms of a mental health disorder or through routine screening of patient populations. The PCP and CM work together to gather enough history to generate a differential diagnosis.

- **Measures:** Consider using standard measures to assess common symptoms, such as depression and anxiety symptoms. Some measurement tools can also be used to track response to treatment.
- **Past mental health history:** Number and severity of previous mental health episodes, and experience with mental health treatments.
- **Current and past history of alcohol or substance use:** Use of prescription or nonprescription drugs or alcohol. History of prior substance abuse treatment.

Common psychological symptoms

Mood and anxiety symptoms, enjoyment/quality of life, relationships, social activities, work or employment status, hobbies, and sex.

Common physical/Somatic symptoms

Physical symptoms such as acute or chronic pain; physical activities such as walking, eating, and sleeping; and side effects of medications.

Common functional impairments

Activities of daily living (how does the patient spend his/her day?). How are symptoms impacting function?

Assessment of safety

All team members should remember this important part of assessment.

- **Self-harm:** Self-harm or suicidal ideation, or history of suicide attempts or other self-harm, such as cutting, or other high-risk behaviors.
- **Thoughts of harming others and other safety risks:** Serious inability to care for self (grave disability) and environmental or social issues posing safety risks: housing/shelter risks, violence (i.e., domestic violence and other dangerous social circumstances).

Team goal: Identify the chief complaint, initial physical exam, gather history, and safety assessment

In most clinics, the PCP will conduct the preliminary steps as part of routine care and then refer to the BHP for additional assessment. Some clinics may opt to routinely screen vulnerable patient populations for common mental health and substance use problems. Especially important will be to plan for consistent safety assessment by all clinic staff.

Working as a team

Patient: Describes symptoms, how symptoms impact daily life, desired treatment goals, and relevant history, such as prior treatments, to the PCP and BHP. Completes measurement tools as part of initial assessment. Shares symptoms of past and current suicidal ideation with the treatment team, informs the team if symptoms worsen. Shares psychosocial and risk factors with the treatment team.

PCP: Gathers health history, conducts physical exam, reviews results from diagnostic studies, and begins to formulate an assessment. Fosters a therapeutic alliance with the patient, introduces the team approach to behavioral health, and provides an introduction to the BHP. Assesses for safety, coordinates with BHP to monitor safety issues and implement treatment plan.

BHP: Completes detailed assessment of psychiatric, social, and substance use history; use of coping strategies; and readiness to engage in self-management. Prompts patient to complete measurement tools. Assesses safety issues and helps with safety planning. Tracks safety plan.

PC: Assists in identifying and evaluating psychiatric symptoms. May suggest additional assessment. Assists in safety planning as needed.

Typical Timeline, Week 1

BHP: Visit 1–2
PCP: Visit 1–2

Case example

31-year-old male, presents to his primary care doctor asking for "sleeping pills." His PCP takes a history and finds out he has not been sleeping well for the last month, he has been struggling to get work and has missed a few days, he has difficulty concentrating, and his wife is frustrated because he has "just checked out." His PCP suspects he may be experiencing depression. Mr. A's PCP introduces him to Collaborative Care and the idea that a team of providers will care for him and treat depression in the primary care clinic. That first day he meets his BHP/care manager, who starts a mental health assessment, including a safety evaluation. Mr. A's team makes sure he completes a depression measure (in this case, the PHQ-9) to measure his symptoms. Mr. A's BHP/care manager enters him into the clinic patient registry. Mr. A is also scheduled for a close follow-up appointment to make sure he quickly is engaged in care.

Differential diagnosis and identifying a provisional diagnosis

Rule out common contributing medical problems and substance-related conditions

Some medical conditions can cause, contribute to, or mimic symptoms of mental illness.

- **Medical conditions:** Identify possible medical symptoms that present as psychological symptoms. In general, lab tests are indicated only if there is concern about a particular medical diagnosis.
- **Substance-related conditions:** Consider that substance abuse, withdrawal, or intoxication may present as psychological symptoms.

Develop and refine the differential diagnosis as a Collaborative Care team

A good differential diagnosis is needed to inform decisions regarding evidence-based treatment for behavioral health disorders. Chief complaint, associated somatic and psychological symptoms, and current level of functional impairment related to any symptoms must be assessed. This information helps teams develop an informed provisional diagnosis, which leads to an appropriate integrated-care treatment plan. However, developing a differential diagnosis as a team differs from developing one as an individual clinician. Each team member has an important role in developing differential and provisional/working diagnoses. Table 1.1 illustrates key questions and team goals helpful in generating differential diagnosis.

Table 1.1 Generating a differential diagnosis

Question	Key team goals	Further assessment
Are presenting symptoms caused by a medical problem?	PCP should consider medical causes for all presenting problems. Other team members may also identify medical problems for the PCP to consider.	Refer back to PCP for any medical concerns. Acute concerns are referred for urgent evaluation as appropriate.
Is this distress or a mental health disorder?	Functional assessment helps differentiate life distress from a mental health disorder. All mental health disorders cause significant functional impairment as criteria for diagnosis.	A patient with psychological distress but no formal mental disorder may only need brief supportive engagement and treatment instead of ongoing care management.
Is there a mood disorder?	Depressed mood is a common presentation. The team must work together to differentiate unipolar depression from bipolar disorder. Screening for mania or mixed bipolar disorder symptoms is an important part of assessment of every patient presenting with depression. • The PHQ-9 is widely used to screen for depression and to monitor treatment response. • The CIDI-3 brief structured interview for bipolar disorder can be used to assess for bipolar disorder in patients with depression.	Depression alone → Major Depression chapter Depression + history concerning for bipolar disorder → Bipolar Disorder chapter
Is there an anxiety- or trauma-related disorder?	Anxiety symptoms, including somatic symptoms of anxiety restlessness or feeling of fast heart rate, are common presentations in primary care. • Generalized anxiety disorder (GAD): Have you been worrying excessively for greater than six months? Are you a worrier?	See Anxiety and Trauma Disorders chapter for additional assessment.

(Continued)

Table 1.1 (*Continued*)

Question	Key team goals	Further assessment
	• Panic disorder: Do you experience sudden attacks of anxiety or unexplained physical symptoms, such as rapid heartbeat, shortness of breath, or chest tightness? • Social anxiety disorder: Are you uncomfortable in or do you avoid social situations? • Post-traumatic stress disorder (PTSD): Do you have a history of trauma or abuse with nightmares and flashbacks? • Obsessive-compulsive disorder (OCD): Do you have any repetitive or intrusive thoughts or behaviors that bother you?	
Is there a substance use disorder?	Asking about substance use and considering urine toxicology can be helpful to identify substance use disorders in primary care. Symptoms can be caused by intoxication or withdrawal from substances as well. • For alcohol: Use the Audit-C three-item measure • For other substances: "In the past year have you used an illegal drug or used a prescription medication such as a narcotic pain pill for nonmedical reasons or more often than prescribed?"	See Substance Use chapter for additional assessment.
Is the patient experiencing psychotic symptoms?	Patients may complain of depression or other negative schizophrenia symptoms such as loss of motivation or anhedonia. Active psychotic symptoms can range from patients reporting auditory hallucinations to subtle symptoms such as concrete or disorganized thinking. Delusional thoughts or ideas of reference (patients reading special meaning into common occurrences) or thought broadcasting	See Psychosis chapter for additional assessment.

Table 1.1 (*Continued*)

Question	Key team goals	Further assessment
	(other people can hear the patient's thoughts) can occur and should be assessed for.	
	• Is the psychosis recent in onset or chronic? • Are the symptoms changing or are they fairly stable over time?	
Is there an acute safety concern?	This is a crucial step because suicidal thoughts can lead to a suicide attempt. Safety concerns require development of a safety plan. Common safety concerns: danger to self (suicidal ideation, domestic violence situations), danger to others, grave disability (inability to take care of self due to a mental health condition putting the individual at risk of serious harm).	Every clinic should have a clear active suicide protocol developed as part of implementation. Clearly defining whose role it is to manage acute safety concerns should be part of team building. (See online materials for additional information.)
Is there another mental health presentation?	If the patient has screened negative for all the above disorders but still presents with significant functional distress, consider screening for other common presentations, such as chronic pain, attention-deficit hyperactivity disorder (ADHD), or dysfunctional coping style. Consult with PC or refer for additional treatment as appropriate.	Pain can cause functional impairment. See Chronic Pain chapter for additional assessment. Patient presenting with inability to concentrate and/or focus as an isolated symptom or after other mental health comorbidity is treated could have ADHD. See ADHD chapter for additional assessment. The team is struggling with difficult patient interactions; see Challenging Clinical Situations chapter for additional assessment.

Table 1.2 Common conditions in primary care

Behavioral health care in primary care settings focuses on mental health problems commonly encountered in this setting. In each chapter common ICD10 codes will be listed here for easy reference.

Assessment of comorbid psychiatric disorders and psychological difficulties

Many mental health problems are comorbid with both medical and other mental health diagnoses. Common co-occurring illnesses for each disorder are discussed in individual chapters. These are often identified as part of the differential diagnosis process and treatment planning.

Identifying a provisional diagnosis

The differential diagnosis process results in a provisional/working diagnosis (See Table 1.2). Team members may also identify comorbid medical or psychiatric disorders. This provisional diagnosis will inform recommendations for evidence-based treatment. All team members should understand the provisional diagnosis. Team members will learn additional clinical information about the patient, including observations of the patient, over time. Additional observations and information may lead to changes in diagnosis. Tracking a patient over time and adjusting diagnosis and treatment as needed is one of the strengths of Collaborative Care.

Team goal: Generate differential diagnosis and establish provisional diagnosis

Team members share significant information to ensure treatment planning is patient-centered, appropriate, safe, and effective. Discover the mental health comorbidities that should be addressed as part of a comprehensive and effective treatment plan.

Working as a team

Patient: Describes health and mental health history. Works with PCP and BHP and follows through on recommended diagnostic testing; reports patterns of medication use and potential side effects; tracks and reports physical and social activities as recommended by the BHP.

   PCP: Evaluates possible medical problems using diagnostic testing and medical consultation as appropriate. Considers common diagnoses and refers to

BHP for additional assessment as needed. Continues to provide general medical care and prescribes medications for common mental health disorders as clinically indicated.

BHP: Conducts a thorough psychosocial assessment. Works with the PCP and PC to work through differential diagnoses to refine mental health treatment targets and plan.

PC: Expands medical and psychiatric differential diagnosis and recommends additional assessment as needed. Assists BHP in differential diagnosis.

Typical Timeline Week 1
BHP: Visit 1–2
PCP: Visit 1–2

Case example
Mr. A's team works together to develop a differential for his presenting symptoms of insomnia. The PCP generates an initial diagnosis of depression after excluding obvious medical comorbidity, such as sleep apnea. This diagnosis is further assessed by the BHP/care manager, who assesses for bipolar disorder, anxiety disorders, and substance use disorders, none of which are found. The BHP/care manager focuses on understanding current functional impairments and Mr. A's goals for treatment.

Collaborative Care treatment

Treatment in Collaborative Care can be broken down into three key phases: (a) initiation of treatment, (b) follow-up and treatment to target, and (c) completion of treatment and relapse prevention. Effective treatment strategies for the Collaborative Care team are reviewed in two chapters: Chapter 10, "Evidence-Based Psychopharmacology for the Collaborative Care Team," and Chapter 11, "Evidence-Based Behavioral Interventions for the Collaborative Care Team."

Initiate treatment plan

General approaches
Common treatment approaches are shared by the whole team. These strategies are often important in engaging the patient in treatment.

Patient education
All team members are comfortable in providing basic patient education. Teams can provide this information verbally or by using patient handouts.

High-quality Web resources may also help. Having common resources that team members utilize can lead to providing consistent information for patients.

Examples of patient education include:
- Information about the diagnosis and typical illness course
- Treatment options available to patient, including pros and cons of options
- Self-management strategies
- How the team will work together to provide treatment
- Roles of different team members
- Expectations for participation in treatment

Setting treatment goals
A core feature of Collaborative Care is setting clearly understandable patient-centered goals supported by the whole team. These goals should be clearly noted in the patient's chart. Goals should have observable, measurable outcomes (i.e., behaviors).

Common strategies for setting Collaborative Care treatment goals:
- Functional improvement: Which current symptoms interfere the most in the patient's life? What would the patient be doing if not experiencing symptoms? How will the patient and the team know if the treatment is effective?
- Behaviorally defined and measurable: Goals should be concrete and specific. Goals must be informed by the patient's perspective. Make sure goals reflect what is of high priority for the patient. Be aware of setting goals the patient does not value or feels are impossible to reach.
- Patients must participate in treatment goal development, and should "own" or at least "co-own" the treatment plan. The BHP makes sure the treatment team is patient-centered and advocates for crafting goals in ways that will be most engaging to the patient. If initial plans do not succeed, the BHP can help explore alternatives that are more likely to help the patient achieve his/her goals.
- Consider using a standard measure to track progress: Tracking symptoms using standardized measures, such as the PHQ-9 for depression, can help the team measure both individual patient as well as aggregate population outcomes.

Using evidence-based treatment
Team members delivering Collaborative Care work together to provide high-quality evidence-based treatments. Because team members have different skills, patients can benefit from choosing from a range of

evidence-based medication and behavioral interventions. Each chapter will highlight current evidence-based strategies for common mental health disorders.

In general, the PCP will initiate medication treatments if indicated and the BHP will focus on delivering behavioral or psychotherapeutic interventions. The psychiatric consultant should help guide the effective application of these interventions. Although each treatment section is divided up by these roles, *all* team members should be familiar with *all* treatments to reinforce treatment participation to the patient. For example, although medications will be prescribed by the PCP, the BHP will support medication adherence and may be the first person to hear about side effects. Conversely, although the BHP will set behavioral goals with the patient, a PCP checking in with the patient about these goals can reemphasize the importance of this part of the treatment plan.

Medications: Each chapter will review current medication options for the specific disorder. Chapter 11 will review general approaches to medication management in primary care and more detailed prescribing protocols for commonly used medications

Brief behavioral interventions: Each chapter will review current behavioral interventions and, as available, adaptations for use in primary care settings. Chapter 10 will give a general overview of delivery of brief behavioral interventions in primary care settings and overviews of key evidence-based psychotherapies.

Safety Planning

Safety planning is a team responsibility. Each team member will have a specific role in assessment, triage, and developing a safety plan defined by their organization. Team members should consider safety planning part of the patient-centered care delivered in a Collaborative Care model. Being supported in providing distressed patients with a safety plan is one benefit of working as part of a Collaborative Care team. Each Collaborative Care team will need to develop a protocol to manage safety concerns that is appropriate for the clinic setting and takes into account state laws and available resources. A sample protocol and safety plan is included in the online materials.

Team goal: Initial treatment planning

Create an initial treatment plan aligned with the patient's treatment goals and appropriate to the biopsychosocial assessment of the patient's unique presentation. The patient should have an initial understanding of the role of each clinician in the plan, a sense that all clinicians are working together and

(Continued)

with him/her to help achieve the patient's goals, and a clear sense of how the plan addresses his/her concerns and goals.

Working as a team

Patient: Actively participates in exploring treatment options and formulating an initial treatment plan. Voices concerns about the treatment plan. Follows through on initial treatment recommendations, speaks up about issues and concerns as treatment progresses.

PCP: Establishes and maintains therapeutic alliance; educates the patient about components of the treatment plan, in particular the use of medications and other medical treatments; emphasizes the importance of addressing psychosocial contributors to depression and other problems, such as chronic pain and working closely with the BHP; sets and reviews medical treatment goals and monitors progress; prescribes and monitors medications; and makes medical referrals as needed.

BHP: Establishes and maintains therapeutic alliance; addresses crisis management and safety planning strategies; reviews the full treatment plan with the patient and addresses questions and concerns; provides brief behavioral interventions addressing comorbid mental health issues and promoting chronic pain self-management; facilitates communication between team members; and makes and supports referrals (e.g., disability, vocational rehab, social services, chemical dependency, additional psychotherapy).

PC: Resource for diagnosing and treating psychiatric comorbidities; informs treatment planning; supports safety planning; and medication and behavioral management recommendations.

Typical Timeline Week 1

BHP: Visit 1–2
PCP: Visit 1–2
PC: Available for initial case review.

Case example

Mr. A's main focus is on sleeping and he is interested in taking medications. Both the PCP and BHP/care manager feel that input from the psychiatric consultant would be helpful to find a good medication treatment. Mr. A's BHP/care manager discusses his case with the psychiatric consultant by presenting his case over the telephone and after obtaining a basic history, the psychiatric consultant recommends mirtazapine, an antidepressant that is mildly sedating. The PCP prescribes this medication and the BHP/care manager provides psychoeducation about this choice with a special emphasis on why this is a good choice for the patient goal of improving sleep and how depression treatment will also support this goal. The BHP/care manager again schedules close follow-up by telephone (to assess tolerability of the medication in a week) and a future visit in person in three weeks.

Follow-up and treatment adjustment to achieve treatment to target

Measurement-based practice

Principles of Collaborative Care include regular assessment of symptoms and progress toward clinical goals, as well as adjusting treatment to achieve treatment targets. Collaborative Care teams will schedule regular follow-up to track patient progress toward goals. This proactive approach to patient care often involves outreach to patients who do not attend scheduled follow-up visits. At each follow-up visit, patient response to treatment is assessed by both interview and standardized measures. This approach helps team members quickly identify patients needing treatment adjustments, so patients do not stay on ineffective treatments for too long.

PCP approaches: Focus on common follow-up questions, important monitoring for common medications, common next steps.

BHP approaches: Focus on common challenges encountered in brief behavioral interventions and how to address them. Also, patient engagement strategies discussed.

PC approach: Will evaluate entire active caseload and work with BHP to provide case reviews for patients not improving as expected.

Stepped-care approach

A key principle of Collaborative Care treatment is that care is intensified or changed if patients are not responding to initial treatments. If patients are not achieving treatment goals, the treatment plan should be adjusted. This process is repeated until a patient demonstrates clinical improvement, or until resources in the clinic have been exhausted and a referral to more intensive treatment is needed. Sometimes this involves the psychiatric consultant providing additional case review, via in-person or televideo consultation, to help the team consider other evidence-based approaches.

Referring for additional services: Some patients will need more intensive services than can be offered in primary care. Each chapter will review commonly used criteria for each disorder for when to increase level of care. These will be listed for the typical primary care situations, although availability of resources will vary depending on your practice setting.

Team goal: Be prepared to adjust the treatment plan until treatment targets are achieved

Adjust medications and behavioral treatments as appropriate to step up care. As patients become more engaged in treatment and move toward treatment goals, self-management strategies can begin, and comorbid psychiatric disorders can continue to be treated.

Working as a team

Patient: Participates as a partner in trying treatment strategies and communicates concerns with treatment.

PCP: Addresses therapeutic alliance concerns as needed; consults with the BHP as needed; follows through on medical treatment goals and outcomes of medical referrals as needed; continues to monitor progress; and adjusts prescriptions as needed.

BHP: Continues to address engagement, crisis management, and safety planning as needed. Steps up brief behavioral interventions as needed to address comorbid mental health issues or persistent mental health symptoms.

PC: Informs treatment planning; supports safety planning; advocates for stepping up care and altering medication recommendations as needed; and supports and suggests behavioral management recommendations.

Typical Timeline ~6–12 months

BHP: Every two weeks until completion of treatment.

PCP: Every four to six weeks while adjusting medications, then less often.

PC: Case review at least every eight weeks until improvement and more frequently if needed.

Case example

Mr. A reports having tolerated mirtazapine when contacted by phone a week after his initial appointment. He reports improved sleep but no change in depressed mood. The BHP/care manager provides reassuring psychoeducation that it was a good sign that he was tolerating the medication and experienced improved sleep. The BHP/care manager also explains that typical response for antidepressant treatment occurs at six to eight weeks. The BHP/care manager introduces the idea of patient activation and helps Mr. A set a goal to call one friend a week to reduce social isolation. Mr. A is reminded to attend his follow-up appointment. At his follow-up appointment, Mr. A reports a little less depression when his PHQ-9 behavioral rating scale is administered. His PCP decides to increase his dose to the middle of the dosing range as previously suggested by the psychiatric consultant note. The BHP/care manager continues to set goals for patient activation. This proactive treatment approach continues for eight weeks until patient has experienced a significant reduction in depression symptoms.

Completing treatment and relapse prevention
Caseload management
Typically, an active caseload in Collaborative Care will only include symptomatic patients. Managing the size of the active caseload will be important as BHPs have to meet with patients regularly and can only mange a specific size caseload at any one time. The decision to graduate a patient should be made as a team. Often the psychiatric consultant and the BHP will discuss patient progress as part of psychiatric consultation.

Completion of treatment
The concept of a defined treatment episode may be new to a treatment team, but it is an important concept for caseload management in Collaborative Care. Ideally, each patient completes treatment by accomplishing improvement in clinical symptoms and daily functioning. Sometimes patients may complete treatment by referral to outside resources.

Relapse prevention
As an episode of treatment ends, relapse prevention planning should be started. Relapse prevention is important for long-term sustainability of a patient's clinical improvement. The patient and the team should work together to identify the treatments and interventions that have supported improvement and the ways in which they can maintain these gains. Ideally this should involve the completion of a written relapse prevention plan (a sample is included in the online materials).

All team members should contribute to this plan:
PCP: Will outline for the patient a medication plan and clear instructions to request reevaluation; frequency of follow-up for regular visits.

BHP: Is primarily responsible for working with patient to complete relapse prevention plan. Will document this plan in medical record, and will identify warning signs and behavioral approaches to address these with the patient.

PC: Will provide the patient with monitoring, guidance about medications, and clear instructions regarding when to request reevaluation.

Self-help books and Web resources: Each chapter has a section with books and websites to be used for further information and to share with patients as part of the psychoeducation delivered by the Collaborative Care team.

References: Each chapter lists a short bibliography of key papers and resources used to develop the content for the chapter. These may be interesting for members of the team who desire deeper knowledge about a key clinical area.

Team Goal: Relapse prevention

The relapse prevention plan should capture the key treatment strategies that the patient used to improve. This should include both medical and psychotherapeutic approaches that were helpful. The relapse prevention plan should also include recommendations for duration of medications treatment and symptoms to monitor, including when to represent to clinic if symptoms reappear.

Working as a team

Patient: Participates in establishing a relapse prevention plan with the BHP and the PCP; tracks the ongoing plan and reengages in additional care if symptoms or functional impairment significantly worsen.

PCP: Provides plan for ongoing medication management and clear instructions to the patient to request reevaluation if symptoms recur.

BHP: Reviews successes and gains in treatment, as well as the ongoing behavioral changes and treatment plan; clarifies team roles, including with whom the patient should reengage if function declines or symptoms worsen.

PC: Clarifies to the team recommendations for long-term use of medications and supports the BHP in creating a treatment summary and relapse prevention plan as needed.

Typical Timeline After 6–12 months

BHP: Start preparing six to eight weeks before last visit.

PCP: Will convert to care as usual by PCP.

PC: Case review with final recommendations for PCP.

Case example

Mr. A achieves remission of his depression in 10 weeks. At that time the BHP/care manager works with Mr. A to develop a relapse prevention plan. This plan includes early warning signs, effective treatments, and clear instructions for follow-up. The psychiatric consultant includes final medication recommendations. The BHP/care manager continues to meet with Mr. A monthly for three months. As Mr. A continues to experience minimal depression symptoms, he returns to care as part of his PCP's general patient panel, allowing for new patients to be seen by the BHP and receive Collaborative Care treatment.

Part 1

Collaborative Care for Common Primary Care Presentations

Chapter 2 **Mood Disorders—Major Depression**

Amy Bauer and Patricia Areán

Clinical impact

Depressive disorders are among the most common psychiatric conditions in primary care settings. Depression is often a recurrent condition that may become chronic over time or if untreated.

- Lifetime prevalence is 17 percent (2:1 female:male).
- Point prevalence is 10 percent in primary care settings (versus 2–4 percent in the general population).
- Among socioeconomically disadvantaged groups, depression is more prevalent and persistent.
- Thoughts of death and suicide are common in depression, but active suicidality is less common. Over half of people who commit suicide in the United States have depression.

Depression and chronic diseases have adverse bidirectional associations. Depression is a risk factor for development of many common medical illnesses, such as type 2 diabetes, dementia, and coronary heart disease. Depression may also be precipitated by the functional impairment and adverse symptoms associated with these illnesses, such as chronic pain. Depression is more prevalent among people with chronic diseases—diabetes mellitus (DM), coronary artery disease (CAD), cerebrovascular accident (CVA), chronic obstructive pulmonary disease (COPD), rheumatoid arthritis (RA), systemic lupus erythematosus (SLE), multiple sclerosis (MS), epilepsy, Alzheimer disease, Parkinson's disease, human immunodeficiency virus (HIV), cancer, obesity, and others. Depressed patients experience greater physical-symptom burden from comorbid medical conditions and have more unexplained physical symptoms. Depression is more disabling

Integrated Care: Creating Effective Mental and Primary Health Care Teams, First Edition.
Anna Ratzliff, Jürgen Unützer, Wayne Katon, and Kari A. Stephens.
© 2016 John Wiley & Sons, Inc. Published 2016 by John Wiley & Sons, Inc.

than many chronic medical conditions, has a greater impact on quality of life, and starts earlier in life. In addition, depression is associated with:
- increased health risk behaviors (tobacco, alcohol, illicit substance use, unsafe sexual practices, inactivity, poor diet)
- less adherence to medical treatment and poorer self-management
- increased risk for developing chronic diseases and complications
- increased medical costs
- early mortality

Assessment

Identify chief complaint, associated somatic and psychological symptoms, functional impairment, and safety concerns
Patients with depression may present with one of two core symptoms: persistently depressed mood or lack of interest and pleasure (anhedonia). Depressive disorders are diagnosed only when there is significant psychosocial distress and functional impairment related to depression. If such impairment is present, a depressive disorder should be diagnosed even if the symptoms are in the context of a stressful life event or medical illness. Bipolar disorder usually presents with depression instead of mania but requires different treatment, so it is important to rule out bipolar disorder as part of the initial assessment (see Chapter 3).

Common psychological symptoms
Most depressed patients will acknowledge mood or cognitive symptoms of depression when asked; however, not all patients with depression experience sadness or depressed mood. Social withdrawal is particularly common among older adults. Other symptoms may include:
- sadness, low mood, hopelessness, helplessness, tearfulness
- irritability, anger, worrying, feeling overwhelmed
- loss of interest, low motivation
- guilt, rumination, low self-esteem, negative thought distortions
- poor concentration, executive dysfunction (planning, decision making)
- mood-congruent psychotic symptoms can complicate severe major depression. These include delusions of low self-worth, somatic delusions, and auditory hallucinations.

Always ask about thoughts of self-harm or suicide in evaluation of all patients with psychiatric conditions, particularly depression. Asking about suicidal thoughts does not trigger suicidal thoughts.

Common physical/somatic symptoms

Somatic symptoms, such as pain, are not part of the formal criteria for depressive disorders, but they are as common as other presenting symptoms of depression in primary care.

- Chronic pain: neck, back, joint, limb, and abdominal pain; headaches; and body aches.
- Neurovegetative symptoms: fatigue, malaise, low energy, sleep disturbance, appetite changes, weight gain/loss, psychomotor agitation, and retardation.
- Gastrointestinal symptoms: nausea/indigestion and bowel symptoms.
- Sexual: low libido, sexual dysfunction, and anorgasmia.
- Other: palpitations, dyspnea, and dizziness.

Common functional impairments

Depression can affect every domain of a person's life. When severe, patients may have poor hygiene or self-care, inability to cook or feed themselves, and inability to get out of bed or leave the home. Even mild to moderate depression can affect functioning in different domains:

- Education/work: disinterest, inability to focus on tasks, low motivation or poor follow-though on tasks, and absenteeism.
- Relationships: isolating oneself, avoidance of intimacy, and sexual dysfunction.
- Social: isolation and withdrawal.

Assessing for safety

As many as 20–40 percent of patients with major depression have suicidal ideation, but suicidal plans and behavior are less common. The lifetime rate of suicide among all people with depression is about 6 percent. Rates are much lower among individuals with treated depression. Additional risk factors for suicide include:

- male gender
- older age
- alcohol or substance abuse
- history of prior suicide attempts
- chronic pain
- medical illness
- anxiety, impulsivity, or psychotic symptoms

Primary care providers (PCPs) have an important role in suicide assessment. Nearly half of patients who complete suicide have seen a PCP within the last month. When conducting a safety assessment, pay close attention to the following indicators of risk:

- Severe major depression can be complicated by mood-congruent psychotic symptoms, including somatic delusions, paranoia, or auditory hallucinations.
- Patients with severe major depression can become gravely disabled if they are unable to get out of bed for basic self-care and feeding. When oral intake is severely impaired, hospitalization may be required for intravenous fluids and nutrition.
- When uncertainties exist regarding patient safety, team members should seek additional consultation (e.g., PCP may enlist the behavioral health provider, or BHP, who may enlist the psychiatric consultant or PC) to ensure that adequate evaluation has occurred and that relevant state laws regarding referral for treatment, including involuntary treatment, are followed.
- Violence among patients with depression is more likely when patients experience hostility, angry outbursts, or psychotic features.

Team goal: Identifying the chief complaint, initial physical exam, gathering history, and safety assessment

Recognize patients with depressive disorders who present with differing clinical symptoms. Engage patient in treatment. Initiate appropriate evaluation for possible comorbidities. Compassionately assess for active suicidality/safety concerns at initial evaluation and throughout treatment for depression.

Working as a team

Patient: Participates in assessment of symptoms and functioning, including completion of relevant screening instruments and measures; authorizes collateral information from medical or mental health providers or family/friends. Answers questions about safety.

    PCP: Primary role in identifying a possible depressive disorder, often basic screening, e.g., PHQ-9. Assesses safety and coordinates with BHP to monitor safety issues.

    BHP: Completes detailed assessment; often develops a more complete understanding of the functional impairment related to depressive disorder; obtains collateral information. Assesses safety.

    PC: When indicated for more complex presentations, broadens psychiatric differential diagnosis and suggests strategies for BHP to obtain additional information to inform diagnostic assessment through evaluation or collateral information.

Case example

A 53-year-old Caucasian man presents to his PCP with a chief complaint of "not sleeping enough, having headaches, and feeling run down." For the last four months, he has been waking up too early in the morning and cannot get back to sleep. During the day he is exhausted and is having trouble focusing when he's at work. His chronic back pain has increased so he has been staying at home and has stopped exercising. He has tried everything he can think of to "break out of this rut" but feels it is pointless and is ready to give up.

The PCP administered a PHQ-9 (the patient scored 18) and then asked the patient about suicidality. After discussing the symptoms on the PHQ-9, the patient said that he never thought of himself as depressed before. At the first visit, the PCP conducted a safety assessment to follow up on the patient's thoughts of giving up. The patient revealed he has thought about jumping off a local bridge but he feels he does not have the courage to go through with it. The patient had never told anyone this but felt relieved that his PCP knows about this, so they could start to address this. The PCP expressed confidence to the patient that he would be able to improve and introduced the patient to the BHP for further evaluation and treatment.

The BHP conducted a comprehensive assessment of the patient and learned that he has been more irritable at home with his wife and children for the past six months. He has also stopped going out with friends. In the last two weeks he has been late to work four times because he can't get himself to get started in the morning. Additional history revealed he had a similar episode in the past when he was about 20 years old when he was having trouble with his coursework at the college; he described it as a very stressful time. He talked with a college counselor for several months, and then things improved before he graduated. To manage his stress recently, the patient reports he has started smoking cigarettes again after having quit four years ago. The PCP had conveyed the patient's thoughts of suicide to the BHP who also assessed the patient's safety as part of the comprehensive assessment. With the patient's permission, the BHP contacted the patient's wife in his presence. Together they discussed his passive suicidality, which she had not known about. She was grateful to be included in the assessment and had no additional concerns. The BHP invited the wife to contact the treatment team should she have new concerns about the patient's safety and the patient felt reassured that everyone was on the same page.

Differential diagnosis and identifying a provisional diagnosis

Rule out common contributing medical problems and substance-related conditions

In general, lab tests are not indicated routinely for evaluation of depression and should only be considered if the patient history, review of systems, or physical exam suggests relevant medical issues. Routine thyroid screening (TSH) among depressed patients has a low yield, but may be worthwhile among women over 50 years of age who have a higher baseline prevalence of thyroid disorders. When major depression is severe, patients may not eat or drink adequately to maintain their nutritional status and may require medical evaluation and intervention for serious metabolic problems. For patients who have none of the mood or cognitive symptoms of depression, it is particularly important to reevaluate for potential medical causes. Symptoms of depression overlap with symptoms of many types of medical conditions.

- Medical Conditions Causing Symptoms of Depression

  Cardiovascular: congestive heart failure

  Hematologic/oncologic: anemia, cancer

  Endocrine: diabetes, hypothyroidism, hypogonadism (men), polycystic ovary syndrome, hypo/hyperadrenalism

  Infectious: HIV, hepatitis B or C, tuberculosis, neurosyphilis, neurocysticercosis, prion disease, urinary tract infection

  Immunological: multiple sclerosis, lupus, rheumatoid arthritis, autoimmune or paraneoplastic encephalopathy

  Metabolic: Vitamin D, B12, folate, or thiamine deficiency, hyponatremia, hypocalcemia, hypokalemia, heavy metal poisoning, Wilson's disease, porphyria, hepatic or metabolic encephalopathy, uremia

  Neurological: delirium, dementia, Parkinson's disease, Huntington's disease, epilepsy, traumatic brain injury, postconcussive syndrome, stroke, CNS tumor, subdural hematoma

  Respiratory: COPD, obstructive sleep apnea

Use of psychoactive substances including some prescription medications can cause symptoms of depression. Assessing the contribution of such substances is important because treatment for depression will be less effective if a patient's substance use is not also addressed.

- Substance-Related Conditions Causing Symptoms of Depression

  Withdrawal: cannabis, cocaine, amphetamine, ecstasy, caffeine, stimulants (such as bath salts and khat)

  Intoxication: opioid, sedative

  Chronic use: alcohol, marijuana

Prescribed medications: corticosteroids, chemotherapy agents, digoxin, gonadotropin-releasing hormone agonists, interferon-alpha, interleukin-2, levetiracetam, levodopa, mefloquine, opioids, progestin-containing contraceptive implants, propranolol, sedatives. Anecdotal reports have suggested that depressive symptoms can occur with isotretinoin, acamprosate, and other immune system suppressants, although the evidence is limited.

Develop and refine differential diagnosis

Use the chief complaint and core presenting symptoms to generate a broad differential diagnosis (Tables 2.1 and 2.2). Standardized tools can be helpful both for clarifying diagnosis, assessing severity and tracking symptoms over time.

- The Patient Health Questionnaire-9 (PHQ-9) is widely used to screen for depression and to monitor treatment response.
- As part of the initial assessment of depression, it is important to assess for bipolar disorder because bipolar depression requires a different treatment approach (see Chapter 3).
- Postpartum depression is assessed and treated similarly to other depressive disorders and has similar response. Among postpartum patients, it is especially important to rule out bipolar disorder because postpartum depression and psychosis are more common among women with a history of bipolar disorder.

For patients with recurrent major depression, assess for a seasonal pattern which may suggest seasonal affective disorder.

Assessment of comorbid psychiatric disorders and psychological difficulties

Most patients with depressive disorders have comorbid psychiatric conditions. Comorbidity is a common reason for treatment-resistance among patients with depression. Patients are at increased risk of comorbid major depression if they have any of these preexisting conditions:

- Persistent depressive disorder (dysthymia)
- An anxiety disorder (GAD, panic disorder, social phobia)
- PTSD, OCD
- Substance use disorders
- Somatic symptom disorders
- Eating disorders
- Borderline personality disorder
- Chronic medical conditions
- Chronic pain

Table 2.1 Generating the differential diagnosis for depressive disorder

Diagnosis	Key questions	Differentiating symptom	Behavioral health measure
Major depressive disorder	Have you been feeling depressed or having difficulty enjoying things in your life?	Depressed mood, anhedonia	PHQ-9
Bipolar disorder, depressed	Do you have periods of time with extra energy and much less sleep than usual and not really miss it the next day?	History of hypo-mania/mania	CIDI-3
Somatic symptom disorders	Have you been bothered by multiple physical problems such as pain of any kind, nausea, dizziness, fainting, palpitations, shortness of breath, diarrhea, or constipation?	Multiple somatic symptoms	PHQ-15
Substance use disorders	Do you currently drink alcohol or use street drugs? Have you in the past?	Evidence of substance use	AUDIT DAST CAGE-AID
Anxiety disorders	Have you been worrying excessively for greater than six months? Are you a worrier?	Excessive worry	GAD-7
PTSD	Do you have a history of trauma or abuse with nightmares and flashbacks (daytime vivid memories of trauma)?	Reexperiencing trauma	PCL-C
Delirium	Cognitive assessment of orientation, digit span forward and reverse, days of the week [months of the year] in reverse, backward spelling.	Acute/subacute onset of inattention, level of alertness, psychomotor retardation	Confusion Assessment Method (CAM)
Dementia	Do you have difficulty keeping track of things or remembering things or finding your way home?	Cognitive deficits	MOCA

Table 2.1 (*Continued*)

Diagnosis	Key questions	Differentiating symptom	Behavioral health measure
Premenstrual dysphoric disorder	Do you have mood or behavior changes that are regularly worse before your period and go away in the first few days after your period?	Luteal-phase mood symptoms relieved by menses	

Other disorders to consider: Adjustment Disorder, Borderline personality disorder, Demoralization, Domestic violence

Table 2.2 Common depressive disorders in primary care (ICD-10)

- Major depressive disorder (Single episode F32.x; Recurrent episode F33.x; Add severity/course specifier)
- Adjustment disorder with depressed mood (F43.21)
- Alcohol-induced depressive disorder (F10.x)
- Bipolar disorder, depressed (Bipolar I depressed F31.3x, F31.4, F31.5, F31.75, F31.76, F31.9 or Bipolar II depressed F31.81)
- Depressive Disorder due to [Another Medical Condition; specify name of the condition] (F06.3x)
- Persistent depressive disorder (Dysthymia; F34.1)
- Substance/Medication–induced [Specify name of the substance or medication] depressive disorder (Opioid F11.x, Sedative/hypnotic/anxiolytic F13.x, Cocaine F14.x, Other Stimulant F15.x, Hallucinogen F16.x, Inhalant F18.x, Other/unknown substance F19.x)
- Unspecified depressive disorder (F32.9)

Team goal: Differential diagnosis and identifying a provisional diagnosis

Comprehensively identify conditions that may mimic depression but require different treatment approaches, as well as factors that may interfere with or contraindicate standard depression treatment.

Working as a team

Patient: Discloses medical and substance use issues and participates in their assessment; authorizes collateral information from medical or mental health providers or family/friends; participates in medical evaluation (e.g., labs, imaging, specialty referrals) as indicated. Discloses additional psychiatric issues

(*Continued*)

and prior treatment history; authorizes coordination with other medical or psychiatric providers; participates in evaluation; tracks symptoms.

PCP: Primary role in evaluating possible medical etiology for presenting complaints. Performs a thorough differential diagnosis and establishes a working diagnosis of depression; orders labs, tests, and medical consultation as appropriate; coordinates care with other medical providers and mental health providers. Coordinates with BHP to refine differential diagnosis.

BHP: Important role in noting any concerning physical symptoms and connecting patient to PCP for evaluation. Considers and screens for comorbidities and conducts psychosocial assessment; obtains collateral information; assists PCP in coordinating care with other medical providers; supports client in following through on medical recommendations such as getting lab work. Consults with PC as needed to clarify diagnosis.

PC: Expands medical differential as needed; recommends additional assessment. Refines differential; provides provisional diagnosis.

Case example

In the PCP's initial assessment, the patient's review of systems was notable for headaches along with exacerbation of his chronic back pain. He reported minimal alcohol use on the CAGE and does not use opioids. He has hypertension, but his blood pressure was in the normal range on hydrochlorothiazide and his physical exam including neurological exam were unremarkable. No lab tests were indicated. The BHP screened for substance abuse with the DAST, which was negative and confirmed that the patient did not have a prior history of drug or alcohol problems.

At the initial visit the PCP conducted additional screening for anxiety, which revealed that the patient's GAD-7 score was 6. As part of the BHP's initial comprehensive assessment, the BHP administered screening instruments for PTSD (PCL-C) and bipolar disorder (CIDI-3), both of which were negative. The BHP and patient discussed the provisional diagnosis of major depression and its treatment, as well as the connections between depression and chronic pain.

Treatment

Initiate treatment

General principles

It is important to differentiate major depression and dysthymia from other conditions presenting with depressed mood (such as demoralization or adjustment disorders) because the treatment approaches differ. Assess prior treatment response to inform treatment planning. Talk to patients about their treatment preferences and concerns about different treatments and engage patients in shared decision-making.

Collaborative Care for depression

More than 80 studies (e.g., see Archer et al., 2012) have demonstrated that Collaborative Care programs in which PCPs are supported by a care manager and systematic psychiatric consultation to facilitate treatment adjustment if patients are not improving as expected are more effective than care as usual.

The PCP should assure the patient that the PCP will be working closely with the care manager to help the patient. The PCP should:

- emphasize to patient that primary care provider and care manager work closely together;
- explain to patient that care manager is an expert in helping patients with treatment planning;
- alert care manager to any medical contraindications for behavioral interventions;
- communicate regularly with care manager about patient engagement and progress.

Introducing the care team

The way we help people with the symptoms you are having is by having you meet regularly with an expert in our clinic, called a care manager. The care manager and I will be working closely together and with you to come up with the best treatment plan we can to help you recover. It will be important in the first couple of months for you to check in with us regularly about how the treatment is working for you, because if it's not helping, we will want to make changes to the treatment plan as soon as possible. So, the care manager will be checking in with you and then reporting to me about how you are doing. If things are going well, you just keep checking in with the care manager until our next appointment. If the treatment isn't really working, then we will discuss other treatment options. How does that sound? Do you have any questions?

Psychoeducation

Use psychoeducation to provide an explanatory model in specific phrases that might be helpful for the primary care team. Examples of psychoeducation about mood and treatment options include:

- what depression, including its causes and its course, is;
- how depression affects the patient's thoughts, feelings, and behaviors;

- treatment options available to patient;
- pros and cons of each option;
- self-management strategies;
- how team will work together to support treatment.

Safety planning
Recognizing and treating depression is the most important step in reducing suicide risk. In patients presenting with depression, treatment of risk factors contributing to suicidality (e.g., anxiety, substance abuse, insomnia, agitation, persistent pain) can reduce the depressed patient's risk of suicide.

General treatment principles
The majority of patients with depression experience significant improvement when treated. The goals of treatment are symptom remission and improved functioning. Psychosocial interventions such as evidence-based counseling and psychotherapies are the first-line approach for patients who do not have major depression but present with some depression symptoms, as in the case of demoralization or adjustment disorders. Evidence-based psychosocial interventions and antidepressant pharmacotherapy are equally effective for mild to moderate major depression. For patients with severe (PHQ-9 $\geq$ 20) or chronic ($\geq$2 years) depression, combination therapy is recommended (Table 2.3).

Medication treatment
Ask patients about their beliefs about medications and expectations for treatment. Provide relevant education to patients with concerns that antidepressants are addictive or who expect immediate improvement.
- Prior to initiating an antidepressant, screen for bipolar disorder (CIDI measure listed in Appendix).
- For patients with severe major depression with psychotic features, initial management should consist of an antidepressant medication plus an antipsychotic medication.
- Treating depressed patients over 25 years of age with antidepressant reduces suicidal ideation and behavior. Among adults under age 25, there is conflicting evidence regarding whether there is a small risk of treatment-emergent suicidal behavior; however, this is generally not considered to be a reason to withhold antidepressant medications. All patients and especially young adult patients should be monitored closely for suicidality, particularly in the initial stages of treatment.
- For patients who have seasonal pattern to recurrences of major depression (seasonal affective disorder), consider phototherapy.

Table 2.3 Team-based treatment for depression in primary care

		PCP approaches	BHP approaches
Biological		**Evidence-Based Medication Treatment:**	**Evidence-Based Medication Treatment:**
		• Medications are safe and effective but patients will likely need adjustment in antidepressant treatment to achieve remission.	• Support assessment of past medication trials.
		• First-line medications are **SSRIs, SNRIs, bupropion, and mirtazapine**, which all have comparable efficacy but have different side effect profiles.	• Assess for potential barriers to engaging in medication management (e.g., cost or cultural barriers).
			• Support patients through making medication changes and troubleshoot adherence challenges.
Psychosocial		**Evidence-Based Behavioral Treatment:**	**Evidence-Based Behavioral Treatment:**
		• Validate behavioral interventions are treatment; consider giving the patient a prescription for these treatments.	• There are a number of evidence-based behavioral interventions for depression that can be delivered briefly in primary care medicine.
		• Assess engagement with and reinforce behavioral treatment during medical visits.	• First-line treatments include BA, CBT, IPT, and PST.

Brief behavioral interventions

There are a number of evidence-based behavioral interventions for depression that can be delivered briefly in primary care settings. Almost all the evidence-based behavioral interventions can be done in individual or group therapy, and most can be delivered in less than 30 minutes; some as little as 15 minutes. The evidence-based therapies are:

- Cognitive behavioral therapy (CBT for Depression). CBT is a 12-session intervention that teaches patients mood regulation strategies, helps patients reengage in valued activities, and teaches communication skills.
- Problem solving therapy (PST). PST is a four- to eight-session treatment that focuses on helping patients develop solutions to overcome the problems they feel are contributing to poor mood.
- Behavioral activation (BA). BA is a 6–12 session intervention that focuses on identifying activities that patients have stopped engaging in because of their mood, and gradually reexposes the patient to the activities.
- Interpersonal therapy (IPT). IPT is a 12-session intervention that helps patient identify interpersonal communication problems and works toward helping patients have more fulfilling interpersonal relationships.

In addition to these evidence-based treatments for depression, Motivational Interviewing (MI) can be used as a tool to engage and motivate patients into treatment (i.e., for psychotherapy or antidepressant treatment). MI focuses on helping patients move toward change by helping clarify ambivalence about making changes and can be a useful tool to foster understanding of patient centered goals.

Most people feel the effect of behavioral treatment by the second or third week of treatment. It will be important for clinicians to explain how the therapies work so that the patient is prepared for their first meeting with the treating clinician. When explaining behavioral treatment to a patient, the clinician should cover the following points:

- Behavioral treatments are an effective alternative or augmentation to medication.
- Treatment usually consists of 4–12 meetings by phone or in person, which last about 30 minutes.
- At each meeting, the patient will be learning new ways to cope with their mood and any problems they feel contribute to their mood.
- The treatments are active, so instead of just talking about how the patient feels, the patient will be working to improve their mood.
- In general, patients should start to feel better in about two to three weeks.

PCP approaches to treatment
Prescribing principles
Antidepressant medications may take 8–12 weeks at a therapeutic dose for full therapeutic effect. Only about 40–50 percent of patients will have an adequate response to initial treatments such as medications or psychotherapy. The majority will require dose escalations and many will require medication switches or augmentation with additional medications or psychotherapy to achieve an adequate treatment response. With appropriate changes in treatments based on persistent symptoms, approximately 80 percent of patients can achieve remission. Older adults and patients with significant comorbid anxiety may be more sensitive to medication side effects and require slower dose titration.

Choice of medication
First-line medications are **SSRIs, SNRIs, bupropion, and mirtazapine**, which all have comparable efficacy. (Table 2.4) Choice of an agent should be guided by side effect profile and tolerability, and history of positive response in the patient or first-degree relative (when applicable). If a patient has previously been treated successfully for depression, reinitiation of the same

Table 2.4 Medications commonly used in the treatment of depression

---

Bupropion (Wellbutrin)
Citalopram (Celexa)
Duloxetine (Cymbalta)
Escitalopram (Lexapro)
Fluoxetine (Prozac)
Mirtazapine (Remeron)
Paroxetine (Paxil)
Sertraline (Zoloft)
Venlafaxine (Effexor)
Nortriptyline (Pamelor)

For prescribing details and protocols, please see Chapter 11, "Evidence-Based Psychopharmacology for the Collaborative Care Team."

agent is a reasonable initial strategy. The dose of the initial agent should be escalated to optimize the dose. Because many antidepressants (except mirtazapine) cause minor GI side effects, it is often helpful to take them with food.

- Bupropion and mirtazapine do not cause sexual side effects.
- Bupropion and fluoxetine are weight-neutral.
- SNRIs are effective at reducing pain (particularly neuropathic pain) independent of their antidepressant effects.
- Although nortriptyline and other tricyclic antidepressants are effective for pain, they are not considered first-line antidepressants; see below.
- Paroxetine: Category D pregnancy, most sedating, increased weight gain, discontinuation syndrome.
- Venlafaxine, particularly in the immediate-release formulation, has a higher incidence of discontinuation symptoms, which can be uncomfortable for patients who miss even a single dose.
- Immediate-release bupropion lowers seizure threshold in a dose-dependent manner and is contraindicated among patients with epilepsy or with other risk factors for seizures, such as comorbid eating disorders or alcohol dependence, or history of significant head trauma.
- Mirtazapine is sedating, particularly at low doses; it stimulates appetite and often causes weight gain.
- Trazodone is less effective than other second-generation antidepressant medications but is an effective medication for insomnia when used at low doses (i.e., 25 to 50 mg).

Although similarly efficacious to newer antidepressant medications, **tricyclic antidepressants** are used less frequently due to their potential cardiac toxicity and side effects (anticholinergic symptoms, orthostatic hypotension, sedation). For patients who have failed *adequate* trials (at least 12 weeks at maximum dose) of two or more first-line antidepressants, a tricyclic may be considered. Compared to other tricyclics, nortriptyline has fewer side effects and therefore is a good first choice, whereas side effects with amitriptyline are greater than others which make it less desirable.

- The dosing required for antidepressant effect is considerably higher than doses that are used off-label for pain or insomnia.
- Initial dosing for tricyclics is not at full therapeutic doses, and therefore gradual dose escalation is required early in treatment.

Safe prescribing

SSRIs interact with St. John's wort and tamoxifen and are associated with a slight increase in bleeding risk that may be relevant for patients who are on anticoagulation or have clotting disorders. Linezolid, isoniazid, and hydralazine have weak MAO inhibitor activity and thus should be avoided among patients taking antidepressant.

- Serotonin syndrome is a rare but dangerous potential complication associated with serotonergic antidepressants when patients are taking other medications that increase serotonin or in overdose. Risk is increased in the presence of high-dose or multiple serotonergic medications (other antidepressants, triptans, St John's Wort, odansetron and others) or illicit substances.

Pregnancy: Consider psychotherapy or phototherapy for women with mild to moderate depression. Antidepressant medication is indicated for severely depressed women and women who don't respond to nonpharmacological interventions. Risks of untreated depression include increased risk of preterm labor and low birth weight, reduced fetal growth and delayed infant language development. Paroxetine should be avoided during pregnancy. Transient neonatal effects can occur among newborns exposed to SSRIs in utero. For severe cases of depression, consider electroconvulsive therapy (ECT).

Breast-feeding: Infant exposure to first-line antidepressants is slight or negligible among breastfeeding women. Because sertraline has a short half-life, it is the preferred antidepressant for breastfeeding women. Switching antidepressants among women who have been stabilized on another agent is not generally recommended.

Managing side effects

- Minor side effects (nausea, headache, jitteriness, insomnia) are common early in the course of antidepressant treatment and when doses are increased. Most minor side effects dissipate with time, so patients should be encouraged to continue if side effects are not serious.

- Sexual side effects occur with many antidepressants and are dose-related. They generally do not improve with time and are a common reason for discontinuing an antidepressant. Sexual side effects may respond to lowering the antidepressant dose or may be able to be targeted by addition of a phosphodiesterase inhibitor such as sildenafil.
- Serious side effects include emergence of hypomania/mania, increase in suicidal ideation, development of psychotic symptoms, or akathisia (restless legs).

Symptomatic management

- For patients with significant insomnia, **trazodone** may be used off-label in low doses (25–50 mg) as a hypnotic and has some evidence to support this use. Trazodone is not habit-forming and patients do not develop tolerance. It can be used for patients with chronic insomnia. Unlike benzodiazepines, it is unlikely to cause problems with cognition. Monitor for orthostasis and counsel male patients about the rare occurrence of priapism.
- **Benzodiazepines** are *not* effective in the treatment of depression and may exacerbate social withdrawal, avoidance, and inactivity. There is some evidence that time-limited coadministration of a low-dose benzodiazepine (e.g., two weeks) may help improve adherence to a new antidepressant medication, especially among anxious patients, but this strategy is not generally recommended due to the many problems with benzodiazepines.

Psychosocial approaches

- Being familiar with some brief behavioral interventions helps when pitching psychosocial treatments to patients and increasing patient follow through with referrals to the BHP.
- To jump-start patients beginning psychosocial treatment for depression, PCPs can prescribe patients to work on small behavioral targets that can help either increase rewarding behaviors and/or interrupt depressive maintaining behaviors.
- A key to helping patients in short but often frequent visits, PCPs can break down behavioral targets into very small doable steps, making sure to reinforce engagement in these behaviors by asking patients to commit to a small goal and checking in at next visits to promote follow through, supporting any attempt to try the behaviors.

BHP approaches to treatment

Psychosocial approaches

Cognitive Behavioral Therapy (CBT) for Depression. This is a 12-session intervention that teaches four different mood management strategies. These strategies include:

- scheduling enjoyable or valued activities during the week
- reevaluating social perceptions and expectations
- learning to communicate positively
- challenging cognitions that perpetuate depression (i.e., "I am a failure because I have depression")

Problem Solving Treatment (PST). This is a four- to eight-session treatment that identifies key problems patients are struggling with and develops action plans based on a seven-step strategy:

- Define the problem.
- Choose a realistic goal.
- Identify strategies to reach the goal.
- Evaluate the feasibility of each strategy.
- Choose a strategy.
- Create an action plan.
- Implement and evaluate the plan.

Behavioral Activation (BA). This is a 6–12 session intervention focused on helping patients to reengage in work, social, health, and family activities they have abandoned because of depressed mood. The intervention follows these steps:

- Create a list of activities patient is not engaged in that can promote more pleasure and mastery.
- Decrease activities that promote or maintain depression.
- Create a hierarchy of activities from easiest to hardest and target avoidance that perpetuates behaviors that maintain depression.
- Develop and maintain an action plan that includes identification of obstacles, triggers, and consequences.

Interpersonal Therapy for Primary Care (IPT). This intervention is a 12-session treatment that helps patients solve interpersonal and social problems. It focuses on four key social problems and works with the patient to discuss their feelings and engage in more proactive behavior around these problem areas. The four key areas are:

- Grief (e.g., death, divorce, loss of function)
- Role transition (e.g., becoming a new parent, leaving school)
- Interpersonal dispute (e.g., family arguments)
- Interpersonal deficits (e.g., anger management)

Selecting treatments. All these interventions have a strong evidence base for the treatment of mood disorders. PST is particularly useful for older adults, people with chronic illnesses (e.g., diabetes), and people with serious illnesses (e.g., cancer). CBT is useful for depression in younger and older adults. IPT has been found to be effective for older adults and new mothers with postpartum depression.

Working with medications

Prepare patients for antidepressant trials by educating them that it can take 2–6 weeks for an initial effect and up to 12 weeks for maximum benefit from a given antidepressant dose. Prepare patients to monitor and report concerns and side effects. Working through patient ambivalence related to taking medications can also be helpful.

Team goal: Initial treatment planning

Engage patient in discussion of evidence-based depression treatment, including both psychosocial treatments and antidepressant medication management. Negotiate an individualized treatment plan that accounts for patient's preferences, limitations, resources, access, and any other social or environmental factors that may have implications for the successful implementation of a specific evidence-based treatment plan.

Working as a team

Patient: Learns about diagnosis and treatment; participates in negotiation of treatment plan. Monitors relevant symptoms such as mood or sleep; participates in behavioral interventions and regular follow-up. Participates in safety planning; authorizes coordination between treatment team and relevant supports (e.g., family members, friends); seeks crisis services appropriately when indicated.

PCP: Engages and plans for safety; prescribes and monitors medications; monitors baseline and follow-up labs and vital signs; maintains general health care; makes medical referrals as needed.

BHP: Engages and plans for safety; develops full treatment plan; conducts brief behavioral interventions; supports medication adherence and helps monitor for side effects; facilitates communication between team members; makes and supports referrals (disability, vocational rehab, social services, chemical dependency, additional psychotherapy) and safety planning; develops plan to monitor safety issues and track plan; when indicated, refers to crisis services.

(Continued)

PC: Is a resource for safety planning; supports treatment planning; makes medication recommendations and prescribing details; makes behavioral recommendations.

Other providers: Some patients may benefit from referral to other providers for more intensive or specialized psychotherapeutic approaches.

Case example

The BHP and PC discussed the patient's presentation. The PCP had asked whether fluoxetine would be appropriate for the patient. The PC suggested considering bupropion as an initial antidepressant given its efficacy in supporting smoking cessation. A titration schedule was provided to escalate the dose to the therapeutic range and monitor response with a PHQ-9 over four to six weeks.

The PC and BHP determined that the BHP would offer behavioral activation to the patient and help support the antidepressant management. BA was selected because the brief nature of the intervention (30-minute visits) fit the patient's desire to keep meetings short. Additionally, the patient reported that he would like to focus on reengaging in work and social activities but was having a hard time getting started.

In the first BA meeting, the BHP explained the rationale behind BA and what to expect from treatment. The BHP first described how when one is depressed and in pain, the tendency is to avoid physical, social, and work activities because these activities either seem too hard to start or there is an expectation that they will not be successful or enjoyable. Unfortunately, the less one does, the more depressed and pain one feels, something the patient had reported in his initial evaluation. The BHP then explained that to correct the course, the patient would have to start doing activities he has stopped engaging in, but that they would work together to consider which activities the patient felt he could reasonably engage. The BHP was already familiar with the activities the patient had stopped engaging in and thus was able to immediately help the patient identify activities that were enjoyable and easy to implement. In discussing the various activities he had stopped doing, the patient indicated he felt he could do two things: extending his walks with his dog beyond what he was already doing and inviting a friend along with him on these walks. The BHP consulted with the PCP about the activities the patient could safely engage in, given his chronic back pain, and also worked with the PC regarding the analgesic effects his antidepressant might confer to assist in gradual increase in physical activity.

Following the BHP's recommendation, the patient scheduled a follow-up visit with his PCP. The BHP updated the PCP about the treatment plan and the PC's recommendations for antidepressant medication. The PCP prescribed bupropion SR 150mg daily. The PCP arranged follow-up with the patient, and reinforced the role of the BHP in coordinating care and the value of BA for depression.

Follow-up and treatment adjustment to achieve treatment to target

General principles

During the acute phase, treatment response should be monitored closely and adjustments to treatment should be made every four to eight weeks until substantial improvement occurs. Team members, especially the BHP, can consult with the PC to discuss the case and how to adjust treatment.

- Assess adherence to initial treatments (medications, behavioral interventions, or both). If adherence is low, assess reasons for low adherence and address these.
- For patients who are adherent to initial treatment approaches, treatment adjustments may be indicated.
- Make adjustments to treatments already initiated (e.g., adjustments in psychotropic medication or behavioral intervention strategies).
- Or, add psychotropic medication or behavioral interventions for patients who initially are not receiving these.

When to consider referral

Consider referring a patient for direct psychiatric evaluation and/or management if the patient has not responded adequately to primary care management, particularly if they have failed to respond to two or more trials of antidepressant medication at maximum dose for at least 12 weeks' duration. Referral for specialty care is also appropriate for patients with conditions requiring longer term, more intensive, or specialist psychotherapy, long-term case management, or evaluation for ECT.

- Active suicidality is a psychiatric emergency and requires referral for emergency evaluation.
- Major depression with psychotic features is a severe condition and earlier specialty referral may be beneficial.

Certain patients with depression may also benefit from referral for other community-based services:

- Employment services: especially if people have developed avoidance patterns

- Disability: more severe cases, especially if anticipate inability to work for greater than a year

PCP approaches

Acute phase: Treatment response should be monitored closely and adjustments to treatment should be made every four to eight weeks until substantial improvement occurs.

No response: Escalate medications incrementally to maximally tolerated dose. If no benefit after eight weeks, switch to another first-line agent in the same or different class. One-fourth of patients who fail to respond to an initial SSRI will respond to a different SSRI.

Partial response: Escalate incrementally to maximally tolerated dose. If inadequate, consider augmentation in consultation with the team PC (see below).

Augmentation strategies
There are a number of options for medications to augment antidepressants for patients with incomplete treatment response.

Antidepressants.
- SSRI or SNRI antidepressants can be combined with an antidepressant from a different class (e.g., bupropion, mirtazapine) or with buspirone for augmentation.

Mood stabilizers.
- Lithium can be used off-label as adjunctive treatment for patients with depression.

Atypical antipsychotics.
Due to their adverse metabolic profiles, use of an atypical antipsychotic for major depression without psychotic features should generally be reserved for patients who have failed two or more adequate trials of antidepressant medications.
- Aripiprazole and quetiapine (as monotherapy) and olanzapine (in combination with fluoxetine) have FDA approval for treatment-resistant depression.
- See Chapter 5 for further information about use of antipsychotic medications.

Other augmenting agents.
- Tri-iodothyronine is effective as augmentation of antidepressant medications. It is better tolerated than lithium and carries fewer long-term adverse risks than lithium or atypical antipsychotic medications.

- Stimulants (atomoxetine, modafanil, or amphetamines), lamotrigine, folate, omega-3 fatty acids, and testosterone are occasionally used adjunctively, but evidence supporting their use is limited.

BHP approaches

During the acute phase, treatment response should be monitored closely (ideally every two weeks) and adjustments to treatment should be made every four to eight weeks until substantial improvement occurs. If there is little or no response by 6 weeks of treatment, consider adding medication or switching behavioral treatments. Consult with the psychiatric consultant to discuss the case and how to adjust treatment.

Brief behavioral treatments continuation phase

Active treatment contains both acute and continuation phases. The number of prescribed sessions is based on the average number of sessions needed to induce behavior change and practice that change until it becomes fluid. As an example, PST is four to eight sessions, and assumes most patients will respond to treatment by four weeks. The remaining sessions are then considered opportunities to practice solving problems until the patient can solve problems without the care managers' help.

Working with medications

Premature discontinuation of antidepressants is common in primary care settings, so it is especially important to ask about medications at every session. Support patients through making medication changes and troubleshoot adherence challenges. There are several other strategies that care managers can use to support medication management:

- Be responsive to concerns and side effects (see above regarding specific side effect issues).
- Help patient schedule an appointment with PCP to address medications.
- Help patient write down questions.

Team goal: Be prepared to adjust the treatment plan until treatment targets are achieved

Monitor progress every two to four weeks with standardized measurement tools (e.g., PHQ-9). Because depressed patients can have difficulty keeping appointments, provide proactive outreach to keep patients engaged in treatment. When patients are not improving as expected, address adherence and/or adjust treatment with ongoing monitoring until adequate

(Continued)

improvement occurs. Depressed patients may become discouraged, so it is important to instill hope while treatment adjustments are under way.

Working as a team

Patient: Notifies treatment team of medication side effects or any barriers or problems in treatment; renegotiates treatment plan with treatment team as needed.

PCP: Retains overall responsibility for patients' treatment. Makes adjustments to psychotropic medications when needed to address tolerability (i.e., side effect management) or lack of efficacy. Continues to monitor for contributions from medical or substance use conditions.

BHP: Provides behavioral interventions; monitors patients' progress in treatment, treatment adherence to medications and psychosocial treatments, and treatment side effects; facilitates communication between team members; provides ongoing assessment of need for additional supports and makes indicated referrals (disability, vocational rehab, social services, chemical dependency, additional psychotherapy); consults with PC regularly, with emphasis on adjusting treatment for patients not improving as expected.

PC: Through regular psychiatric case reviews, provides additional suggestions for treatment changes for patients not improving as expected; may conduct direct patient assessment (in-person or by telemedicine) for patients who do not improve despite changes in treatment.

Case example

After four weeks in treatment, the patient's sleep was improving and his energy improved, but his PHQ-9 score remained elevated at 14. The BHP notified the PCP and the patient's bupropion SR dose was increased to 150mg twice daily (morning and afternoon) as suggested by the psychiatric consultant. By week eight, the patient reported his concentration was improving at work, his back pain had improved, and his PHQ-9 score was down to 8. The patient continued on bupropion 150mg twice daily and ongoing follow-up with the BHP for behavioral activation. The BHP taught the patient ways to manage his negative thoughts.

At week 12, the patient's PHQ-9 dropped to a 4 and he reported that his pain was more manageable. The patient indicated that he had added to his walking routine with his dog and twice-weekly aquarobics class at his local community center. He reported feeling better connected socially, and while he occasionally had bad pain days, he felt he had a plan to manage them well. The patient also reported a decrease in irritability, which resulted in better relationships with his family. The BHP recommended that the follow-up meetings be reduced to every month.

Completing treatment and relapse prevention
General principles
The goal of depression treatment is symptom remission. Patients who have residual depressive symptoms have had incomplete treatment and are at risk for relapse. Once remission of symptoms has been achieved, patients can complete a relapse prevention plan and return to standard primary care panel monitoring, typically every three to six months. Such monitoring should include the use of the standardized depression tool (e.g., PHQ-9) as well as clinical assessment of symptoms, functioning, and use of maintenance pharmacotherapy (if applicable).

Ongoing medication management
Continuation phase: For patients with a first episode of major depression, antidepressant medications should be continued for four to nine months following symptom remission at the same dose used to achieve symptom remission.

Maintenance phase: For patients with recurrent major depression (three or more lifetime episodes) or chronic depression, maintenance antidepressant treatment should be provided for at least two years at the same dose as the acute phase treatment. Consider maintenance treatment for patients with other risk factors for relapse including: persistent residual symptoms or negative cognitions, early onset or strong family history of mood disorders, history of childhood trauma, current psychosocial stressors, and active psychiatric comorbidities.

Discontinuation: When discontinuing antidepressant medications, patients who taper medications gradually over at least several weeks have a lower rate of relapse. Tapering also lowers the likelihood that patients will experience discontinuation symptoms which are bothersome but not dangerous.

Ongoing psychosocial interventions
Maintenance phase: There is limited data on the necessity for maintenance phase for behavioral interventions, however clinical experience suggests that once a month visits with the care managers over one year after treatment response to reinforce the newly learned behaviors is helpful to maintain treatment gains.

Discontinuation phase: One of the assumptions underlying the effects of behavioral interventions is that treatment response is due to practiced changes in behavior that over time become permanent changes. As a result there is no such thing as discontinuation because the expectation is that patients continue to employ the strategies that helped them overcome their depression for the rest of their lives.

Team goal: Relapse prevention
Consolidate gains made during the acute phase of treatment; identify specific strategies to recognize and address early warning signs of relapse.

Working as a team
Patient: Identifies early warning signs; participates in routine monitoring for such signs, enlisting family members or other supports when possible.

PCP: Follows up for continuation phase of antidepressant management and considers need for maintenance antidepressant management. Considers long-term medication consequences.

BHP: Offers psychoeducation about recurrence of depression. Assists patient in developing relapse prevention plan that identifies and summarizes strategies to prevent a depression relapse, early warning signs, and steps to take if depressive symptoms to worsen. Monitors ongoing adherence to psychotropic medications, behavioral activation strategies, and other approaches to preventing depression recurrence. Reinforces the use of behavioral strategies the patient found most useful in their recovery.

PC: Assists evaluation of need for maintenance antidepressant management. Assists BHP in identifying other residual risks for relapse that have not yet been addressed or referral for additional specialty mental health services.

Case example
After an additional four months, the patient's PHQ-9 score dropped to a 1 and he reported continued success in social engagement, even when his back bothered him. The patient and BHP began to discuss relapse prevention plans. He understood the need to remain on his antidepressant medication for a minimum of four months even though he was feeling better, but that he might consider a longer course given his prior history of a depressive episode. At the final meeting, the BHP and patient developed a detailed relapse prevention plan that included continuation of his medication for another year, and a plan to continue his pleasant activities (walking, swimming, socializing with family and friends, volunteering at the local church on Sundays). The plan also included the patient continuing to track his symptoms on his own as well as a plan to monitor his "hot" symptoms, depression symptoms he felt are an indication he may need to check in with his doctor. The plan specified that if his PHQ-9 was above 5 for two weeks, he experienced unremitting pain for one week, or began to drop his activities, he would contact his PCP for follow-up.

Special considerations for adolescent depression

Depression is common among adolescents, and frequently unrecognized or undertreated. Although the US Preventive Services Task Force recommends screening for depression among adolescents, screening alone will not improve outcomes.

Collaborative Care has been shown to be an effective model for treating depression among adolescents. While the principles of Collaborative Care for adolescents are unchanged from programs for adults, adaptations are made to ensure that care is developmentally appropriate. Engaging parents as active supports through structured involvement in the adolescent's care is a key factor for success. Other adaptations include the use of educational materials that are developmentally appropriate for teens, and including a team member with expertise in adolescent development.

Resources for providers

Websites:
- American Psychiatric Association Practice Guideline for Treatment of Patients with Major Depressive Disorder, 3rd Edition http://psychiatryonline.org/pb/assets/raw/sitewide/practice_guidelines/guidelines/mdd.pdf
- PHQ measures (translated into many languages) http://www.phqscreeners.com/overview.aspx
- IMPACT Depression Care: http://impact-uw.org/
- DAWN Care: http://www.dawncare.org/
- TEAMcare: http://www.teamcarehealth.org/
- Reach Out 4 Teens: www.reachout4teens.org

Videos:
- Care manager demonstrating medication education (video) http://uwaims.org/files/videos/antidepressant_education.html

Resources for patients

Books:
- Katon, W., Ludman, E., & Simon, G. (2002). *The Depression Helpbook*. Boulder CO: Bull Publishing Company.

Websites:
- National Suicide Prevention Lifeline http://www.suicidepreventionlifeline.org/
- NIMH http://www.nimh.nih.gov/health/topics/depression/index.shtml
- American Psychiatric Association http://www.psychiatry.org/patients-families/depression

- National Alliance on Mental Illness (NAMI) http://www.nami.org/
- Depression and Bipolar Support Alliance (DBSA) http://www.dbsalliance.org/site/ PageServer?pagename=home
- Right Direction http://www.rightdirectionforme.com/

Videos:
- Depression in older adults (including patient stories) http://uwaims.org/files/ videos/patient_education.html
- Discovery Health Depression in teenagers (website with video) http://health .howstuffworks.com/mental-health/depression/facts/depression-cure.htm
- How Antidepressants Work http://www.mayoclinic.com/health/antidepressants/ MM00660
- Defense Centers of Excellence Depression http://www.afterdeployment.org/ topics-depression
- Electroconvulsive Therapy (ECT) http://www.mayoclinic.com/health/electro convulsive-therapy/MM00606

Self-management tools:
- Mood Gym (interactive Web program for depression management) https:// moodgym.anu.edu.au/welcome
- Life Armor mobile app (depression education, management tools, and videos) http://t2health.org/apps/lifearmor#.UjODz3_g1Js

References

Archer, J., Bower, P., Gilbody, S., Lovell, K., Richards, D., Gask, L., Dickens, C., & Coventry, P. (2012). Collaborative care for depression and anxiety problems. *Cochrane Database Syst Rev.* Oct 17;10:CD006525. doi: 10.1002/14651858. CD006525.pub2, 2012

American Psychiatric Association. (2010). *Practice Guideline for the Treatment of Patients with Major Depressive Disorder, 3rd Edition.* Washington DC: American Psychiatric Association.

Cipriani, A., Furakawa, T. A., Salanti, G., Geddes, J. R., Higgins, J. P., Churchill, R . . . . Tansella, M. (2009). Comparative efficacy and acceptability of 12 new-generation antidepressants: a multiple-treatments meta-analysis. *Lancet, 373,* 746–58.

Qaseem, A., Snow, V., Denberg, T. D., Forciea, M. A, & Owens, D. K. (2008). Using second-generation antidepressants to treat depressive disorders: a clinical practice guideline from the American College of Physicians. *Annals of Internal Medicine, 149,* 725–33.

Richardson, L. P., Ludman, E., McCauley, E., Lindenbaum, J., Larison, C., Zhou, C . . . . Katon, W. (2014). Collaborative care for adolescents with depression in primary care: a randomized clinical trial. *Journal of the American Medical Association, 312*(8), 809–16.

Sussman, N. (2007). Translating science into service: Lessons learned from the Sequenced Treatment Alternatives to Relieve Depression (STAR*D) Study. *Primary Care Companion Journal of Clinical Psychiatry, 9,* 331–37.

Chapter 3 **Bipolar Disorder**

Joseph Cerimele, Lydia Chwastiak, and Evette Ludman

Clinical impact

- Bipolar disorder I or II occurs in approximately 0.5–4 percent of primary care patients but can be as high as 9 percent in some clinical settings such as safety net clinics. Bipolar disorder causes significant functional impairment. Depressive symptoms are more frequent and contribute more to functional impairment than manic symptoms. Patients experience mood symptoms approximately 50 percent of days, not just during major mood episodes.
- Occurs in at least 10 percent of patients presenting to primary care with a psychiatric complaint
- Often a delay of 10 years between onset of symptoms and bipolar disorder diagnosis
- Approximately 17 percent of patients with bipolar I and 24 percent of patients with bipolar II attempt suicide, compared to 12 percent in unipolar depression

Patients with a long history of bipolar disorder have significantly increased risk of chronic medical illnesses. Since age of onset for bipolar disorder is in late teens to early 20s, this means that many patients with bipolar disorder will have co-occurring medical problems such as hypertension and type II diabetes in late 30s to early 40s.

Integrated Care: Creating Effective Mental and Primary Health Care Teams, First Edition.
Anna Ratzliff, Jürgen Unützer, Wayne Katon, and Kari A. Stephens.
© 2016 John Wiley & Sons, Inc. Published 2016 by John Wiley & Sons, Inc.

Assessment

Identify chief complaint, associated somatic and psychological symptoms, functional impairment, and safety concerns

Patients with bipolar disorder are most likely to present in primary care with a depressive episode or subsyndromal depressive symptoms.

- Depressive symptoms occur 3–4 times as often as manic symptoms in bipolar I disorder, and approximately 20 times as often in bipolar II disorder.
- Subthreshold symptoms (mood symptoms not meeting full criteria for a mood episode) occur 3 times as often as a full episode in bipolar I and II disorder.
- Over 2/3 of patients with bipolar depression experience at least 1 co-occurring manic symptom during the depressive episode.
- The most common co-occurring manic symptoms are: distractibility, racing thoughts, and psychomotor agitation.
- Many women with bipolar disorder experience a postpartum mood episode.

Common psychological symptoms

Patients with bipolar disorder commonly present with depression. Patients will acknowledge mood or cognitive symptoms of depression when asked; however, not all patients with depression have sad or depressed mood.

Depressive symptoms: depressed mood, anhedonia, guilt, retardation, impaired concentration, suicidal ideation. Hypersomnia, hyperphagia, significant guilt, any psychotic feature (i.e. pathological guilt) or co-occurring manic symptom increases likelihood that depressive episode is bipolar, rather than unipolar, depression

Manic symptoms: irritability (more common than elevated mood), elevated mood, racing thoughts, distractibility, increased activity, impulsive behavior, inflated self-esteem

Hypomanic symptoms: same symptoms as manic episode, though occurring for a shorter time; usually does not result in hospitalization as manic episode often does

Mixed symptoms: manic and depressive episode occurring concurrently

Cyclothymia symptoms: chronic dysthymia and hypomania

Common physical/Somatic symptoms

Physical symptoms occur often in individuals with bipolar disorder, particularly during bipolar depression:

- Depression—sluggish feeling, "heavy" limbs, fatigue
- Mania or hypomania—Overenergized, restless, can't sleep or less need for sleep

- Pain symptoms or syndromes such as headache (see Chapter 2: Depression for additional details)

Common functional impairments

Severity of functional impairment is similar in patients with bipolar disorder seen in primary care and specialty care settings. Functional impairment can be chronic, and independent of severity of current mood episode.

- Unemployment, loss of relationships, financial losses, illegal activities, and homelessness can all occur in patients with bipolar disorder.
- Chronic medical problems, substance use, smoking, and obesity are associated with lower quality of life in patients with bipolar disorder. Comorbid alcohol and substance use and other high-risk behaviors are common.

Assessing for safety

Suicide attempts in bipolar disorder are associated with: being single, history of childhood abuse, bipolar disorder onset before age 25, presence of current depressive symptoms or mixed state, progressively worsening mood episode, co-occurring substance use or anxiety disorders, and family history of suicide. Mania can be associated with high risk of harm to the patient due to impulsivity and associated psychosis. Co-occurring substance use increases risk of harm to the patient or to others.

Team goal: Identifying the chief complaint, initial physical exam, gathering history, and safety assessment

Recognize that patients with depressive disorders may have bipolar disorder. Engage in treatment by providing empathetic care and hope, and initiate appropriate evaluation of possible comorbidities. Compassionately assess for active suicidality/safety concerns at initial evaluation and throughout treatment for depression.

Working as a team

Patient: Provide information to the clinical team. Provides the names of friends and family to provide collateral information about mood history. Works with BHP to generate a safety plan.

    PCP: Recognize depressive symptoms in patient and ask about co-occurring manic symptoms. Conducts suicide risk assessment.

    BHP: Further assess patient's history of mood symptoms and episodes. Generates safety plan with patient.

    PC: Recommends assessing for key historical points or examination findings that differentiate major depression from bipolar disorder. Consider assessing for co-occurring disorders such as anxiety. Advises BHP and PCP on risk assessment and risk mitigation.

Case example

A 35-year-old woman presented to primary care "to get her thyroid checked out" because she has gained 20lbs over the previous six months. Further questioning by the primary care clinician revealed that the patient has also experienced low energy with associated "heavy sleeping," depressed mood, anhedonia, guilt, trouble concentrating, distractibility, and intermittent racing thoughts.

The patient reports being hospitalized to a psychiatry ward when she was 24 "because I started acting like my mom—I couldn't think straight or sleep at all, spent all my money, drove really fast and just couldn't slow down." The patient is currently overweight and smokes 10 cigarettes per day—her most recent primary care note reported "follow-up on slightly elevated blood pressure."

The patient is introduced to the clinic BHP and reported to the BHP that she was intermittently experiencing preoccupations with death but denied any intent or wish to injure herself or attempt suicide. The BHP then assessed the patient's prior experiences with suicidal ideation, suicide attempts, and assessed current risk factors for suicide using a standardized clinical assessment. The BHP called the psychiatric consultant to discuss the patient's current risk for suicide, and the BP communicated the PC's impression and recommendations to the PCP and the patient. The BHP then created a safety plan with the patient.

Differential diagnosis and identifying a provisional diagnosis

Rule out common contributing medical problems and substance-related conditions

Symptoms of depression overlap with symptoms of many types of medical conditions and these are discussed in Chapter 2. Medical conditions and substance-related conditions that mimic mania are listed below.

- Medical conditions that mimic mania

    Endocrine: hyperthyroidism, hypercorticolism (Cushing's disease)
    Immunological: autoimmune disorders such as lupus
    Metabolic: hypercalcemia
    Neurological: multiple sclerosis, seizure, brain tumor

- Substance-related conditions that mimic mania

    Withdrawal: alcohol, benzodiazepine, opioid,
    Intoxication: anticholinergics, alcohol, phencyclidine (PCP), amphetamine, cocaine
    Prescribed medications: steroids, stimulants

Develop and refine differential diagnosis

Use the chief complaint and core presenting symptoms to generate a broad differential diagnosis (Table 3.2). Standardized tools can be helpful both for clarifying diagnosis, assessing severity, and tracking symptoms over time.

- Bipolar disorder should be considered in all patients presenting with depression; however, most patients with depression will have unipolar, not bipolar, depression.
- The Mood Disorder Questionnaire has a very low positive predictive value in primary care, meaning that most patients with a positive MDQ actually do not have bipolar disorder.
- The CIDI brief structured interview for bipolar disorder can potentially be used as a screening instrument in patients with depression or other psychiatric complaints. The CIDI involves asking initially about whether a patient has ever experienced a time of prolonged euphoria or irritability, with concurrent associated manic symptoms. A recent paper by Kessler, et al. describes using the CIDI in primary care (http://journals.cambridge.org/abstract_S0033291712002334).
- However, it is necessary to follow up with key questions and ask about differentiating symptoms listed below to narrow the differential diagnosis.

Assessment of comorbid psychiatric disorders and psychological difficulties

- Many patients with bipolar disorder have comorbid psychiatric conditions.
- Comorbidity is a common reason for treatment-resistance among patients with depression.
- Anxiety disorders co-occur in approximately 75 percent of patients with bipolar disorder
  - Approximately 25 percent have PTSD
  - Approximately 30 percent have GAD
- Substance use disorders co-occur in over 40 percent of patients with bipolar disorder
- Pain symptoms can also occur in about 50 percent of patients with bipolar disorder
- Impulse control disorders may also occur
- Cigarette use occurs in up to 50 percent of patients with bipolar disorder

Table 3.1 Generating the differential for bipolar disorder

Diagnosis	Key questions	Differentiating symptom or history	Behavioral health measure
Major depressive disorder	• Does the patient have a history of mania or hypomania? • Is patient experiencing manic symptoms such as distractibility or racing thoughts during depressive episode? • What was age of onset of depression? • What is patient's prior response to antidepressant medication?	• The presence of prior mania or hypomania is consistent with bipolar, not unipolar, depression • Manic symptoms during depressive episode are more suggestive of bipolar disorder • Onset before age 18 is more suggestive of bipolar disorder • Prior adverse response to antidepressant medication including increased activity (i.e., onset or worsening of racing thoughts or irritability), development of suicidal thoughts are suggestive of bipolar disorder	PHQ-9 (Note—PHQ-9 can be used in bipolar depression as well)
Borderline personality disorder	• How long do the hypomanic/manic symptoms last? • How often do hypomanic/manic "episodes" occur?	• Episodes lasting a few hours and/or a few times a week are more indicative of a personality and/or substance use disorder	None

Generalized anxiety disorder	• Does patient have inability to control worry? Is patient a "worrier"?	• Inability to control worry is more indicative of generalized anxiety disorder	GAD-7
Posttraumatic stress disorder	• Did patient experience traumatic event? • Does patient have symptoms of: re-experiencing, avoiding, or hyperarousal?	• Reexperiencing traumatic events, avoiding reminders of the traumatic event and hyperarousal are more suggestive of PTSD	PCL-C
Substance use disorders	• Does patient use substances? (i.e., alcohol, cocaine, opioids, cannabis)	• Substance use often co-occurs in bipolar disorder; however, accurate diagnosis of manic or depressive episode can be clouded by current substance use, since substances can cause or worsen mood episodes	AUDIT DAST CAGE-AID

Other disorders to consider: schizoaffective disorder, schizophrenia, traumatic brain injury, ADHD, panic disorder, impulse control disorders

Team goal: Differential Diagnosis and Identifying a Provisional Diagnosis

Differentiate unipolar depression and bipolar depression as these require different treatment approaches. Complete a thorough assessment to identify any other conditions that may affect treatment.

Working as a team

Patient: Agrees to undergo examination and provide history of symptoms. The patient completes some of the measures on own time. May supply mood charts.

PCP: Recognizes that patients with psychiatric illness often have co-occurring general medical illnesses, and assess for these illnesses. Uses follow-up questions to further assess history. Considers co-occurring illnesses and refers to BHP for additional assessment as needed.

BHP: Communicates PCP findings to PC, and PC recommendations to PCP. Describes process to patient. Communicates results of screening tools and follow-up questions. Obtains the necessary information related to co-occurring illnesses.

PC: Suggests alternate diagnoses that could account for the current presentation. Suggests certain follow-up questions or screening tools that can help differentiate disorders. Consider which co-occurring illness to assess; offer a diagnostic interview if differential diagnosis is complex and challenging.

Case example

The primary care clinician completes a full examination including a TSH measurement that is within normal limits. A urine toxicology study is negative. The PCP further assessed the patient and recognized that the patient was experiencing two manic symptoms (distractibility and racing thoughts) in the context of a depressive episode. The PCP had also elicited a history that "sounded like mania." The PCP referred the patient to the Collaborative Care program.

The BHP conducts a detailed assessment using a combination of structured clinical questions and standardized measures. The patient provides the information to the BHP, and the BHP relays this information to the psychiatric consultant. The PC then reviews the results of the structured clinical questions and standardized measures. (See Table 3.1 for a list of questions and measures commonly used in the assessment of patients with bipolar disorder.)

The psychiatric consultant advises the BHP to assess the patient for co-occurring substance use and psychiatric symptoms and disorders using the measures in Table 3.1 and a detailed clinical assessment. The BHP also discovered that the patient has a difficult time controlling her worries and is often preoccupied with uncertainty about future events. The BHP obtained additional information including a lifetime mood episode chart. The patient had experienced one manic episode at 24, then six subsequent depressive episodes, and possibly one hypomanic episode that occurred in the context of alcohol use. The patient had demonstrated improvement in depression and mania with lithium treatment in the past. Because substance use is common in bipolar disorder, the BHP then used the AUDIT scale to screen for alcohol use problems, and the DAST to screen for other substance use disorders. It is learned that the patient smokes 10 cigarettes daily and wants to quit, and has had episodes of binge alcohol use in the past.

Treatment

Initiate treatment plan

General principles
There are three domains of treatment for bipolar disorder: treatment of acute mania (and acute hypomania), treatment of acute depression, and maintenance treatment. The mood episodes of bipolar disorder are treatable. (see Table 3.3) Once remission from an acute mood episode occurs, maintenance treatment can improve functioning and help prevent mood episode recurrence. Evidence supports continuing successful acute phase treatments for subsequent maintenance treatment.

Table 3.2 Common bipolar disorders in primary care (ICD-10)

- Bipolar I disorder: F31.x (Add severity/course specifier)

  Bipolar disorder, current episode hypomanic: F31.0x
  Bipolar disorder, current episode manic without psychotic features F31.1x
  Bipolar disorder, current episode manic severe with psychotic features F31.2x
  Bipolar disorder, current episode depressed, mild or moderate severity F31.3x
  Bipolar disorder, current episode depressed, severe, without psychotic features
    F31.4x
  Bipolar disorder, current episode depressed, severe, with psychotic features F31.5x
  Bipolar disorder, current episode mixed F31.6x
  Bipolar disorder, currently in remission F31.7x

- Bipolar II disorder: F31.8x
- Bipolar disorder, unspecified F31.9
- Cyclothymia: F34.0

Table 3.3 Team-based treatment for bipolar disorder

	PCP approaches	BHP approaches
Biological	**Evidence-Based Medication Treatment:**	**Evidence-Based Medication Treatment:**
	• Mood stabilizer medications are the first line treatment. • Different phases of treatment may require different treatments. • First-line mood stabilizing medications include lithium, divalproex and atypical antipsychotics.	• Medication adherence is the foundation of treatment for bipolar disorder treatment and addressing any potential barriers to engaging in medication management. • Support patients through making medication changes and troubleshoot adherence challenges. • Help gather collateral information from family and friends as the opportunity arises to help with treatment planning.
Psychosocial	**Evidence-Based Behavioral Treatment:**	**Evidence-Based Behavioral Treatment:**
	• Validate behavioral interventions that augment medication treatment by explaining and encouraging patients to try this type of treatment. • Assess engagement with and reinforce behavioral treatment during medical visits by asking patients about utility and progress in treatment and checking in with the BHP about treatment progress.	• Delivering evidence-based sleep hygiene approaches may be an important target for initial brief behavioral intervention. • Provide evidence-based therapies in primary care or helping patients connect to community resources. • Evidence-based behavioral interventions that have shown to be helpful in bipolar disorder include CBT, family-focus therapy, interpersonal therapy and social rhythm therapy.

However, most patients experience mood episode recurrence. Therefore, managing bipolar disorder is similar to managing other chronic diseases (i.e., focusing on adherence, self-management and other chronic illness principles). Subsyndromal symptoms (i.e., one to two depressive symptoms or one to two manic symptoms) often precede a full mood episode and should be treated. Subsyndromal symptoms also significantly impair functioning.

Medication principles
- Mood stabilizer medications are the first line treatment.
- The role of antidepressant agents in the treatment of bipolar depression is controversial. Some, but not all, evidence suggests that antidepressants added to mood stabilizing medications do not improve treatment of acute bipolar depression, and that antidepressants may worsen manic symptoms. There may be a role for antidepressant medications in the maintenance treatment of some patients with bipolar II disorder. However, in general, use of antidepressant medications in patients with bipolar disorder should generally be done in consultation with the psychiatric consultant.
- Many patients require treatment with more than one medication (i.e., "augment rather than substitute"). If a patient's previous mood episode was successfully treated with combination therapy (i.e., more than one medication) then combination therapy will likely be better at preventing mood episode recurrence in that patient.

Brief behavioral interventions
- Studies have shown that when medication is combined with psychotherapy patients were more likely to get well faster and stay well longer.
- For a patient with bipolar disorder, regularity and consistency in day to day activities can help reduce the risk of mood episode recurrence, and this is an important target for BHP support.
- Sleep hygiene and consistent sleep/wake times are important behavioral interventions that can easily be delivered in primary care.
- Patients can track symptoms, functioning, treatments, and life events using a mood chart.
- Behavioral interventions for depression are helpful augmentations during depressive episodes. Problem-solving treatment, cognitive behavioral therapy, behavioral activation, and interpersonal therapy (see Chapter 2) can be helpful as early as the second or third week of treatment.
- Motivational Interviewing can be particularly helpful for medication or behavioral treatment adherence issues.

Psychoeducation

• About one half of patients with an acute bipolar disorder episode treated to remission will experience recurrence of a mood episode within two years. Clinical factors associated with shorter time until relapse include: co-occurring anxiety or substance use disorder, residual depressive or manic symptoms at remission, female gender, and greater number of prior mood episodes.

• Medication nonadherence is common in patients with bipolar disorder. Stigma, limited insight, complicated medication dosing, limited social support, cost, and perception of treatment ineffectiveness all contribute to nonadherence.

• Consider describing illness as a chronic disease (similar to hypertension or diabetes) that requires ongoing assessment, treatment and follow-up—even during "symptom-free" times.

• Evidence supports the use of group psychoeducation in preventing mood episode recurrence in bipolar I and bipolar II patients treated effectively with medications.

PCP approaches to treatment
Choice of medication

• *Acute mania*: The treatment of acute mania is generally straight-forward (Table 3.4). However, mania is not as commonly encountered as acute bipolar depression. First-line treatment is usually lithium carbonate or divalproex plus an antipsychotic medication. Carbamazepine plus an antipsychotic is also an effective treatment for acute mania.

• *Acute depression*: Generally the agent(s) that successfully treated a prior episode is (are) the first choice for the current episode. Evidence supports the use of lithium monotherapy in acute bipolar depression; however, quetiapine (FDA indication for bipolar depression) and lurasidone (FDA indication for bipolar depression) are also first-line treatment options. Olanzapine-fluoxetine combination also has an FDA indication for bipolar depression. Divalproex is a reasonable first-line choice. Lamotrigine monotherapy has mixed evidence in bipolar depression; however, there is evidence supporting the addition of lamotrigine to lithium when treating bipolar depression.

• *Maintenance*: Some patients will present with a history of bipolar disorder but no current symptoms. The next section describes approaches to medications during maintenance phases.

• Additional information:
  • The role of antidepressant medications in the treatment of bipolar depression is controversial.

- Anticonvulsants such as divalproex and carbamazepine are usually more effective in treating rapid cycling bipolar disorder compared to lithium. [Rapid cycling bipolar disorder is the occurrence of 4 or more mood episodes in the previous 12 months, with either remission between episodes lasting 2 months or more, OR switch to a mood episode of opposite pole (i.e., from mania to depression)].

Table 3.4 Medications commonly used in the treatment of bipolar disorder

Acute bipolar depression
Quetiapine
Olanzapine-fluoxetine combination
Divalproex
Lithium carbonate
Lamotrigine
Lamotrigine plus lithium carbonate
Lurasidone

Acute mania
Severe (i.e., with psychosis):
Lithium carbonate or divalproex plus an antipsychotic
Antipsychotics to choose from:

Haloperidol
Risperidone
Aripiprazole
Olanzapine
Quetiapine

Moderate (i.e., without psychosis):
Lithium carbonate monotherapy
Divalproex monotherapy
Lithium carbonate plus divalproex

Maintenance
Lithium carbonate
Divalproex
Carbamazepine
Quetiapine
Lamotrigine
Lurasidone
Lithium carbonate plus divalproex
Lithium carbonate plus lamotrigine
Lithium carbonate plus quetiapine
Lithium carbonate plus lurasidone

For prescribing details and protocols, please see Chapter 11, "Evidence-Based Psychopharmacology for the Collaborative Care Team"

Safe prescribing
- Most medications used to treat bipolar disorder require laboratory monitoring (i.e., serum levels for lithium and divalproex, thyroid and kidney functioning for lithium, metabolic monitoring for antipsychotics).
- Medication discontinuation in bipolar disorder should be approached with caution, and generally accompanied by consultation with a psychiatric consultant.
- Consider providing limited supplies (i.e., prescriptions for just one week rather than one month) of medications with high lethality such as lithium in suicidal patients.

Support engagement in psychosocial approaches

As the BHP will play an important role to support medication adherence and patient engagement, the PCP can play an important role in promoting a team approach.
- Validate behavioral interventions that augment medication treatment by explaining and encouraging patients to try this type of treatment.

BHP approaches to treatment
Psychosocial approaches
In the acute phase of treatment the BHP will often prioritize supporting medication management because the need to establish good medication adherence is critical to stabilize mood.
- Basic psychoeducation that teaches people about the disorder, its treatments, and self-management strategies are cornerstones of care for patients with bipolar disorder. Ideally, this is accompanied by family and caregiver education about bipolar disorder symptoms, relapse, and treatment.
- Regular daily routines and sleep schedules may help protect against manic episodes.
- Helping patients fill out daily planners to guide their activities is a useful brief behavioral activation strategy.
- It is often useful to have patients track daily symptoms with a mood chart so that the patient, family, and clinicians can recognize early if the patient is experiencing symptom relapse.
- Mood charts can also help patients understand that life experiences (and behaviors and cognitions) can sometimes influence symptom severity. Mood charts are easily downloaded from mental health consumer advocacy organizations online. A mood chart is provided by the Depression

and Bipolar Support Alliance here: http://www.dbsalliance.org/pdfs/tracking.pdf.

- Nonjudgmental exploration of the positive and negative effects ("upsides" and "downsides") of one's coping responses to mania or depression (e.g., taking drugs, avoiding work or friends) may help patients identify coping responses more in line with their life goals and values.
- Peer support and psychoeducation for patients and their families may be available locally or through online consumer advocacy organizations (e.g., Depression and Bipolar Support Alliance).

Evidence-based psychotherapeutic approaches

Most psychotherapeutic approaches for bipolar disorder emphasize education, symptom identification, relapse prevention, and adherence to medications. Please see Chapter 2 for more information about using behavioral interventions that may be helpful to augment mood stabilizers for depressive symptoms.

Evidence-based approaches to consider:

- Cognitive behavioral therapy (CBT): helps people with bipolar disorder learn to change negative thought patterns and behaviors. (strong evidence)
- Family-focused therapy: includes family members in the treatment. It helps enhance family coping strategies, such as recognizing new episodes early and helping their loved one. This therapy also focuses on improving communication among family members, as well as problem-solving. (strong evidence)
- Other evidence-based treatments include interpersonal and social rhythm therapy, which helps people with bipolar disorder improve their relationships with others and manage their daily routine such as improving sleep hygiene.

Working with medications

Prepare patients for mood stabilization trials by educating them that it can take several weeks and often adjustments in medications for maximum benefit from a mood stabilizer.

- Ask if they have questions about medication treatment and help them get information on common misconceptions.
- Remind them that in the initial days to weeks of a trial of medication the focus is tolerability.
- Prepare patients to monitor and report concerns and side effects.
- Troubleshoot common barriers to medication adherence including cost and need for a system to remember to take medications.

Team goal: Initial treatment planning
Provides psychoeducation about the diagnosis of bipolar disorder and identify patient goals and preferences to guide the decision making about mood stabilizers. Engage the patient in dialog about the importance of long-term mood stabilization to treat bipolar disorder.

Working as a team
Patient: Participates in a discussion on treatment options and makes an informed decision regarding treatment with the help of the clinicians.

PCP: Leads discussion of initiating treatment with patient and BHP. Potentially communicates directly with the psychiatric consultant to enhance understanding of treatment options.

BHP: Accurately communicates the psychiatric consultant's recommendations to the PCP and the patient. Additionally, the BHP can help coordinate a consultation with the PC.

PC: Supports establishing a diagnosis based on available information and provide detailed information on reasonable treatment options. Considers directly consulting on the patient if needed, and remains available to talk directly to the PCP.

Case example
The PC supported the team in establishing a diagnosis of bipolar depression, and recommended obtaining laboratory studies (urinalysis with specific gravity, electrolyte panel including serum calcium, BUN, and creatinine, and a TSH and free T4 level) prior to initiating lithium carbonate. The PCP hesitated to initiate lithium and asked the BHP to talk with the PC again. The PC acknowledged that quetiapine and olanzapine-fluoxetine combination have FDA indications for bipolar depression, and that lithium carbonate does not. However, the PC was reassured by the extensive literature demonstrating effectiveness of lithium in treating all phases of bipolar disorder and shared this information with the team. The patient had also previously experienced full remission of a manic and depressive episode with lithium treatment. The BHP relayed this information to the PCP and the lithium therapy was initiated.

Follow-up and treatment adjustment to achieve treatment to target

General principles

It is important to closely follow symptoms of depression and mania during treatment of bipolar disorder. In additional to assessment of current functioning, there are several mood scales that can support assessment of response to treatment. The PHQ-9 can be useful for tracking depressive symptoms over time. The Internal State Scale (ISS) Version 2 can be used to assess bipolar disorder symptom severity over time and can also be used to determine the need for treatment intensification. Research studies on bipolar disorder often use the Young Mania Rating Scale to assess the severity of mania and track it over time, though that scale has not been studied in primary care settings.

When to consider referral

- Persistent symptoms despite treatment with two or more mood stabilizer medications
- Diagnostic clarification
- Psychoeducation for patient regarding diagnosis or treatment
- Psychosis in the context of mania or depression
- Family history of completed suicide
- Patient history of numerous suicide attempts
- Question of whether to discontinue treatment

PCP approaches

Adjusting and Augmentation Strategies

A partial response with some ongoing mood symptoms is common for patients in an acute phase of treatment, so the following strategies can be helpful to facilitate prompt mood stabilization.

- Patients will need to be scheduled for close follow-up, ideally weekly, to allow for timely adjustment of medications.
- For lithium and divalproex, monitoring blood drug levels frequently will allow for rapid optimization of dose.
- For antipsychotics, if mood symptoms continue to be disturbing and impair functioning, gradually increase the dose while monitoring for problematic side effects.
- If significant symptoms persist and a patient cannot tolerate a higher dose of the medication, consider a slow cross taper to another mood stabilizer. The psychiatric consultant can provide guidance about cross tapers between medications.

Managing side effects

- *Lithium*: Patient should be assessed for both symptomatic and asymptomatic side effects.
  - Common SYMPTOMATIC side effects: Nausea, sedation, weight gain, tremor, loose stools, apathy, polyuria, and thirst.
  - Common ASYMPTOMATIC side effects: Hypothyroidism, hyperparathyroidism, hypercalcemia, reduced urinary concentrating ability.
  - Additional information on tremor: Postural tremor associated with lithium may be managed by dividing the lithium dose (note that dividing the dose will generally reduce the serum lithium level by about 20 percent), or administer Vitamin B6 up to 1200mg/day which has reduced lithium tremor in some cases, or treatment with propanolol. Other modifications such as cessation of caffeine consumption, can help.
- *Divalproex*: Common side effects include weight gain, nausea, vomiting, hair loss, and tremor.
- *Antipsychotics*: Please refer to Chapter 5 for management of side effects associated with antipsychotic medications

BHP approaches
Brief Behavioral Treatments Continuation Phase
Between four and six weeks after treatment initiation it is helpful to evaluate whether the behavioral treatments are helping with symptom improvement and patient satisfaction and confidence in managing their condition.

- Help patients become effective collaborators in their treatment. Ask them to identify if there are parts of their treatment that are particularly helpful and parts that don't seem to help.
- Confirm that patients and providers are working toward consistent goals.
- Help patients voice concerns about something a provider said or didn't say and consistently set between visit activities for patients to work on.
- If patients and providers do not think a particular modality is working or acceptable to patients consider adding or switching modalities. Consider helping patients find peer support from others with lived experience with bipolar disorder. This can be particularly helpful for patients who are feeling demoralized.

Working with medications
Patients with bipolar disorder are likely to stop taking medications at some point when in remission because symptoms are not always present and

because lack of insight is a symptom of bipolar disorder (specifically a symptom of mania).

- Troubleshoot adherence challenges
- Be responsive to concerns and side effects
- Support patient through making medication changes
- Help patient schedule an appointment with PCP to address medications
- Help patient write down questions

Team goal: Revising treatment planning and stepping up care
Supports the patient with bipolar disorder to stay engaged with care while medications are adjusted to target mood stabilization, and use behavioral interventions to support patient goals.

Working as a team
Patient: Attends follow-up appointments, discusses concerns and treatment goals, and completes standardized symptom assessment measures.

PCP: Follows up with patient and obtains necessary laboratory studies. Continues managing the medication treatment. Reviews results of standardized symptoms measures and discusses results with the patient.

BHP: Reaches out to patient to maintain close follow-up and assesses symptoms. Monitors medication adherence and side effects. Provides education and coaching about lifestyle modifications such as consistent sleep-wake cycles and stress management. Continues relaying information between PCP and PC. Delivers psychotherapeutic interventions aiming to enhance treatment adherence, reduce symptom burden, and reduce impairment associated with symptoms.

PC: Continues to consult with the BHP on the patient's care. Advises PCP and BHP on chronic mental health disease management. Gives direct recommendations on when to step up care in the context of nonresponse or partial response to the initial treatment plan. Can provide alternative treatments if first choice is not tolerated or ineffective.

Case example
The patient attended a follow-up appointment and was found to still be experiencing significant depressive symptoms. The BHP learned that the patient had misunderstood the dosing instructions for lithium and was only taking one-half of the recommended dose of 600mg per day, and had a serum lithium level of

(Continued)

0.3mEq/L. The BHP consulted with the PC to determine how to move ahead, and the PC advised increasing the dose to 600mg by mouth at bedtime and to obtain a serum lithium level one week later with the goal serum lithium level of 0.8–1mEq/L measured 12 hours after the last dose. The PCP agreed with this plan and provided the patient with these instructions.

Completing treatment and relapse prevention

General principles

Collaborative Care treatment for acute episodes can be used to monitor symptom severity and intensify treatment when nonresponse to treatment occurs. Bipolar disorder is a chronic illness and individuals with bipolar disorder will likely benefit from ongoing treatment monitoring even after resolution of acute episodes. Patients with bipolar disorder should be educated about identification of subsyndromal symptoms such as worsening irritability or sleep disturbances that can precede full mood episode but also indicate to patients and clinicians that closer monitoring or more intense treatment is needed.

Ongoing medication management

- Patients with bipolar disorder are likely to stop taking medications because symptoms are not always present and because lack of insight is a symptom of bipolar disorder (specifically a symptom of mania)
  - Troubleshoot adherence challenges
  - Be responsive to concerns and side effects
  - Support patient through making medication changes
  - Help patient schedule an appointment with PCP to address medications
  - Help patient write down questions
- Maintenance for Bipolar I: The goals of maintenance treatment are to prevent depressive and manic episode recurrence, minimize functional impairment and improve overall quality of life. If an acute manic or depressive episode has just been successfully treated, then it is generally preferable to continue the successful treatments as maintenance treatment. Otherwise, lithium carbonate or divalproex should be considered first-line treatment for maintenance treatment in most patients with bipolar disorder who have not just had a successfully treated acute mood episode.
- Maintenance for Bipolar II: Evidence suggests that lithium or divalproex plus an antipsychotic medication (such as quetiapine) is more effective

than lithium or divalproex monotherapy in preventing mood episode recurrence for some patients. Lithium and divalproex can also be used together. Lamotrigine plus lithium may also be used.

- Benzodiazepine use in bipolar disorder maintenance and depression treatment is associated with increased risk of depression recurrence. Alternative interventions for insomnia or anxiety should be considered.

- Unlike major depressive disorder where treatment may be stopped for some patients after 9–12 months, the treatment of bipolar disorder is generally much longer. Many patients are treated for decades, since the risk of mood episode recurrence, functional impairment, and co-occurring illnesses does not lessen with time in bipolar disorder.

- Notable common interactions with lithium carbonate: Thiazide diuretics, ACE inhibitors, and NSAIDS increase serum lithium levels.

Ongoing psychosocial approaches

- Encourage patients to create, update, and maintain a self-care plan to maintain gains and prevent recurrences. An example self-care plan would include the following sections:
  - Medication plan: names, doses, daily reminder activity, MD checkback date, coping suggestions for side effects
  - Stress reduction plan: list of daily activities to help prevent daily hassles from adding up
  - High risk situation plan: identify situations, negative coping reactions that might occur, is there any way to prevent situation? What is the plan for coping/reacting in a different way?
  - Self-monitoring plan: what tool? When and where?
  - Personal warning signs
  - Emergency or booster plan: who to contact on care team, friends and family

- Linking patients with bipolar disorder to a peer support specialist for support can also be helpful. Many peer support specialists have personally experienced bipolar disorder and can help patients set meaningful life and recovery goals, and coach patients in action-planning and problem-solving as they move toward the identified goals. Being linked to a peer support specialist can also reduce the stigma associated with bipolar disorder, which can enhance treatment adherence. The Depression and Bipolar Support Alliance provides information on connecting patients with peer support specialists (http://www.dbsalliance.org/site/PageServer?pagename=home).

Team goal: Relapse prevention

For bipolar disorder, relapse prevention is particularly important as patients without symptoms often think about stopping medications. Team works together to send a strong message about the need for long-term medication management and engagement in care.

Working as a team

Patient: The patient continues attending appointments at the primary care clinic, and may still meet with a peer support specialist. Ongoing monitoring of symptoms is a key part of relapse prevention.

PCP: The PCP continues with medication management and with conducting necessary laboratory and other monitoring such as weight and waist circumference.

BHP: The BHP supports the patient's recovery and helps the patient set functional goals. Enhancing adherence to treatment is also an ongoing part of relapse prevention.

PC: The PC remains available to consult on the patient.

Case example

Over the next six months the lithium dose was increased to 1200mg/day in divided doses (i.e., 600mg po twice daily) to achieve a serum lithium level of 0.8mEq/L measured 12 hours after the most recent dose of lithium. The patient experienced reduction in depressive symptoms evidenced by a 50 percent reduction in PHQ-9 score, and complete resolution of manic symptoms. The patient continued attending appointments with the BHP to identify goals and problem-solving techniques necessary for achieving the goals. The BHP also connected the patient with community support. As active treatment phase came to a close, the patient and the BHP completed a relapse prevention plan with clear behavioral indications for need to seek an appointment with a PCP and medication recommendations for maintenance treatment from the PC. The patient then returned to care as usual with the PCP, scheduling visits quarterly for medication check-ins and refills.

Resources for providers

- American Psychiatric Association Practice Guidelines http://psychiatryonline.org/content.aspx?bookid=28&sectionid=1682557
- STABLE Toolkit http://www.cqaimh.org/stable.html

Resources for patients

- National Institute of Mental Health http://www.nimh.nih.gov/health/publications /bipolar-disorder/index.shtml
- The Depression and Bipolar Support Alliance is an online resource for patients and their families http://www.dbsalliance.org/site/PageServer?pagename=home
- Bauer MS, Kilbourne AM, Greenwald DE, Ludman EJ. (2008.) *Overcoming Bipolar Disorder*. Oakland CA: New Harbinger Publications, Inc.

References

Belmaker, R. H. (2004). Bipolar disorder. *New England Journal of Medicine, 351*, 476–486.

Benyon, S., Soares-Wesier, K., Woolacott, N., Duffy, S., & Geddes, J. R. (2008). Psychosocial interventions for the prevention of relapse in bipolar disorder: systematic review of controlled trials. *British Journal of Psychiatry, 192*, 5–11.

Calabrese, J. R., Farley, P. A., Kessler, R. C., et al. (2012). Composite International Diagnostic Interview screening scales for DSM-IV anxiety and mood disorders. Psychological Medicine, Available on CJO 2012 doi:10.1017/S003329171200234

Cerimele, J. M., Chwastiak, L. A., Chan, Y. F., Harrison, D. A., & Unützer, J. (2013). The presentation, recognition and management of bipolar depression in primary care. *Journal of General Internal Medicine, 28*, 1648–1656.

Frye, M. A. (2011). Bipolar disorder—a focus on depression. *New England Journal of Medicine, 364*, 51–59.

Ludman, E., Von Korff, M., Katon, W., Lin, E., Simon, G., Walker, E., Bush, T., & Wahab, S. (2000). The design, implementation and acceptance of a primary care-based intervention to prevent depression relapse. *International Journal of Psychiatry in Medicine, 30*(3), 229–245.

Price, A. L. & Marzani-Nissen, G. R. (2012). Bipolar disorders: a review. *American Family Physician, 85*, 483–493.

Querques, J. & Kontos, N. (2010). An approach to the patient with dysregulated mood: major depression and bipolar disorder. *Medical Clinics of North America, 94*, 1117–1126.

Simon, G. E., Bauer, M. S., Ludman, E. J., Operskalski, B. H., & Unützer, J. (2007). Mood symptoms, functional impairment, and disability in people with bipolar disorder: specific effects of mania and depression. *Journal of Clinical Psychiatry, 68*, 1237–1245.

Chapter 4 **Anxiety and Trauma Disorders**

David A. Harrison, Kari A. Stephens, Anna Ratzliff, and Jennifer Sexton

Clinical impact

Anxiety disorders are highly common, have a higher lifetime prevalence than mood disorders (28.8 percent vs. 20.8 percent in the National Comorbidity Study Replication), and are comorbid with mood disorders the vast majority of the time. Because of the multitude of somatic symptoms frequently occurring in anxiety disorders, anxiety disorders complicate diagnosis and treatment and can lead to significantly increased medical costs. Anxiety disorders, like mood disorders, are highly associated with impaired general health and psychosocial functioning, can worsen suicidal thinking, and can be a significant risk factor for suicide attempts. Although the majority of patients with anxiety disorders are treated in the primary care setting, anxiety disorders are commonly underrecognized and undertreated in this setting.

Assessment

Identify chief complaint, associated somatic and psychological symptoms, functional impairment, and safety concerns

Somatic symptoms are a very common feature of anxiety disorders, and need to be recognized along with psychological symptoms and functional impairment in making the diagnosis of anxiety disorders. Listed below are common somatic and psychological symptoms seen in the major anxiety disorders together with common functional impairments.

Integrated Care: Creating Effective Mental and Primary Health Care Teams, First Edition.
Anna Ratzliff, Jürgen Unützer, Wayne Katon, and Kari A. Stephens.
© 2016 John Wiley & Sons, Inc. Published 2016 by John Wiley & Sons, Inc.

Common psychological symptoms

Generalized Anxiety Disorder (GAD): excessive worry or fears, worry difficult to control, irritability, poor concentration and attention

Panic disorder: fear of going crazy, fear of losing control, sense of impending doom or death

Social anxiety disorder/social phobia: excessive fears of scrutiny, embarrassment, and humiliation in social or performance situations, anticipatory anxiety

Post-Traumatic Stress Disorder (PTSD): feeling "keyed up" or on edge, hypervigilance, exaggerated startle, nightmares, flashbacks, irritability, anger, poor concentration, emotional numbing, avoidance, detachment or estrangement, restricted emotional range

Obsessive-Compulsive Disorder (OCD): persistent and intrusive thoughts, ideas, and images (fear of contamination, need for ordering things), repetitive intentional behavior

Common physical/Somatic symptoms

GAD: muscle tension, feeling "keyed up" or on edge, fatigue and sleep problems

Panic disorder: chest pain, palpitations, shortness of breath, trembling or shaking, sweating, nausea, abdominal pain, diarrhea, dizziness

Social anxiety disorder/social phobia: blushing, sweating, trembling, palpitations

PTSD: problems with sleep, night sweats

OCD: Physical signs of compulsive behavior (i.e., skin chapping, bald spots, scabs from picking)

Common functional impairments

Education/work: early difficulty in school, separation anxiety, missed work due to fear and avoidance

Relationships: history of trauma, risk for domestic violence, conflict due to irritability

Activities of daily living: inability to leave home

Assessing for safety

Anxiety disorders are significant independent risk factors for suicide attempts, more than doubling the risk (OR 2.2). In addition, comorbid anxiety has been found to amplify the risk of suicidal ideation (SI) in patients with mood disorders. Due to this elevated risk, any patient presenting with anxiety should be screened for SI and monitored at follow-up visits.

Team goal: Identifying the chief complaint, initial physical exam, gathering history and safety assessment

Use the initial visit with the PCP and BHP to understand the functional impairment related to anxiety which will shape the goals for treatment. All team members must share the responsibility of the safety assessment and communicating the risks to the team.

Working as a team

Patient: Describes both physical and emotional symptoms, the impact of these anxiety symptoms on their life, and their goals for treatment. Describes past anxiety management strategies or treatments used and treatment preferences for medications, therapy, or both. Provides information about thoughts of self-harm or other safety concerns.

PCP: Recognizes possible anxiety disorders, especially in patients who may present with unexplained physical conditions. Performs basic screening of the patient with the GAD-7, gathering additional history pertinent to the patient's symptoms and performing a focused exam directed by potential medical causes of the patient's symptoms (e.g., signs of hyperthyroidism). Conducts initial safety assessment and safety planning; coordinates with BHP to monitor safety issues.

BHP: Completes a detailed assessment of the patient's anxiety symptoms and their impact on the patient's life. Conducts safety assessment and safety planning; develops plan to monitor safety issues and track plan.

PC: May help refine the differential of different types of anxiety disorders often asking for greater clarification about particular symptoms (e.g., how long the panic symptoms last) which will later guide treatment decision making. May assist in clarifying the patient's risk of self-harm or harm to others or in safety planning.

Case example

A 23-year-old woman presents to her PCP with a chief complaint of "racing heart and shortness of breath." She describes increasing difficulty at work because she has sudden onset episodes, lasting a few minutes of overwhelming fear, shortness of breath, nausea, racing heart, and dizziness. She is worried that something is "wrong with her heart." She notices that she does not have these episodes in the evening when she is drinking wine. She has had one ER visit in the past month, where "heart tests" were normal and she treated with alprazolam with relief of her symptoms. She scored a 12 on the GAD-7, indicating moderate anxiety. The PCP and BHP assessed the patient for safety, and the patient denied any thoughts of hurting herself or others or previous suicidality or self-harm behaviors (e.g., cutting).

Differential diagnosis and identifying a provisional diagnosis

Rule out common medical diagnoses and Substance/ Drug-related conditions

Especially in patients with anxiety who often present with physical symptoms, an essential part of the diagnostic process is to identify potential medical or substance/drug-related conditions that may be causing the anxiety symptoms. Unrecognized and untreated medical or substance/drug related conditions can pose a threat to patient well-being (e.g., untreated cardiovascular disease) and can prevent other treatment modalities from working effectively. It is only after an anxiety disorder due to a medical condition or substance/drug has been effectively treated or ruled out can a clinician confidently and appropriately diagnose a patient with other types of anxiety disorders.

Medical conditions to consider in evaluation of anxiety:
Cardiovascular: angina, arrhythmias, congestive heart failure (CHF), hypotension, myocardial infarction (MI)
Gastrointestinal: gastroesophageal reflux disease (GERD), irritable bowel syndrome (IBS), malignancy
Hematologic: anemia
Endocrine: hyperadrenalism, hypo/hyperthyroidism, endocrine tumor
Immunological: anaphylaxis, lupus, multiple sclerosis (MS)
Metabolic: hyponatremia, hypocalcemia, hypoglycemia
Neurological: encephalopathy, temporal lobe epilepsy, central nervous system (CNS) tumor, traumatic brain injury, vertigo
Respiratory: asthma, chronic obstructive pulmonary disease (COPD), pneumonia, pulmonary embolism (PE)

Substance-related conditions consider in evaluation of anxiety:
Withdrawal: alcohol, opiates, sedatives, hypnotics
Intoxication: digitalis, anticholinergics, caffeine, hallucinogens, cannabis, stimulants

Prescribed medications: selective serotonin reuptake inhibitors (SSRIs) and antipsychotics (both potentially causing akathisia), bronchodilators (e.g., theophylline, sympathomimetics), oral or inhaled steroids

Develop and refine differential diagnosis

Once anxiety symptoms due to a medical condition or substance/drug have been ruled out or effectively treated, the chief complaint together with the core presenting symptoms can generate a differential diagnosis and establish a diagnosis (Table 4.1 and Table 4.2). In addition to the general Differential Diagnosis Table (in Chapter 1), use the key questions and behavioral health measures in Differentiating Symptoms for Anxiety Disorders Table.

Tips for differential diagnosis between various anxiety disorders:

- Assessment of anxiety triggers, can help guide diagnosis:

    GAD: thoughts
    Panic disorder: physical sensations of panic
    Social anxiety disorder/social phobia: social situations
    PTSD: trauma reminders
    OCD: obsessive thoughts

- Don't automatically assume that a trauma history (e.g., a history of child sexual abuse) is the same as a diagnosis of PTSD. Utilize a PTSD screener (e.g., Primary Care PTSD Screen) or symptom measure (e.g., PTSD Check List–Civilian Version) to help identify the diagnosis and intensity of current symptoms to guide diagnosis.

- Ongoing substance use (e.g., opioids, benzodiazepines, marijuana, and alcohol) may mask underlying anxiety issues. If substances are being actively used, ask the patient to describe their anxiety symptoms when they have not been using these substances in the past and ask about benefits they find from using these substances to determine whether they help reduce anxiety in the moment.

- To help distinguish between panic disorder and other anxiety disorders, determine whether the panic attacks come out of the blue, which is consistent with panic disorder, or if they are predictably preceded by a worrisome thought or event of some kind, which would be indicative of another anxiety disorder.

- When avoidance of social situations is present, inquire whether the avoidance is due to fear of embarrassment or intense negative judgment of others, which is consistent with social anxiety disorder, versus the avoidance being related to the patient wanting to avoid the irritability and anger that social situations can often trigger in the context of PTSD.

Table 4.1 Generating the differential for anxiety disorders

Diagnosis	Key questions	Differentiating symptom	Behavioral health measure
GAD	• Have you been worrying excessively for greater than six months? Are you a worrier?	• Worry	GAD-7
Panic Disorder	• Do you experience sudden attacks of anxiety or unexplained physical symptoms?	• Sudden unexpected anxiety or physical symptoms	GAD-7
Social Anxiety Disorder	• Are you uncomfortable in or do you avoid social situations?	• Fear of embarrassment	GAD-7 Mini-Social Phobia Inventory
PTSD	• Do you have a history of trauma or abuse with nightmares and flashbacks?	• Reexperiencing	GAD-7 PC-PTSD PCL-C PCL-5
Obsessive-Compulsive Disorder	• Do you have any repetitive thoughts or behaviors that bother you?	• Repetitive thoughts or behaviors	YBOC
Major Depressive Disorder	• Have you been feeling depressed or having difficulty enjoying things in your life?	• Low mood or anhedonia	PHQ-9
Bipolar Disorder: Hypomania/Mania	• Do you have periods of time with much less sleep than usual and not really miss it the next day?	• Decreased need for sleep	MDQ CIDI-3
Substance Use Disorders	• Do you currently drink alcohol or use street drugs? Have you in the past?	• Evidence of substance use	AUDIT DAST CAGE-AID
ADHD	• Do you have trouble concentrating and/or sitting still?	• Inability to complete tasks and disorganization	UTAH Criteria ASRS–v1.1

Other disorders to consider: Adjustment Disorder, Psychotic Disorder (See Chapter 5), Malingering, Delirium, Traumatic Brain Injury, Personality Disorders, Somatic Symptom Disorders Specific Phobia, Acute Stress Disorder.

Table 4.2 Common anxiety disorders in primary care (ICD-10)

- Acute Stress Disorder: F43.0
- Adjustment Disorder With Anxiety F43.22
- Agoraphobia: F40.00
- Anxiety Disorder Due to Another Medical Condition: F06.4
- Generalized Anxiety Disorder: F41.1
- Obsessive-Compulsive Disorder: F42
- Panic Disorder: F41.0
- Posttraumatic Stress Disorder: F43.10
- Social Anxiety Disorder: F40.10
- Substance/Medication-Induced Anxiety Disorder: highly variable coding—see DSM-V
- Unspecified Anxiety Disorder F41.9

Assessment of comorbid psychiatric disorders and psychological difficulties

Comorbid psychiatric disorders occur in most patients with anxiety disorders. Lack of treatment of these conditions negatively impacts recovery from anxiety disorders, and increases their probability of recurrence. Examples include:

Social anxiety disorder/social phobia: Associated with severe and persistent comorbid mood disorders.

PTSD: 50 percent of patients with PTSD have three or more coexisting psychiatric disorders including: other anxiety disorders, mood disorders, substance abuse, traumatic brain injury, and somatization disorder.

GAD: Frequently associated with other mental disorders, with a lifetime comorbidity of about 90 percent. GAD is often difficult to distinguish from major depression due to the extensive symptom overlap, but the pervasive presence of thoughts associated with high anxiety across many facets of life is unique to GAD.

Panic disorder: Commonly occurs among patients with bipolar disorder and alcohol abuse.

OCD: The impairment in quality of life and the level of shame often lead to comorbidity with other anxiety and depressive disorders.

Team goal: Differential diagnosis and identifying a provisional diagnosis

Once the PCP has evaluated for medical causes for anxiety symptoms, the team will work together to complete screening for common mental health conditions, to identify any comorbid diagnoses, and to make a provisional anxiety or trauma disorder diagnosis.

Working as a team

Patient: Accurately reports all known medical problems, prescribed and nonprescribed medication use (e.g., Adderall from a friend), supplement or herbal use, as well as honestly reporting current substance use. Provides information about potential additional symptoms of anxiety and completely and accurately fills out the behavioral health measure for anxiety disorders and other possible comorbities. Provides information about potential additional nonanxiety psychiatric symptoms and completely and accurately fills out the additional measures.

PCP: Takes the lead in evaluating potential medical etiologies for presenting complaints; ordering labs, tests, and medical consultation as appropriate. Coordinates with BHP to refine differential. Considers comorbidities and refers to BHP for additional assessment as needed.

BHP: Important role in noting any concerning physical symptoms and connecting patient to PCP for evaluation. Screens for substance use. Supports patient in following through on PCP's recommendations such as getting lab work. Considers and screens for comorbidities, including depression. Consults with PC as needed to clarify diagnosis.

PC: Expands medical differential as needed; recommends additional assessment. Refines differential, including considering additional comorbidities for which to screen. Provides provisional diagnosis.

Case example

The patient was further assessed by her PCP and the review of systems was positive for episodes of diarrhea but otherwise negative. Electrolytes, CBC, EKG, and TSH and physical exam were within normal limits. After screening with AUDIT (Score = 8), she reported moderate alcohol intake, particularly in evening after coming home from work. The patient scores a 3 on the PHQ-9, screens negative for bipolar disorder with the CIDI-3, and denies a history of psychotic symptoms. The BHP screened for other anxiety symptoms and took a more detailed history of anxiety symptoms. Due to some past trauma history, BHP had the patient complete a PC-PTSD to screen for PTSD which was negative. Additional history reveals that the patient is still leaving the house regularly, able to go to work but it is a struggle because she often worries about having another "attack." These symptoms have occurred over the last several months up to a couple times a week. She was given the provisional diagnosis of panic disorder without agoraphobia.

Treatment

Initiate treatment

General prinicples

Ideally, identifying a provisional anxiety diagnosis and initiating treatment will occur during the first visit with the team. In putting together a treatment plan, the treatment team should be considering psychoeducation, safety planning, behavioral approaches, and pharmacotherapy. (Table 4.3) As a general rule, each member of the treatment team should participate in psychoeducation and safety planning.

- *Psychoeducation* provides an explanatory model that demystifies and depathologizes anxiety resulting in a better-informed and engaged patient. Examples of psychoeducation are as follows:
  - "Anxiety is a normal part of life: a little is helpful, too much is disabling."
  - "Anxiety is a normal reaction that has just become too intense or is triggered at times when it is not really needed."
  - "Anxiety disorders are a product of genetic makeup, learning, and habit and are most effectively treated with a combination of behavioral approaches and medications."
  - "Behavioral approaches can manage and treat anxiety and medications can help reduce baseline anxiety symptoms."
- *Safety planning* is particularly important in patients with anxiety disorders as the treatment of risk factors contributing to suicidality (e.g., insomnia, agitation, and panic) can reduce the anxious patient's risk of suicide.
- Because of the robust evidence supporting the efficacy of *behavioral treatment* for anxiety disorders, behavioral approaches should always be a top priority when reviewing the overall treatment plan. Despite significant time constraints, brief behavioral interventions can be employed by PCPs with great success.
- The decision-making process for utilizing *pharmacotherapy* should always be collaborative and patient centric, but the final decision about prescribing medications ultimately is determined by the PCP.

PCP approaches to treatment

Treatment is most effective when it includes pharmacotherapy, psychoeducation, safety planning, and supporting behavioral interventions. The PCP has two important roles in treating anxiety: 1) pharmacological approaches and 2) supporting engagement with the BHP and brief behavioral interventions.

Table 4.3 Team-based treatment for anxiety

	PCP approaches	BHP approaches
Biological	**Evidence-Based Medication Treatment:**	**Evidence-Based Medication Treatment:**
	• Pharmacological treatment is most clearly indicated in patients with severe symptoms.	• Help the team consider medications in the context of overall plan as some medications, i.e., high doses of opioids, benzodiazepines, or other sleep and memory disruptive agents can interfere with CBT approaches.
	• As a general rule, serotonergic antidepressants are the first-line therapy, except in patients with bipolar disorder.	
	• Wellbutrin is usually avoided for the treatment of anxiety disorders as it can worsen anxiety due to its activating properties.	• The BHP can also advocate for medication reevaluations as needed, either in the case of anxiety improving and reducing medications, or in the case of anxiety persisting or worsening and needing to step up care (i.e., increase doses).
	• Although benzodiazepines are effective for symptomatic relief, this class of medications should be used with caution.	
Psychosocial	**Evidence-Based Behavioral Treatment:**	**Evidence-Based Behavioral Treatment:**
	• Explain and encourage engagement in cognitive behavioral therapy.	• The BHP should prioritize engagement and crisis management first before launching into CBT based treatments for anxiety.
	• Introduce the concept of exposure and stepping up care to CBT for anxiety.	• Introduce patients to the cognitive behavioral therapy model of anxiety.
		• Identity how anxiety interferes most with activities to developing patient-centered treatment goals.
		• Patients should be screened for readiness to engage in CBT based anxiety treatments, including exposure.

Pharmacotherapy

Prescribing principles:

- Pharmacological treatment is most clearly indicated in patients with severe symptoms, with significant functional impairment, or with safety issues (e.g., suicidality). (Table 4.4)
- As a general rule, serotonergic antidepressants are the first-line therapy, except in patients with bipolar disorder (see below).
- Although benzodiazepines can provide acute symptomatic relief, this class of medications should be used with caution. Benzodiazepines are associated with multiple problems, including dependence, interfering with effectiveness of therapy, cognitive impairment, high street value, and impairment of long-term recovery (e.g., PTSD).
- Ideally, the prescriber should be thinking about the time frame for pharmacological treatment including when and how the medication will be discontinued and the behavioral approaches that will be utilized to facilitate patient recovery.
- "Start low, go slow, but go" when prescribing medications, given greater sensitivity to side effects in anxious patients.
- Generally start at one-quarter to one-half of the initial target dose and try to reach the initial target dose in two to four weeks (e.g., start

Table 4.4 Medications commonly used in the treatment of anxiety disorders

---

Selective Serotonin Reuptake Inhibitors (SSRIs)
Citalopram (Celexa)
Escitalopram (Lexapro)
Fluoxetine (Prozac)
Paroxetine (Paxil)
Sertraline (Zoloft)

Mixed Receptor Antidepressants
Duloxetine (Cymbalta)
Mirtazapine (Remeron)
Venlafaxine (Effexor)

Other Anxiety Medications
Buspirone (BuSpar)
Hydroxyzine (Vistaril)
Prazosin (Minipress)

For prescribing details and protocols, please see Chapter 11, "Evidence-Based Psychopharmacology for the Collaborative Care Team."

sertraline 12.5–25 mg qday and increase by 12.5–25 mg qday per week to 50 mg qday).

- Encourage patients to continue meds in the face of tolerable side effects as they often resolve after one to two weeks. Tell patients that the side effects often resolve quickly and be specific to what these may feel like. Patients with high anxiety often have high somatization and are often hyper aware of side effects and quick to stop medications when these arise.
- Higher doses and longer period of time (12–16 weeks) may be necessary to achieve remission as compared to treatment of depression.
- Start with the best-tolerated medication with the fewest drug-drug interactions (e.g., escitalopram and sertraline)
- Bupropion is usually avoided for the treatment of anxiety disorders as it can worsen anxiety due to its activating properties.
- Other approved treatments include buspirone (takes 4–6 weeks to work) and hydroxyzine.
- In comorbid conditions, consider the following:
  Chronic pain: medications affecting serotonin and norepinephrine (e.g., serotonin-norepinephrine reuptake inhibitors [SNRIs], tricyclic antidepressants [TCAs], and mirtazapine)
  ADHD: medications with potent noradrenergic reuptake inhibition (e.g., duloxetine)
  Insomnia: sedating medications (e.g., mirtazapine and nortriptyline)
  Bipolar disorder: mood stabilizing agents with anxiolytic properties (e.g., quetiapine)

Working with benzodiazepines

When to consider:
- Severe functional impairment (e.g., severe panic disorder with agoraphobia)
- Brief situational anxiety (e.g., before MRIs)
- As a bridging medication during antidepressant titration—use rarely and only if absolutely necessary.

Prescribing Principles (Table 4.5):
- Long-acting benzos are preferred (e.g., clonazepam) over benzos with rapid onset and brief duration (e.g., alprazolam).
- Use as a scheduled medication (vs. PRN) for greater efficacy and fewer withdrawal symptoms.
- Define in advance the anticipated length of treatment and criteria for discontinuation.

Table 4.5 Benzodiazepines commonly used in the treatment of anxiety

---

Alprazolam (Xanax)
Chlordiazepoxide (Librium)
Clonazepam (Klonopin)
Diazepam (Valium)
Lorazepam (Ativan)
Temazepam (Restoril)

For prescribing details and protocols, please see Chapter 11, "Evidence Based Psychopharmacology for the Collaborative Care Team."

- Consider the inclusion of random toxicology screens with a written contract (i.e., a benzodiazepine contract).
- Discuss restrictions on replacing lost scripts and/or early refills.

Discontinuation:
- Aim for gradual reduction in patients who have been on benzos long-term due to potential dangerousness of the withdrawal process and to improve tolerability.
- Aggressive discontinuation protocol: 10 percent every three days or 25 percent every week—if significant/severe withdrawal symptoms appear, then slow down the taper.
- Extended discontinuation protocol (e.g., after months/years of use): 10 percent per month or slower, if necessary.

PCP role in behavioral interventions

Helping patients understand behavioral treatments are first-line treatment for anxiety can greatly increase the likelihood they will engage using this types of treatment. You can also begin helping the patient use these skills and explain the BHP's role in this type of treatment to help with engagement.
- Introducing non-pharmacological treatments for anxiety disorders:
   "Our most effective treatments for anxiety involve psychotherapy, the process of talking about your anxiety with a therapist. In psychotherapy you learn about how your thoughts, feelings, and behaviors impact your symptoms of anxiety, and then learn new skills and approaches to reduce your symptoms of anxiety."
- Introducing Cognitive Behavioral Therapy (CBT) for anxiety:
   "The most commonly used psychotherapy for anxiety is called cognitive behavioral therapy (CBT). CBT focuses on training the patient to be less anxious through management strategies for anxiety and exposure techniques that reduce the effects anxious cues. Engaging patients in CBT

for anxiety and developing treatment targets is best done by aligning treatment with what the patient defines as the most meaningful function goals."

- Introducing basic behavioral anxiety management techniques: targeting the body and brain through physiological relaxation skills:

  "You can manage some of the symptoms of anxiety by learning how to relax your body and challenge the negative thoughts you have when you get anxious."

- Introducing mindfulness strategies for coping with anxiety:

  "Mindfulness is a skill you can learn over time to help you focus your mind and awareness in general and this skill will help you learn the skills you need to treat your anxiety much faster and easier."

BHP approaches to treatment

Patients should be screened for readiness to engage CBT-based anxiety treatment.

- They should have some engagement established with the BHP, namely, be willing and able to return for treatment (i.e., for office visits or via phone).
- They should also be relatively stable from immediate crises (i.e., are they suicidal? is their housing stable? are they in a domestic violence situation in need of immediate safety planning?).
- Patients will need a certain level of stability and engagement with the BHP to effectively benefit from this type of treatment, including having an adequate mental status to lay down new memories (i.e., high doses of opioids, benzodiazepines, or other sleep and memory disruptive agents may interfere with effective treatment).

The BHP should prioritize engagement and crisis management first before launching into CBT based treatments for anxiety. It is important for the BHP to make sure the team is aware of treatment s/he is delivering and that this treatment plan is consistent with the overall plan for care. For example, engaging in exposure therapy that may increase anxiety initially may be disruptive if done during a medication titration or taper. Treatment should be consistent with the patient's goals and team's treatment plan.

Modular anxiety treatment (MAT)

Many evidence-based practices can treat anxiety disorders in adults and children. A movement toward modularizing treatment has begun, to try to distill the most active and effective components of these treatments. This consolidation has led to an understanding of key anxiety management and anxiety reducing behavioral interventions that can be used to treat anxiety disorders in adults, regardless of the anxiety disorder. Modular treatment, a first-line treatment, should be customized to the patient and therapist. However, in severe cases, this type of treatment may not be adequate and stepping up care should be considered, including referring a patient to a higher level of care if possible (i.e., community mental health, anxiety specialist, etc.).

MAT Strategies:
1. Present the cognitive behavioral therapy model of anxiety:
   - The three B's (body, brain, behavior): anxiety interacts as a fear response that is fueled by a body's physical response to fear, a brain's set of negative thoughts, and behaviors that often create avoidance patterns to run away from the perceived danger
   - Helping patients understand this model can frame anxiety as controllable and promote understanding of treatment
2. Assess how anxiety interferes most with activities, developing patient-centered treatment goals:
   - Asking the patient for his/her perspective on how anxiety disrupts their life is key to achieving early and strong engagement, as well as setting the most appropriate treatment targets for exposure. Helping the team understand the patient's priorities for treatment is key to bringing the team in line with creating the most effective treatment plan.
3. Selling exposure-based strategies:
   - Cognitive approaches, psychoeducation, relaxation techniques (e.g., diaphragmatic breathing and progressive relaxation), and/or medications often aren't adequately effective for patients with moderate to severe symptoms of anxiety.
   - The addition of exposure-based strategies, which are evidence based and highly effective, can extinguish anxiety triggers and bring about a lasting and full recovery.
   - Patients may need support in understanding that staying exposed to something they fear will be helpful in stopping their fear in the first place. As such, it is important to pitch this technique as very effective.
   - PCPs can improve treatment outcomes by reinforcing the potential strong effectiveness of exposure therapy and encouraging the patient to participate in treatment.

4. Conduct exposure: develop a hierarchy
   - As exposure treatment begins, it is important to develop exposure targets the patient can tolerate. Inform the team that exposure treatment is occurring and that anxiety may increase during this phase of treatment.
   - Make sure patients measure anxiety before and after exposures to track progress over time with being able to tolerate anxiety cues more easily.

Team goal: Initial treatment planning

Using the provisional diagnosis and patient preference, the team must work together to make sure behavioral and medication treatments are initiated and that the patient is engaged in the overall plan.

Working as a team

Patient: Learns about anxiety disorder and treatment options. Works with the team to develop a treatment plan that fits with their goals to target anxiety. Agrees to close follow-up, monitoring of symptoms, and response to chosen anxiety treatment.

PCP: Completes any medical assessment as needed. Works with the BHP to initiate appropriate treatment for provisional anxiety diagnosis. Prescribes initial trial of medications. Anxious patients may need additional support to engage with the BHP, especially if still concerned that symptoms are due to a medical condition. Addresses any needed safety planning.

BHP: Provides important psychoeducation about anxiety. Coordinates with the PCP and PC to develop an integrated anxiety treatment plan. Engages the patient in brief behavioral interventions (especially for panic, GAD, and social phobia), facilitates communication between team members, and supports referrals (disability, vocational rehab, social services, chemical dependency, additional psychotherapy). Makes sure the patient is clear about follow-up plan for anxiety treatment. Develops safety plan if needed.

PC: Supports treatment planning including making behavioral treatment recommendations for specific anxiety disorder as well as medication recommendations including detailed prescribing instructions. Supports team to focus on first-line treatments and guides team about when to use medications such as benzodiazepines. Provides recommendations, as needed, for safety planning.

Case example

The patient stated she was scared she would lose her job if she couldn't "get her act together" at work, which she felt was mostly due to feeling panicked and out of control at times. The patient was requesting a prescription for alprazolam to help her get through her work day. She was discussed with the PC who supported the PCP plan of starting sertraline with an initial target dosage of 50 mg qday with the plan of titrating this medication to a higher dosage, if needed. As the patient was not in acute crisis, the PC supported the BHP plan to use Modular Anxiety Treatment (MAT) and coached the BHP in performing psychoeducation about issues with the use of benzodiazepines as a long term anxiety treatment. The BHP also used motivational interviewing techniques to create ambivalence around the patient's alcohol intake, and the patient agreed to monitor alcohol use.

Follow-up and treatment adjustment to achieve treatment to target

General principles

The goal of this phase of treatment is to make sure anxiety treatment is adjusted until the patient symptoms and functioning improve. The team should continue to provide psychoeducation about anxiety and the benefits of engaging in treatment. Anxiety may interfere with patient engagement, so involve the whole team in supporting patients to stay connected with treatment until symptoms improve.

When to consider referrals

- Condition not responding to treatment
- Conditions requiring longer term, more intensive, or specialist psychotherapy (e.g., severe PTSD)
- Higher level of need including long-term case management
- Employment services: especially if people have developed avoidance patterns
- Disability: more severe cases, especially if anticipate inability to work for greater than a year

PCP approaches

Behavioral Approaches

As part of the team-based nature of treatment, it is important to inquire about the efficacy of behavioral approaches whether initiated by the PCP or BHP. The PCP can play a powerful role in reinforcing engagement in behavioral approaches and emphasizing the role of behavioral approaches in long-term recovery.

> **TIP:** Some patients may be ambivalent about engaging in treatment but may feel more convinced if the PCP reinforces the potential benefit.

Pharmacotherapy

It is important to evaluate efficacy as well as side effects of a medication, track symptoms with the GAD-7 and other more specific behavioral measures as needed, and to consider functional improvement. It is often helpful to obtain collateral information from someone who is close to the patient about the patient's response to the medication. Many patients don't take medications as prescribed, and a common misconception about anxiety medications is to take them only when anxious. As a result, it is useful to assess whether the patient is taking their medication(s) and if so, how many dosages they estimate that they miss/take per week. It may also be helpful to consult with the BHP about medication adherence issues to help with behavioral support needed to increase adherence. Sleep difficulties with sleep onset and maintenance can significantly interfere with recovery. It is always a priority to ask about sleep and treat problems with sleep with psychoeducation about sleep hygiene and with behavioral and/or pharmacological approaches if needed.

> **TIP:** As a general rule, the anxiolytic effects of antidepressant medication can take longer to show benefit as compared to the antidepressant effect and can also take longer, e.g., 12–16 weeks, to reach their maximum efficacy.

General principles of ongoing medication management:
- Partial responders after four to eight weeks should be titrated to higher doses, if tolerated.
- Try to get to maximum doses AND duration in a partial responder before considering adjunctive treatment with another medication from a different class (e.g., buspirone) or focusing more on behavioral approaches.
- If the initial medication trial fails because of lack of efficacy or intolerable side effects, consider switching to another medication in the same class (e.g., switching from sertraline to escitalopram) or to a medication in another class, e.g., mirtazapine, a SNRI, or a TCA.
- If there is *no response* after four weeks at therapeutic dose, but medication is well tolerated AND the patient is willing to persevere, the dose may be increased (e.g., increasing sertraline from 50 mg qday to 100 mg qday) to assess if a higher dosage is helpful.

BHP approaches

As treatment progresses, the BHP should address any difficulties in team coordination of the overall plan. As the patient becomes more engaged with the BHP, the BHP can often act as an advocate with the medical providers to help mediate alliance issues and instruct the patient and medical team about issues the patient may be struggling with due to anxiety. The BHP can also advocate for medication reevaluations as needed, either in the case of anxiety improving and reducing medications, or in the case of anxiety persisting or worsening and needing to step up care (i.e., increase doses). It is also common for patients to experience unpredictable hardships (i.e., new medical diagnoses, job loss, victimization, etc.) that can also set back anxiety treatment. The BHP can stay in touch with these issues and help the patient engage proper services and care as these issues arise, given they often exacerbate anxiety.

> **TIP:** The treatment plan can be adjusted over time to target tougher anxiety issues as the patient experiences improvement.

Team goal: Revising treatment planning and stepping up care

Monitor progress on the anxiety goals, and adjust treatment to until target and goals achieved.

Working as a team

Patient: Reports symptoms of anxiety, efficacy of the behavioral interventions, and efficacy and side effects of medications if utilized. Honestly appraises engagement in treatment including ability to carry out treatment recommendations.

PCP: Continues the process of engaging the patient in team-based treatment and safety planning. Monitors the patient's response to behavioral interventions and assesses response to medication including side effects, if prescribed. Makes adjustments to the treatment plan as needed and in consultation with the treatment team. Obtains follow-up labs and vital signs, if appropriate. Considers health care maintenance and impact on taking medications long-term. Considers medical and/or mental health referrals as needed (e.g., specialized trauma-focused therapy for a patient with PTSD).

BHP: Continues the process of engaging the patient in team-based treatment and safety planning. Evaluates the patient's response to the treatment plan including utilizing behavioral health measures (e.g., rescreening the patient with the GAD-7). Continues to focus on brief behavioral interventions (especially for panic, GAD, and social phobia) with adjustments to these interventions as needed. Facilitates communication between team members. Makes and supports referrals (disability, vocational rehab, social services, chemical dependency, additional psychotherapy).

PC: Supports treatment planning, including making recommendations for adjusting the behavioral treatment recommendations, as well as medication recommendations including detailed prescribing instructions. Provides recommendations, as needed, for safety planning. May suggest referrals, if needed (e.g., for trauma-focused therapy).

Case example

The patient successfully titrated up to a therapeutic dose of sertraline, with support from the BHP to stay the course, despite anxiety persisting in the early weeks of taking the medication. The BHP targeted exposure to physical panic sensations that the patient recognized occurring at work and within a handful of sessions, she noticed her panic attacks had decreased significantly. Adjustments were made to the exposure to pinpoint specific work situations, resulting in the patient becoming more functional at work. After eight weeks of treatment, the patient's repeat GAD-7 decreased to a 3, she reported decrease frequency of panic symptoms, and was more at ease at work. The patient had reduced her alcohol intake and now had an AUDIT score of 2. The BHP also discussed the availability of more intensive CBT treatment or AA if needed in the future.

Completing treatment and relapse prevention

General principles

The goal of this phase of treatment is to reinforce a clear on-going care plan for the patient to maintain an optimal level of functioning and reduce the risk of relapse; clarify and reinforce self-management strategies, medication use, if needed, and review early warning signs of relapse and develop strategies for what to do if symptoms worsen and when to return for further treatment.

PCP approaches

Behavioral Approaches

Once the patient has achieved a sustained remission, it is valuable to monitor for recurrence (e.g., quarterly) and to reinforce use of behavioral strategies by the patient (e.g., briefly reviewing the principles of treatment). It is important to reinforce that the benefits of these behavioral skills can be more powerful than medications long term, but do not work if they are not used, which takes commitment by the patient. It can be helpful to normalize that negative life events in the future can often cause relapses in anxiety and let the patient know they should come in to potentially reengage care for these issues should they escalate in the future.

> **TIP:** Behavioral therapies tend to be more effective long-term than pharmacological therapies as they involve the acquisition of new behavioral skills and strategies.

Pharmacotherapy

In general, the goal as providers is to have patients achieve full remission from their symptoms. Once this remission is achieved, it is desirable to continue pharmacotherapy for another six to nine months to help consolidate this improvement and to prevent relapse. After this six- to nine-month period and in patients without a history of multiple relapses, patients should be slowly tapered off of their medications in a time frame that is proportional to the length of time the patient has been on their medication.

- Although the optimal process for withdrawing patients from antidepressant medications has not been well defined, a slow taper (e.g., between 25 percent per week to 25 percent per month) is likely to reduce withdrawal symptoms and the risk of relapse.
- With benzodiazepines similar principles apply although it may be appropriate to extend the tapering process to up to a year in length.
- In patients with a history of multiple relapses, it is often wise to consider maintenance treatment with medications at the minimally effective dosages.

BHP approaches

At the end of treatment, it is important to summarize treatment progress and a plan for ongoing behavioral changes and use of skills, as well as review the medical plan for any on-going medications to support medication adherence. Providing a deliberate and written summary or relapse-prevention plan can be helpful to summarize effective anxiety treatment. Often patients need to hear encouragement that they can succeed well on their own, but are welcome to check-in in the future should they feel the need.

> **TIP:** Many patients with high anxiety can find it an anxious experience to disengage treatment, so offering concrete reassurance and resisting the urge to keep a patient in care for longer than is needed is important. Spacing out visits can help patients observe that improvement is sustainable.

Team goal: Relapse prevention

Coordinate across all team members to determine agreement that anxiety treatment is complete and patient goals have been adequately met, with a coordinated message to the patient as they complete treatment.

Working as a team

Patient: Participates in establishing a relapse prevention plan with the BHP and the PCP; tracks the ongoing plan and reengages in additional care if anxiety or functional impairment significantly worsen.

 PCP: Provides a plan for tapering off of medication or on-going medication management as appropriate for the patient, reinforces and reviews successful behavioral strategies, and schedules regular follow-up to assess for relapse.

 BHP: Review successes and gains in treatment, as well as the on-going behavioral changes and treatment plan; clarifies team roles and who to reengage should function decline or anxiety worsen.

 PC: Clarify to the team recommendations relative to the long-term use of medications and supports the BHP in creating a treatment summary and relapse prevention plan as needed.

Case Example

After six months of remission from anxiety symptoms the patient requested that she be tapered off of sertraline. The team decided on a conservative discontinuation strategy and the patient was successfully tapered off of sertraline over a four-month period of time. The PCP and BHP subsequently saw the patient quarterly where the continued use of behavioral strategies and limiting alcohol was reinforced.

Resources

- http://www.adaa.org/
- http://www.nimh.nih.gov/health/publications/anxiety-disorders/introduction
- http://www.nami.org/Content/NavigationMenu/Inform_Yourself/About_Mental_Illness/By_Illness/Anxiety_Disorders.htm
- http://www.ocfoundation.org/
- http://ptsdusa.org/

References

Barlow, D. H., Boisseau, C. L., Carl, J. R., Ellard, K. K., Farchione, T. J., Fairholme, C. P., Ellard, K. K., Gallagher, M. W., & Thompson-Hollands, J. (2012). Unified protocol for transdiagnostic treatment of emotional disorders: a randomized controlled trial.

Behavioral Therapy, *43*(3), 666–78. Epub 2012 Jan 18. PubMed PMID: 22697453; PubMed Central PMCID: PMC3383087.

Barlow, D. H., Ellard, K. K., Fairholme, C. P., Thompson-Hollands, J., & Wilamowska, Z. A. (2010). Conceptual background, development, and preliminary data from the unified protocol for transdiagnostic treatment of emotional disorders. *Depression and Anxiety*, *10*, 882–90. Review. PubMed PMID: 20886609.

Bearman, S. K., Chorpita, B. F., Frye, A., Hoagwood, K. E., Langer, D. A., Lau, N., Ng, M. Y., Ugueto, A. M., & Weisz, J. R: Research Network on Youth Mental Health. (2011). Youth Top Problems: using idiographic, consumer-guided assessment to identify treatment needs and to track change during psychotherapy. *Journal of Consulting and Clinical Psychology*, *79*(3), 369–80. PubMed PMID: 21500888.

Bearman, S. K., Chropita, B. F., Gibbons, R. D., Palinkas, L. A., Schoenwald, S. K.... Weisz, J. Research Network on Youth Mental Health. (2012). Testing standard and modular designs for psychotherapy treating depression, anxiety, and conduct problems in youth: a randomized effectiveness trial. *Archives of General Psychiatry*, *69*(3), 274–82. Epub 2011 Nov 7. PubMed PMID: 22065252.

Berglund, P., Demler, O., Jin, R., Kessler, R. C., Merikangas, K. R., & Walters, E. E. (2005). Lifetime Prevalence and Age-of-Onset Distributions of DSM-IV Disorders in the National Comorbidity Survey Replication. *Archives of General Psychiatry*, *62*, 593–602.

Bystritsky, A., Craske M. G., Edlund, M. J., Sullivan, G., Roy-Byrne, P., Veitengruber, J. P.... Stein, M. B. (2009). Brief intervention for anxiety in primary care patients. *Journal of the American Board of Family Med*, *22*(2), 175–186.

Chapter 5 **Psychotic Disorders**

Carolyn Brenner

Clinical impact

Patients with psychotic symptoms frequently present to primary care. Psychosis occurs in 3–5 percent of individuals. The first presentation of these patients is often in emergency rooms or primary care.

- PCPs may see emerging symptoms of psychotic disorders in untreated patients or may provide ongoing treatment of patients with chronic psychotic disorders on antipsychotic medications requiring the management of common medical comorbidities and psychotropic medication side effects.
- Lack of insight and reluctance of patients to engage in treatment is common and can be challenging to providers.
- Patients with psychosis often refuse referral for mental health care and psychiatric medications. When possible, a psychiatric consultant should see patients with chronic psychosis to aid in diagnosis and treatment recommendations.

Chronic psychotic disorders often contribute to poor medical follow-up and worse health outcomes. People with schizophrenia have a 15–25 year reduction in life expectancy with higher mortality rate from cardiovascular disease, chronic obstructive pulmonary disease (COPD), infections, accidents, and suicide.

- Underdiagnosis of physical problems is a risk due to problems with communication and providers' focus on psychiatric symptoms.
- People with chronic psychotic disorders have high rates of cigarette smoking, alcohol abuse, and illicit substance abuse.

Integrated Care: Creating Effective Mental and Primary Health Care Teams, First Edition.
Anna Ratzliff, Jürgen Unützer, Wayne Katon, and Kari A. Stephens.
© 2016 John Wiley & Sons, Inc. Published 2016 by John Wiley & Sons, Inc.

- Side effects from antipsychotics can be significant and contribute to non-adherence and to medical morbidities, particularly obesity, diabetes, dyslipidemia, and movement disorders.

Assessment

Identify chief complaint, associated somatic and psychological symptoms, functional impairment, and safety concerns

Understand how the patient defines their problems and use these terms to discuss. Lack of insight is common and a patient may deny symptoms that are present or refuse to discuss them. It may take time and gradual building of rapport to determine which symptoms are present and how they affect the patient. Collateral information from family and friends is often needed for diagnosis. Understanding the timeline of symptoms also helps to determine the diagnosis. It's important to determine whether the psychosis has recently started or if it is a chronic condition.

Common psychological symptoms

Hallucinations: False sensory perceptions in any of the five senses. Auditory hallucinations are the most common in psychotic disorders. These are often described as hearing voices that are distinct from an individual's own thoughts. Command auditory hallucinations are of particular safety concern.

   Key questions
   - Do you hear voices or sounds that other people can't hear?
   - Does the voice tell you to do anything?

Delusions: Firmly held false beliefs despite evidence to the contrary that are not consistent with common beliefs among the patient's culture or religion. Common delusions are persecutory, religious, somatic, and ideas of reference (belief that certain environmental cues or comments are special messages directed at the individual).

   Key questions
   - Do you worry that someone is following you or spying on you?
   - Do you think people are trying to harm you?
   - Do you get messages from the television, radio, or computer that are meant just for you?

Disorganized Thoughts and Speech: Thoughts that are not logical or linear.

   Key symptoms
   - Look for difficult to follow speech and jumping between topics that don't appear related to each other.

Disorganized behavior: Bizarre behaviors with unclear purpose.

Key symptoms

- Look for odd behaviors and movements. A patient with little movement or very slow movements may have catatonia.

Negative Symptoms: Poverty or decreased thoughts, speech, movement, motivation, socialization, pleasure, or affect. Negative symptoms are significant contributors to functional impairment.

Key questions

- Do you have interest in having relationships with other people?
- What activities do you participate in?
- What does a usual day look like for you?

Cognitive Deficits: Impairment in multiple cognitive domains is common and often worsens over time in chronic psychotic disorders. Impairments are seen in executive functioning (planning, organizing, problem solving), attention, memory, learning, verbal processing, and visual processing. Cognitive deficits are significant contributors to functional impairment.

Key questions

- Do you have problems with your concentration or memory?

Key assessment

- Montreal Cognitive Assessment (MoCA) or Mini-Mental State Examination (MMSE) for brief cognitive screening test

Common physical/Somatic symptoms

- Insomnia and hypersomnia
- Poor food intake, increased fluid intake, dehydration
- Reports of bizarre physical symptoms such as microchips implanted in the brain or having multiple livers
- Physical complaints without clear medical etiology after work-up such as bugs infesting the skin
- Bizarre behaviors with no clear purpose
- Inappropriate affect—smiling while telling of a sad event
- Neurological abnormalities are more frequent in this population
- Catatonic symptoms of immobility or excitability

Common functional impairments

Education/Work: Gradual impairment in education and work skills, sometimes leading to severe impairment related to delusions, hallucinations, disorganized thoughts and behaviors, cognitive impairment, and negative symptoms.

Relationships: Gradual isolation and difficulties with all social relationships is common. Often there is decreased interest in intimate relationships.

Activities of Daily Living: Varies widely. Can have severe impairment of ability to take care of hygiene, shopping for food, housework, taking medications as prescribed, and managing money.

Assessing for safety

Suicide: People with schizophrenia have a significant increase in suicide risk with studies finding over 25 percent with suicide attempts and over 5 percent with suicide completion. Always ask about suicidal ideation, plan, and intent. If any suicidal ideation is present, assess ongoing and new risk and protective factors.

- Suicide risk is highest early in the course of illness.
- Risk factors include prior suicide attempts, rehearsal of suicide, abrupt clinical change, command auditory hallucinations, first psychotic break, substance abuse, comorbid depression, and multiple psychiatric hospitalizations.
- If imminent risk is present, consider higher level of care including hospitalization.

Violence: Psychosis from any cause is a risk factor for violence, though violent actions in this population are rare and difficult to predict. Always ask about thoughts of hurting others.

- Include assessment of command auditory hallucinations, paranoid beliefs, history of violence, and what triggered last episode of violence in risk assessment.
- If imminent risk is present, consider higher level of care including hospitalization. Consider Duty to Warn laws.

Grave Disability: Assess for medical risk related to delusions and disorganized behavior, most often seen with poor food intake leading to hypokalemia and excessive fluid intake leading to hyponatremia. Failure to take care of acute medical risks such as infection should also be considered. Grossly disorganized behavior can lead to putting self in danger, for example, walking into traffic, leaving the stove on, and taking off clothes in public.

- Always consider if psychosis is causing inability to care for oneself and putting patient at imminent risk. Consider the need for a higher level of care, including staying with family, skilled nursing facilities, medical hospitalization, or psychiatric hospitalization.

Team goal: Identifying the chief complaint, initial physical exam, gathering history, and safety assessment
Recognize psychosis and assess functional impairment, which will help determine level of care needed. All team members must share the responsibility of the safety assessment and communicating the risks to the team.

Working as a team
Patient: Discusses any psychiatric symptoms and changes in behavior with PCP and BHP. Develops a realistic safety plan with team and follow steps when needed.

PCP: Identifies a possible psychotic disorder. Safety assessment and safety planning; coordinate with BHP to monitor safety issues.

BHP: Builds rapport with patient and focuses on patient's concerns. Completes detailed assessment, gathers more information from family and friends as patient allows. Safety assessment and safety planning; develop plan to monitor safety issues and track plan.

PC: Broadens psychiatric differential when indicated. Considers need for referral to more intensive psychiatric care or psychiatric hospitalization if needed for safety and treatment. Assists in safety planning and when to refer for hospitalization. When possible assesses patients with increased safety risk in person.

Case example
A 20-year-old male presents with his mother with her chief complaint of "odd behavior and losing weight." His mother describes dropping grades in college, weight loss over the last few months, and appearing withdrawn and distracted since he returned home for the summer. He reports poor sleep because of worrying about "the cameras everywhere," no interest in seeing friends or playing basketball anymore, and concern about "poison" in the food. He states that nothing is wrong with him and he would be fine if "those people would just leave me alone."

PCP assessed patient for safety and the patient denied any thoughts of hurting himself or others or previous suicidal thoughts. He said he would be able to continue eating and drinking food and water as long as it was packaged so it could not be poisoned. BHP again assessed for safety and developed safety plan. Patient denied thoughts of hurting himself or others. Mother denied any history of suicidal behavior or violence. They agreed that patient would be safe to return home with mother with close follow-up and safety plan to call 911 if patient or family felt unsafe.

Differential diagnosis and identifying a provisional diagnosis

Rule out common contributing medical problems and substance-related conditions.

Medical conditions to consider in evaluation of psychosis

Neurological: delirium, dementia, seizure disorder, migraine, traumatic brain injury, central nervous system (CNS) infection, cerebrovascular accident (CVA; also called "stroke"), Huntington's disease, multiple sclerosis, Parkinson's disease, auditory or visual nerve injury, deafness

Endocrine: thyroid, parathryroid, adrenal dysfunction

Immunological: neurosyphilis, HIV, systemic lupus erythematosus (SLE), infection

Metabolic: hypoglycemia, fluid or electrolyte abnormalities, hypoxia, hypercarbia, Wilson disease

Substance-related conditions to consider in evaluation of psychosis
- Withdrawal: alcohol, benzodiazepines, barbiturates
- Intoxication: hallucinogens, inhalants, amphetamines, cocaine, opiates, marijuana, alcohol, bath salts
- Prescribed medications: steroids, anticholinergics, dopamine agonists, disulfiram
- Toxins: anticholinesterase inhibitors, organophosphate insecticides, nerve gas, carbon monoxide

Medical work-up

Consider appropriate medical work-up for new onset psychosis including history and physical exam. Rule out delirium.
- Studies may include complete blood count (CBC), comprehensive metabolic panel (CMP) (including liver function and renal function), thyroid stimulating hormone (TSH), urinalysis (UA), urine toxicology screen (UTOX), and blood alcohol level (BAL).
- Consider brain imaging if patient has neurological symptoms.
- At times lumbar puncture, adrenal level, and urine copper clearance is appropriate.

Develop and refine differential diagnosis

Questions to help narrow the differential diagnosis (See Tables 5.1 and 5.2)
- Is the psychosis recent in onset or chronic?
- Are the symptoms changing or are they fairly stable over time?
- Are mood symptoms prominent?
- Is there a family history of schizophrenia, bipolar disorder, or depression? There is a strong genetic component to these conditions.

Table 5.1 Generating the differential for psychotic disorders

Diagnosis	Differentiating features	Commonly used screeners
Schizophrenia	Chronic and more severe course of disease	
Schizoaffective Disorder	Prominent depression or mania episodically, psychosis persists when euthymic (not in a depressed or manic state)	
Bipolar I Disorder with Psychotic Features	Episodes of mania and depression, psychosis resolves when euthymic	CIDI-3
Major Depressive Disorder with Psychotic Features	Severe depression often with mood congruent psychotic symptoms, psychosis resolves when euthymic	PHQ-9
Substance/ Medication-Induced Psychotic Disorder	Timeline of psychosis onset coincides with substance use	AUDIT DAST
Delusional Disorder	A delusion for over 1 month, no other symptoms of psychosis	
Major Neurocognitive Disorder (Dementia)	Significant cognitive decline before onset of psychosis	MoCA MMSE
Delirium	Waxing and waning attention and orientation	CAM
Psychotic Disorder Due to Another Medical Condition	Hallucinations or delusions with lack of reality testing in setting of medical illness	

Table 5.2 Possible psychotic disorders in primary care (ICD-10)

- Schizophrenia - F20.9
- Schizoaffective Disorder - F25.0, F25.1
- Bipolar I Disorder with Psychotic Features - F31.5, F31.2
- Delirium F05
- Major Depressive Disorder with Psychotic Features - F33.3, F32.3
- Major Neurocognitive Disorder (Dementia) - F02.8x, G31.9
- Psychotic Disorder Due to Another Medical Condition - F06.2, F06.0
- Substance/Medication-Induced Psychotic Disorder - highly variable coding—see DSM

Assessment of comorbid psychiatric disorders and psychological difficulties

Comorbid psychiatric diagnoses are common and should be assessed and treated as they further impair functioning.

- Depressive disorders occur at a significantly higher rate than in the general population. These can be difficult to distinguish from the negative symptoms of schizophrenia. Consider using PHQ-9 to screen.
- Anxiety disorders, particularly panic disorder, obsessive-compulsive disorder (OCD), post-traumatic stress disorder (PTSD), and social phobia, are significantly more frequent than in the general population. Consider using GAD-7 to screen.
- Substance use disorders are very common comorbidities.
- Tobacco use disorder is extremely common in chronic psychotic disorders.
- Mania should always be screened for when a patient has psychosis.

Team goal: Differential diagnosis and identifying a provisional diagnosis

Once the PCP has completed the appropriate medical work-up for psychotic symptoms, the team will work together to engage the patient in care. The team approach may be especially important if the patient has poor insight to his/her symptoms.

Working as a team

Patient: Discusses any physical symptoms with PCP and BHP. Cooperates with needed lab draws and tests. Discusses any recent drug use openly. Asks questions and learns about possible diagnoses. Discusses mood, anxiety, and substance use with team.

PCP: Primary role in evaluating possible medical etiology for presenting complaints; orders labs, tests, and medical consultation as appropriate. Coordinates with BHP and PC to refine differential. Considers comorbidities and refers to BHP for additional assessment as needed.

BHP: Important role in noting any concerning physical symptoms and connecting patient to PCP for evaluation; supports client in following through on medical recommendations such as getting lab work. Consults with PC as needed to clarify diagnosis. Considers and screens for comorbidities including using PHQ-9 and other screeners as appropriate.

PC: Expands medical differential as needed; recommends additional assessment. Refines differential; provides provisional diagnosis. Evaluates patient in person when possible. Considers additional comorbidities for which to screen.

Case example

The patient was assessed by his PCP and the review of systems was positive for a 10 pound weight loss over the last few months, insomnia, fatigue, and poor concentration. He denied taking any medications. Patient endorsed occasional use of alcohol and marijuana, denied other illicit drugs or change in use recently. CMP, CBC, TSH, UTOX, BAL and physical exam were within normal limits.

The BHP further assessed the patient's symptoms and observed paranoia with no prominent mood symptoms. The patient denied auditory or visual hallucinations. He reported feeling scared that people were watching him and that they might be putting poison in his food. He denied symptoms consistent with a major depressive disorder or manic episode. The patient's mother reported that her brother has schizophrenia. The patient was discussed with the PC who confirmed that schizophrenia was the most likely diagnosis and that further evaluation of the timeline of symptoms was needed as well as continued monitoring for any mood symptoms or possible drug use.

The patient is introduced to the BHP as an important member of the team, and the BHP screened the patient for any psychiatric comorbidities. The patient described feeling anxious and upset about recent events, but said he would feel fine if he was left alone. He was not willing to take the recommended screening tests (PHQ-9 and GAD-7) to evaluate for depression and anxiety.

Treatment

Initiate treatment

General approaches (See Table 5.3)

- Symptoms of psychosis should be treated even if a specific diagnosis is not clear.
- Start with a focus on symptoms that the patient defines as the main problem to have a common treatment goal and foster alliance.
- Antipsychotic medication is the most effective treatment for psychosis.
- Building rapport with the patient, psychoeducation, and carefully monitoring and addressing side effects is essential.
- Always consider whether a more intensive level of care is needed for safety (see Assessing for Safety section above).

Psychoeducation
- Provide education about the diagnosis of a psychotic disorder and symptoms involved with a focus on how medications and behavioral changes can help. Include psychoeducation for family members when possible.

Table 5.3 Team-based treatment for psychosis

	PCP Approaches	BHP Approaches
Biological	**Evidence-Based Medication Treatment:** • Antipsychotic medications, usually atypical antipsychotics, are the most effective treatment for psychosis. • Focus should be on finding an antipsychotic medication that the patient will take consistently and improves functioning. • Monitoring and managing side effects will be importance for maintenance.	**Evidence-Based Medication Treatment:** • Troubleshoot adherence challenges • Help monitor common antipsychotic side effects. • Support client through making medication changes • Review psychoeducation with family as appropriate to support acceptance of diagnoses and adherence to treatment
Psychosocial	**Evidence-Based Behavioral Treatment:** • Provide education (including to family when possible) about the diagnosis of a psychotic disorder and symptoms involved with a focus on how medications and behavioral changes can help. • Assess a patient's understanding of symptoms and discuss behavioral strategies to reduce distress. • To build alliance, focus first on whatever symptom the patient states as the main concern.	**Evidence-Based Behavioral Treatment:** • Use specific communication strategies to discuss psychosis symptoms with patients • Consider using cognitive behavioral therapy (CBT) for psychosis when appropriate and available. • Other strategies: Behavioral activation, social skills training, motivational interviewing and chemical dependency treatment, smoking cessation strategies, weight management education and monitoring

• Emphasize that psychotic disorders are medical illnesses that can be chronic and require long-term treatment.
• Symptoms usually improve, but do not always resolve.
• Discuss variability of illness course and offer hope that many people who live with a psychotic disorder are able to lead fulfilling lives and may be able to volunteer, work, live independently, and have social relationships.

Table 5.4 Medications commonly used in the treatment of psychosis

---

Aripiprazole (Abilify)
Asenapine (Saphris)
Haloperidol (Haldol)
Iloperiodone (Fanapt)
Lurasidone (Latuda)
Olanzapine (Zyprexa)
Olanzapine and fluoxetine (Symbyax)
Paliperidone (Invega)—oral formulation
Perphenazine (Trilafon)
Quetiapine (Seroquel IR, Seroquel XR)
Risperidone (Risperdal)
Ziprasidone (Geodon)

For prescribing details and protocols, please see Chapter 11, "Evidence Based Psychopharmacology for the Collaborative Care Team."

PCP approaches
Choice of medication
To pick an initial antipsychotic, it is important to review any past medication trials and past side effects, get patient input and preference, consider cost of medication (this varies widely as some are generic), and try to minimize risk of side effects that will be most bothersome for an individual patient (See Table 5.4). Starting or changing antipsychotics can be co-managed with the PC. When indicated and available, a PC may evaluate the patient in person to discuss the best choice of medication, dosing recommendations, and side effects to monitor.

Risperidone: If no antipsychotics have been tried in the past, consider starting with risperidone.

Aripiprazole: If obesity, dyslipidemia, or diabetes are present, consider starting with aripiprazole which has significantly less weight gain and metabolic side effects than most atypicals.

Quetiapine: If extra pyramidal symptoms (EPS) have been problematic in the past with antipsychotics, consider starting with quetiapine. Quetiapine can be quite sedating (which is sometime helpful for a patient with insomnia) and does have significant metabolic side effects that will need to be monitored closely.

Black box warning

All antipsychotics have an FDA black box warning for increased risk of death when used for elderly patients with dementia-related psychosis.

Brief behavioral interventions for the PCP

Even with a 15 minute appointment, a PCP can assess a patient's understanding of symptoms and discuss behavioral strategies to reduce distress. To build alliance, focus first on whatever symptom the patient states as the main concern. This may mean starting with a focus on insomnia, "stress," or "being followed." Explore hallucinations and delusions without colluding with them or directly challenging the patient's beliefs. See how these affect patient's quality of life and safety.

Use brief reality testing if the patient is willing to consider other explanations for a delusion. Work with the patient to come up with coping strategies with a goal of making symptoms less distressing. For example, listening to music through headphones if auditory hallucinations are disturbing, riding the bus with a friend if paranoia is high in public, checking with someone they trust over the phone when feeling unsafe.

- Discuss importance of taking medications as prescribed and behavioral strategies to help with this, including medisets, setting alarms, using a chart, or help from family or housing staff.
- Always assess for safety and ensure the patient has a clear plan of how to get help if it is needed.
- Work in collaboration with BHP by supporting the same behavioral goals and asking the BHP to work more in depth on particular symptoms with cognitive behavioral therapy (CBT).

BHP approaches

In the initial phase of treatment the main role of the BHP is engagement in medication management of psychotic symptoms. Focus should be on understanding and linking treatment to patient goals. Communication strategies to work with patients with psychosis are listed in Table 5.5.

Working with medications

Prepare patients for antipsychotic trials by educating them that it can take several weeks and often adjustments in dose for maximum benefit from an antipsychotic.

- Remind patients that in the initial days to weeks of a trial of medication the focus is tolerability.
- Prepare patients to monitor and report concerns and side effects.
- Troubleshoot common barriers to medication adherence:
  - Work with patient to come up with ways to help adherence (medisets, setting alarms, using a chart, support from family or housing staff)
  - Help patient schedule an appointment and write down questions to discuss with PCP

Table 5.5 Communication strategies with patients with psychosis

Challenges	Strategies
Paranoia and mistrust	Work in a collaborative manner focusing on the patient's goals and spend time building a therapeutic alliance.
Lack of insight	Use gentle guided questions to explore the patient's understanding and increase insight when possible.
Psychotic beliefs	Explore delusional beliefs without directly challenging or supporting.
	Patient: "It's this computer chip in my brain that is causing the voices."
	BHP: "How can we find out more about what's happening?"
Cognitive deficits	Use repetition and multiple modalities to teach concepts such as writing down important points or recording a session on their phone.
Disorganized thoughts	Use a structured format and guide patient. If a patient's speech is difficult to follow, ask questions about how different comments relate and check your understanding.

Team goal: Initial treatment planning

Team creates a plan to engage patient in medication treatment with focus on psychotic symptoms that are the most concerning to the patient and/or functionally impairing.

Working as a team

Patient: Engage in discussion about treatment options.

PCP: Prescribe antipsychotic medication after discussing options and side effects with patient.

BHP: Facilitate communication between team members; develop full treatment plan to include evaluating medication adherence and brief behavioral interventions such as CBT for psychosis.

PC: Support treatment planning; medication recommendations and prescribing details; support behavioral treatment.

Case example

BHP provided psychoeducation to the patient and his mother including possible behavioral interventions, such as working on delusions so he could sleep. PCP discussed antipsychotic options with patient. Patient agreed to start risperidone 1 mg by mouth twice a day with his mother's encouragement after the PCP said it would help him cope better with the stress of recent events and allow him to sleep.

Follow-up and treatment adjustment to achieve treatment to target

When to consider referral

Consider referral to specialty mental health so the patient can be followed in an ongoing manner if a patient has chronic symptoms, does not respond to medications tried by PCP with support from PC, or has difficult-to-manage side effects from the psychotropic regimen.

Patients who are more severely impaired by a chronic psychotic disorder will likely need ongoing support through a community mental health center. Exploring funding options and helping coordinate applications for programs such as Medicaid or disability is an important way to assist if more intensive treatment may be needed. In many areas community mental health center treatment is not available without particular funding. Consider referral to a community mental health center if a patient is disabled from a chronic psychotic disorder and needs ongoing case management: including assistance with managing symptoms, activities of daily living, money management, employment, or housing.

Other referrals to consider in this population include CBT psychotherapist, spiritual support, nutritionist, podiatrist, dentist, CD treatment, housing support, supported employment program, volunteer organizations, and National Alliance on Mental Illness (NAMI) for education and support of patients with mental illness and their families.

When to consider psychiatric hospitalization

If there is concern that a patient is not able to be safe in the community due to danger to self, danger to others, or inability to adequately care for basic needs (such as not eating or drinking adequately, walking into traffic, or not taking medications that put health at risk), consult with team members (BHP, PCP, PC) and family when possible to determine what higher level of care may be available. Consider if staying with a friend or family may be an option and be sufficient for patient's needs. Some communities have crisis diversion beds that may be an option if no imminent danger to self or others is of concern. When there are imminent safety concerns, evaluation in an emergency room for possible psychiatric hospitalization is indicated. If a patient is agreeable to treatment then a voluntary admission is advised. If a patient is not agreeable to hospitalization then refer for involuntary evaluation; sometimes this requires sending the police or a county mental health evaluator to their home for evaluation.

PCP approaches
Medication adjustment
- A partial response with some ongoing psychotic symptoms is common for patients treated with antipsychotics.
- If psychotic symptoms continue to be disturbing and impair functioning, gradually increase the antipsychotic dose while monitoring for problematic side effects that may not be tolerable.
- If significant symptoms persist and a patient cannot tolerate a higher dose of the medication, consider a slow cross taper to another antipsychotic medication to see if it is better tolerated at an effective dose. Consult with PC to discuss the best medication to try next and how to cross taper to minimize decompensation.
- When medication treatment is complex, patient has severe functional impairment, or patient has chronic safety risks, consider referral to specialty mental health for ongoing care or to a community mental health center for more intensive team care including a psychiatric prescriber and case manager.

Prescribing principles
- Adjust dose to balance efficacy and side effects.
- Optimize dose of one antipsychotic before changing or augmenting.
- Avoid multiple antipsychotics in most cases except when cross tapering.
- To switch antipsychotics, the preferred method is to keep the first antipsychotic near full dose while gradually increasing the new antipsychotic to a therapeutic dose, then tapering off the first antipsychotic. If side effects from poly-pharmacy, the first antipsychotic may have to be reduced more quickly.
- Consider switching the antipsychotic if metabolic side effects are severe to minimize long-term health risks.

Managing side effects
Side effects typically worsen with increasing dose and can be intolerable at a dose needed for efficacy. Side effects are a frequent reason for medication nonadherence. Common side effects of typical antipsychotics include extrapyramidal symptoms (EPS), anticholinergic effects, sexual side effects, and weight gain (less than atypicals). Common side effects of atypical antipsychotics include weight gain, excess body fat around the waist,

hyperglycemia, and dyslipidemia. All antipsychotics have some increased risk for seizure, QTc prolongation, and neuroleptic malignant syndrome.

Metabolic Side Effects: Common in atypical antipsychotics. Symptoms include weight gain, excess body fat around the waist, hyperlipidemia, and hyperglycemia with risk of diabetes. Some evidence for success of weight management programs with focus on monitoring calories and exercise. Consider referral to nutritionist. If severe, consider decrease in dose or switch to a different antipsychotic.

- In order from least to most likely to cause: ziprasidone < aripiprazole < risperidone < quetiapine < olanzapine < clozapine

Extrapyramidal Side Effects: More common in typical antipsychotics. Symptoms include tremor, psychomotor retardation, increased muscle tone, akathisia (motor restlessness), and dystonia (prolonged muscle contraction). Treatment options include benztropine for dystonia and pseudoparkinsonism, propranolol for akathisia and tremor, and clonazepam for akathisia and dystonia. If severe and nonresponsive to side effect medication, consider decrease in antipsychotic dose or switch to a different antipsychotic. Medications used in the management of side effects are listed in Table 5.6.

- In order from least to most likely to cause: clozapine<quetiapine< olanzapine<aripiprazole<ziprasidone<risperidone< haloperidol

Tardive Dyskinesia (TD): Involuntary dyskinetic movements that may develop with antipsychotic use—sometimes irreversible. Much higher risk with typicals and increasing risk with higher doses and amount of time on medication. Watch for repetitive abnormal movements of the lips, tongue, jaw, and face including excessive blinking and grimacing. Jerking or writhing movements of the extremities are less common. TD can be assessed and monitored using the Abnormal Involuntary Movement Scale (AIMS). If TD is detected, consult with PC and consider change to a different antipsychotic.

Neuroleptic Malignant Syndrome (NMS): A rare but potentially life-threatening syndrome related to dopamine blockade that includes confusion, fever, autonomic dysregulation, rigidity, and elevated creatine phosphokinase. NMS is a medical emergency. Antipsychotics and

Table 5.6 Medications to treat extra pyramidal symptom side effects

Propranolol	10–40 mg bid to treat akathisia or tremor
Benztropine	0.5–2 mg qhs or bid to treat pseudoparkinsonism and dystonia
Clonazepam	0.5–2 mg bid for akathisia and dystonia.

anticholinergics should be stopped immediately and patient should be hospitalized for acute medical care. Most cases of NMS occur within a month of starting an antipsychotic or increasing the dose.

QTc Interval Prolongation: The cardiovascular side effect of severe QTc interval prolongation is rare but can be life-threatening if it progresses to polymorphous ventricular tachycardia. Consider what other medications the patient takes that may cause QTc interval prolongation and possible drug interactions before starting an antipsychotic. It is recommended that QTc interval prolongation be evaluated with an electrocardiogram (EKG) when starting ziprasidone and then monitored as indicated.

- In order from least to most likely to cause: haloperidol<olanzapine< iloperidone<risperidone<palperidone<quetiapine<ziprasidone

Special considerations when treating

Issues with Medication Adherence: consider medication monitoring (at clinic, with family, or at housing), long acting intramuscular (IM) medication given every two weeks or every month, or dissolvable medications. Also discuss with the patient if a side effect is making the medicine intolerable, and whether a trial of a different antipsychotic is warranted.

Treatment Resistance: Consult with the PC if the patient has failed to improve on two or more antipsychotics. This may be a patient that will need to be referred for more intensive treatment. A trial of clozapine should be considered. ECT can also be effective for treatment resistant psychosis.

Schizoaffective Disorder: Consider adding a mood stabilizer; lithium is first line.

Delusional Disorder: Medications tend to be less effective. Antipsychotic trial is warranted if delusion is causing significant problems. If not effective, taper off medication and try CBT.

Bipolar Disorder with Psychotic Features: During acute episodes of mania or depression with psychosis, an antipsychotic is indicated. For maintenance, a mood stabilizer alone may be sufficient.

Major Depressive Disorder with Psychotic Features: During acute episode of depression with psychosis, an antipsychotic is indicated. For maintenance, an antidepressant alone may be sufficient.

Substance Induced Psychotic Disorder: Try slow taper off antipsychotic 1–2 months after psychosis resolves. Motivational Interviewing is recommended. Consider chemical dependency treatment.

Psychosis Secondary to Another Medical Condition: Treat underlying medical condition. Try slow taper off antipsychotic one month after psychosis resolves.

Psychosis in Dementia: Antipsychotics have a Black Box warning in this population. Evaluate for possible behavioral interventions first. If antipsychotic is warranted after weighing risks and benefits, use a low dose of antipsychotic and monitor closely. Consider starting with risperidone 0.5 mg po bid or quetiapine 50 mg po qhs.

Psychosis in Delirium: Treat underlying cause of delirium. Use behavioral strategies to reorient. Start with lower dose of antipsychotic. Consider starting with risperidone 0.5 mg po bid and increasing as needed. Try slow taper off antipsychotic one month after psychosis resolves.

Psychosis in Pregnancy and Lactation: Consult with PC and obstetrician. This is usually an indication for direct evaluation and specialty care treatment. Discuss individual risks, benefits, and side effects of medications for both patient and fetus. If the patient has severe chronic psychosis, it is often a greater risk to stop antipsychotics. Haloperidol and all the atypical antipyschotics are class C. If an antipsychotic is warranted, it is advisable to use those that have been most studied: haloperidol, risperidone, olanzapine, or quetiapine.

Comorbid depression, anxiety, or substance abuse: Treating comorbid disorders is often needed. Treat these disorders in the same manner as for individuals without psychosis. Discuss with PC as some antipsychotics are recommended for comorbid depression.

BHP approaches
Working with medications

Medication adherence can be a challenge in this population due to side effects from antipsychotics, lack of insight into mental illness, paranoia about medication, thought disorganization, and cognitive deficits.

- Troubleshoot adherence challenges
  - Work with patient to come up with ways to help adherence (medisets, setting alarms, using a chart, support from family or housing staff).
  - If adherence is a consistent problem discuss issue with PC as dissolvable medication or long acting intramuscular (IM) antipsychotics may be considered.
  - Be responsive to patient concerns and side effects; bring these to the attention of PC and PCP.
- Help monitor common antipsychotic side effects such as weight gain, feelings of restlessness, involuntary muscle movements, lightheadedness when stands, and rigidity of movement.

- Alert the PCP immediately if patient describes difficulty moving, feeling "stuck" physically, severe lightheadedness leading to falls, severe distress from feeling restless, fever, or sudden confusion or disorientation.
- Support client through making medication changes. Help patient schedule an appointment and write down questions to discuss with PCP.

Cognitive behavioral therapy for psychosis—Brief interventions
- Working with delusions
  - Start with a less firmly held belief
  - Explore delusion and elicit patient's evidence
  - Generate alternative explanations to weigh the evidence
  - Hypothesis testing
  - Construct new understanding of events
- Working with hallucinations
  - Thorough assessment of frequency, content, and distress with interviews and hallucination diaries
  - Elicit beliefs about the hallucinations and the context in which they occur
  - Identify and reduce precipitants
  - Develop alternative perspectives
  - Test hypotheses
  - Develop coping strategies to reduce distress
- Working with negative symptoms
  - Behavioral self-monitoring
  - Activity scheduling
  - Mastery and pleasure ratings
  - Graded task assignment
  - Assertiveness training

Team goal: Revising treatment planning and stepping up care
Adjust antipsychotic medication to maximize effect and minimize side effects. BHP will help support medication adherence, engagement in treatment, and consider evidence-based behavioral intervention.

Working as a team
Patient: Keep team informed about symptoms and medication side effects.

(Continued)

PCP: Monitor medications and adjust as needed; use medications to treat side effects from antipsychotics when appropriate. Monitor baseline and follow-up labs and vital signs; consider referral to psychiatrist for ongoing care when needed.

BHP: Adjust treatment plan as necessary with consultation from PC. Focus on behavioral interventions and medication adherence strategies. Make referrals when appropriate (community mental health center, disability, vocational rehab, social services, chemical dependency, additional psychotherapy).

PC: Advises PCP and BHP on changes to medication and behavioral treatment. Evaluates patient in person if symptoms not improving or side effects of current medication not tolerable.

Case example

At the follow-up appointment with the BHP, the patient said that he was feeling a little better with improved sleep and less worry since starting the medication. He denied any side effects except for increased appetite and said he was eating more now. In addition to paranoia he now endorsed hearing a man saying, "You're no good" and commenting on his activities. He denied any command auditory hallucinations. Repeated safety assessments found no increased risk.

After discussion with the BHP, the PC recommended increasing the risperidone to 2 mg by mouth twice a day. This was initiated at the patient's next PCP appointment after the PCP had evaluated for possible medication side effects including orthostasis, weight gain, rigidity, and tardive dyskinesia.

Completing treatment and relapse prevention

General principles

Unlike depression or anxiety in which symptoms will often completely remit with treatment, patients with psychotic disorders will need ongoing medication management and support to maintain functional gains.

- Patients with minimal symptoms and good medication adherence may be able to be followed long term with several visits annually with PCP to complete appropriate monitoring and evaluate symptoms.
- Patients with moderate to severe symptoms will likely need ongoing support of a community mental health clinic and the goal of the primary care team will be to support connection with community resources and coordinate physical and mental health care.

Ongoing medication management

- Psychotic symptoms often improve, but do not always resolve with medications. The goal of treatment is improved functioning and decreased distress.

- Allow adequate time (several months) for full therapeutic response.
- It often takes a higher dose of antipsychotic to stabilize a patient. Longer term, a lower dose may be adequate for maintenance and a very slow decrease in dose with close monitoring for worsening of symptoms should be considered to minimize side effects.
- Patients with schizophrenia or schizoaffective disorder often require long-term use of an antipsychotic. Psychosis from another etiology may only need to be treated until the acute episode has resolved with slow taper off of the antipsychotic over the next one to six months. Consult with PC to discuss optimal time to start tapering antipsychotic and have BHP monitor for any recurrence of psychotic symptoms.

Monitoring guidelines for antipsychotics
- Baseline chemistry 7, fasting lipids, and weight. Monitor weight regularly.
- At least once a year: Abnormal Involuntary Movement Scale (AIMS), weight, waist circumference, lipid profile, and HgA1c.
- Consider yearly EKG to monitor QTc interval prolongation.

Ongoing Psychosocial Approaches

Evidence-based psychosocial treatments to consider
- CBT for psychosis (see above)
- CBT for comorbid depression and anxiety, including PTSD
- Behavioral activation
- Social skills training
- Motivational interviewing and chemical dependency treatment
- Smoking cessation strategies
- Weight management education and monitoring

Brief behavioral interventions for the PCP
- Follow-up on reality testing skills, medication taking behavioral regimen, regular safety assessment, and coordinate with the BHP on treatment goals that can be reinforced and incorporated in the overall communication and plan with the patient.

Team goal: Relapse prevention
The team will develop a long term treatment plan with appropriate level of care in either the primary care clinic or a community mental health clinic to support the patient's long term goals.

(Continued)

Working as a team
Patient: Engages in medication adherence strategies, CBT, and willing to consider referrals to help with ongoing symptoms.
PCP: Health care maintenance and consideration of long-term medication consequences; makes medical referrals as needed.
BHP: Considers appropriate psychosocial treatments, facilitates communication of team.
PC: Considers possible longer term side effects of medication and need for further dose adjustment.

Case example
After four weeks of treatment, the patient was evaluated by the PC due to continued paranoia and auditory hallucinations. The PC reviewed the history of symptoms with the patient and his family and diagnosed schizophrenia. The PC also discussed the need for ongoing treatment with medications and recommended the BHP focus on CBT to increase insight and decrease distress. PCP continued to prescribe antipsychotic medication and monitor for possible side effects from antipsychotic medication, including metabolic syndrome. The BHP worked with the family to discuss resources and options for more intensive ongoing treatment with a psychiatric provider and a case manager at a community mental health center.

Web resources

- APA Practice Guidelines on schizophrenia http://psychiatryonline.org/guidelines.aspx
- National Alliance on Mental Illness (NAMI) http://www.nami.org/
- APA patient and family information http://www.psychiatry.org/schizophrenia

References

Beck, A. T., Dudley, R., & Turkington, D. (2004). Cognitive-behavioral therapy for schizophrenia: a review. *Journal of Psychiatric Practice, 10*(1), 5–16.
Buchanan, R. W., Boggs, D. L., Fischer, B. A., Keller, W., Kelly, D. L., Kreyenbuhl, J. … Noel, J. M. Schizophrenia Patient Outcomes Research Team (PORT). (2010). The 2009 schizophrenia PORT psychopharmacological treatment recommendations and summary statements. *Schizophrenia Bull, 36*(1), 71–93.
Cassisi, J. E., Deavers, F., Mueser, K. T., & Penn, D. L. (2013). Psychosocial treatments for schizophrenia. *Annual Review of Clinical Psychology, 9*, 465–97.

Cipriani, A., Davis, J. M., Leucht, S., Mavridis, D., Orey, D., Richter, F. ... Spineli, L. (2013). Comparative efficacy and tolerability of 15 antipsychotic drugs in schizophrenia: a multiple-treatments meta-analysis. *Lancet, 382*(9896), 951–62.

Druss, B. G., Zhao, L., Marcus, S. S., Morrato, E. H., & Von Esenwein, S. (2011). Understanding excess mortality in persons with mental illness: 17-year follow up of a nationally representative US survey. *Medical Care, 49,* 599–604.

Everitt, B., Tarrier, N., & Wykes, T. (2008). Cognitive behavior therapy for schizophrenia: effect sizes, clinical models, and methodological rigor. *Schizophrenia Bulletin, 34*(3), 523–37.

Chapter 6 **Substance Use Disorders: Alcohol, Stimulants, and Opioids**

Susan E. Collins, Mark H. Duncan, Andrew J. Saxon, Joseph O. Merrill, and Richard K. Ries

Clinical impact

Substance-use disorders are common and are important to consider in the primary-care setting. In 2011, an estimated 20.6 million people in the United States (8 percent of the population) aged 12 or older had a substance use disorder. Of these individuals, 6.5 percent had an alcohol use disorder, 2.5 percent had a substance use disorder involving other drugs, and about 1 percent of individuals had both. Among substance use disorders involving drugs other than alcohol, marijuana is the most common, followed by opioids and cocaine. More than one-third of individuals who are seen in primary care and the ER engage in risky or heavy episodic drinking or have a substance-use disorder. In 2011, approximately 3.8 million people received treatment in self-help groups (55 percent), outpatient treatment centers (39 percent), outpatient mental health centers (26 percent), inpatient treatment centers (26 percent), hospital inpatient units (21 percent), private physician's offices (18 percent), emergency departments (15 percent), and prison/jail (11 percent).

Substance use disorders are important to track and treat in primary-care settings:

- Although consequences vary by substance, intoxication, withdrawal, and substance use disorders are often associated with both acute (e.g., accidents, interpersonal violence, suicide, falls) and longer-term (e.g., cancer, liver disease, HIV, hepatitis C, cardiovascular disease) health problems for the individual.
- They are often comorbid with and may complicate treatment for other psychiatric and medical disorders.

Integrated Care: Creating Effective Mental and Primary Health Care Teams, First Edition. Anna Ratzliff, Jürgen Unützer, Wayne Katon, and Kari A. Stephens.

- Primary care physicians prescribe medications that have the potential for misuse or abuse:
  - Almost 20 percent of individuals using prescription pain relievers for nonmedical reasons reported getting the medications from a single physician.
  - Although rates of prescription misuse, addiction, and diversion in adults prescribed stimulants for ADHD is not known, prescription stimulants are commonly misused by adolescents and young adults. One out of every six high school students has been exposed to prescription stimulants.
- Risky substance use and substance use disorders are also associated with secondary problems experienced by individuals' social network and the larger community such as accidents.
- Substance use disorders are often characterized as chronic and relapsing in nature and must therefore be continually assessed and treated appropriately over the lifespan.

Assessment

Identify chief complaint, associated somatic and psychological symptoms, functional impairment, and safety concerns

General principles
According to the ICD-10 and DSM-5, substance use disorders are characterized by psychosocial, behavioral, and physical symptoms, including perceived loss of control over substance use, craving, difficulty fulfilling socially sanctioned roles, continued risky substance use even in hazardous situations, and/or despite ongoing problems, and manifestations of physiological dependence (tolerance and withdrawal).

- Clinical symptoms are often hidden and present late, thus regular screening and a high index of suspicions are important.
- Substance use disorders are diagnosed if there is significant clinical impairment. However, it is also important for those working in primary care to monitor risky use or hazardous use, because these can denote risk for subsequent development of substance-use disorders as well as other psychosocial, behavioral, and health-related consequences.
- Although many drinkers consume enough alcohol to feel intoxicated, only a minority develop an alcohol-use disorder. Other substances may be used recreationally on an occasional basis. Thus, substance use alone should prompt screening and/or assessment but does not automatically imply disorder.

Common behavioral indicators
General

- Substance is used in larger amounts or over longer periods of time than intended.
- There are a persistent desire and unsuccessful efforts to cut down.
- A great deal of time is spent obtaining, using, and recovering from substances.
- Substance use results in failure to fulfill role obligations (e.g., work, school, family).
- Continued use despite persistent and recurrent substance-related problems.
- Reducing/stopping important social, occupational, or recreational activities due to substance use.
- Recurrent use in risky situations.

Alcohol: inappropriate sexual behavior, aggression
Opioids: psychomotor agitation or retardation
Stimulants: restlessness, talkativeness
Cannabis: increased appetite, risky sexual behaviors

Common psychological symptoms
Alcohol: craving (i.e., desire/urge for a substance), depression, anxiety, sleep disturbances, aggression, blackouts/memory lapses, cognitive deficits, suicidal ideation, impaired judgment
Opioids: craving, apathy, low mood, impaired judgment, anxiety
Stimulants: craving, paranoia, delusions, auditory, visual, and tactile hallucinations, memory and executive function deficits, euphoria or affective blunting, changes in sociability, hypervigilance, interpersonal sensitivity, anxiety, tension, anger, impaired judgment
Cannabis: craving, impaired short-term memory, impaired judgment, cognitive impairment, paranoia and psychosis, anxiety

Common physical/Somatic symptoms
Intoxication and related symptoms can precipitate behaviors that put individuals at risk for traumatic accidents (e.g., falls, fractures, burns), interpersonal problems/violence, suicide, and unwanted/risky sexual encounters.
Alcohol: slurred speech, coordination problems, unsteady gait, nystagmus, impairment in attention or memory, stupor, or coma
Opioids: slurred speech, drowsiness or coma, constricted pupils
Stimulants: tachycardia or bradycardia, pupillary dilation, elevated or lowered blood pressure, perspiration or chills, nausea or vomiting, evidence of

weight loss, muscular weakness, respiratory depression, chest pain, cardiac arrhythmias, confusion, seizures, dyskinesias, dystonias, coma

Cannabis: tachycardia, elevated blood pressure, elevated respiratory rate, conjunctival injections, dry mouth, symptoms of chronic bronchitis/chronic cough, sinusitis, pharyngitis, orthostatic hypotension, impaired motor coordination

Withdrawal syndromes can induce risky behavior and can cause physical symptoms that range in severity from uncomfortable to life-threatening (e.g., alcohol delirium tremens, falls precipitated by seizures).

Alcohol: autonomic hyperactivity (sweating, tachycardia, hypertension); increased hand tremor; insomnia; nausea/vomiting; transient visual, tactile and/or auditory hallucinations/illusions; psychomotor agitation; anxiety; generalized tonic-clonic seizures.

Opioids: dysphoric mood, nausea/vomiting, muscle aches, lacrimation/rhinorrhea, pupillary dilation, piloerection, sweating, diarrhea, yawning, agitation, tremor, insomnia

Stimulants: fatigue, depressed mood, vivid/unpleasant dreams, insomnia/hypersomnia, increased appetite, psychomotor retardation/agitation

Cannabis: fatigue, yawning, hypersomnia, psychomotor retardation, anxiety, depression, anorexia, irritability, restlessness, strange dreams, tremor, diaphoresis, abdominal pain, headaches, fever, chills

Symptoms associated with substance-use disorders can indicate their effects on various body systems. **Clinicians should assess for organ system damage related to chronic substance use such as cardiovascular and hepatic damage caused by alcohol.**

Alcohol: enlarged, shrunken, or tender liver, signs of alcoholic liver disease: hepatitis, encephalopathy, asterixis, caput medusa, edema, ascites, spider nevi, weakness, paresthesias, decreased peripheral sensation, sleep disturbance, Dupuytren's contracture, parotid enlargement, nystagmus, ataxia, hypertension, gastroesophageal reflux, pancreatitis, elevated risk of multiple forms of cancer.

Opioids: nasal septum perforation, abdominal pain, constipation, hyperalgesia

Stimulants: stroke, chest pain, tachycardia, hypertension, choreoathetosis, akathisia, buccolingual dyskinesias, tardive dyskinesia, acute dystonic reactions, arrhythmias, cardiomyopathy, rhinitis, left ventricular hypertrophy, myocarditis, hemoptysis, asthma exacerbation, nasal septum perforation, chronic rhinitis, bruxism, ulcers, skin lesions and ulcerations, rhabdomyolysis.

Cannabis: Symptoms of chronic bronchitis, myocardial infarction, stroke, transient ischemic attack, hyperemesis syndrome

Symptoms specific to IV drug use: symptoms of HIV infection, skin abscesses, new heart murmur due to infective endocarditis, epidural abscess and unexplained weakness or numbness, needle marks, sclerotic veins, lymphadenopathy, symptoms related to hepatitis C virus (HCV)

Common functional impairments

Education/Work: use of substances on the job, loss of employment, withdrawal from classes (if in school), unable to keep up with demands

Relationships: interpersonal violence, interpersonal problems, neglect of partnership and/or family responsibilities

Activities of daily living: poor hygiene, missing meals, incontinence

Assessing for safety

There are many safety risks associated with substance use disorders that should be considered and taken into account during assessment. It is important to consider intoxication, with its inhibition reduction, and withdrawal-related dysphoria as these may be associated with suicidal ideation.

Alcohol

According to the World Health Organization, alcohol-related problems are the world's eighth largest killer, and alcohol is the third leading global risk factor for disease and disability. Thus, alcohol misuse and alcohol use disorders can pose safety risks.

- Intoxication can lead to alcohol poisoning among younger, less experienced drinkers. Thus, providers should screen not only for alcohol-use disorders but also risky or hazardous use.
- Among patients with alcohol-use disorders, physical dependence should be assessed. Alcohol withdrawal can precipitate more serious conditions such as seizures and delirium tremens, the latter of which carries a 20 percent mortality rate when left untreated.
- People with alcohol use disorders also have higher rates of suicidal ideation and death by suicide than the general population, and therefore suicidality screens are recommended.
- Screening for alcohol use among pregnant women is important given its potential teratogenic effects.

Opioids

- Heavy involvement in buying and/or selling drugs in the underground economy can lead to significant risks to the individual (e.g., robbery, sexual abuse, forced prostitution). Lifestyle risk factors should be assessed and discussed.
- Overdose with opioids has become increasingly common—particularly due to increases in diversion of medical-grade opioids as well as uneven

concentrations of street drug formulations. The risks of overdose should be discussed, and naloxone should be prescribed to patients who use opioids as well as their friends and family to prevent overdose deaths.

Stimulants

- Heavy involvement in buying and/or selling drugs can lead to significant risks to the individual (e.g., robbery, sexual abuse, forced prostitution). Lifestyle risk factors should be assessed and discussed.
- Intoxication may precipitate aggressive or violent behavior and traumatic injuries, which should be considered and discussed with patients during assessment.
- Screening for stimulant use among pregnant women is important given potential teratogenic effects.
- Active substance use and uncontrolled psychiatric illness should be addressed before initiating treatment with prescription stimulants.
- Special note regarding medical use of stimulants in screening:
  - Treatment of attention-deficit hyperactivity disorder (ADHD) with a stimulant does not necessarily lead to a substance use disorder; however, it is difficult to identify individuals who are feigning ADHD in order to obtain prescription stimulants.
  - Misuse and diversion of prescription ADHD medications range from 5 percent to 35 percent. This is most prevalent among adolescents and college-age populations among whom they are commonly used for concentration, alertness and intoxication.
  - A more comprehensive assessment including obtaining outside information about the patients' childhood, including neuropsychological testing, and a full psychiatric assessment can be very useful.
  - Misuse can be minimized through the development of a treatment agreement, limiting prescriptions, regular follow-up, reviewing prescription monitoring programs, and checking urine screens for the prescribed substance.

Cannabis

- Risky sexual behaviors precipitated by cannabis intoxication can lead to increased risk of sexually transmitted diseases.
- Impairment in motor coordination can lead to increased risk of injury and death due to motor vehicle accidents.
- Screening for cannabis use among pregnant women is important given its potential teratogenic and neurodevelopmental effects.

- Screening for use in adolescence and young adults are important due to its association with declines in IQ and development of psychoses in susceptible individuals.
- Special note regarding medical cannabis in screening:
  - Some patients in primary care will be using medical cannabis to ease symptoms of various medical conditions (e.g., glaucoma, AIDS-associated anorexia and wasting, chronic pain, inflammation, multiple sclerosis, epilepsy, side effects of chemotherapy), and these uses should be acknowledged and supported, as appropriate.
  - Evidence supporting long-term use of medical cannabis for these conditions, however, is limited, and ongoing study is needed to assess side effects of longer-term use. In addition, the current varied forms of medical cannabis can result in unpredictable dosing and side effects.
  - As with any medication, it is important to collaboratively discuss with the patient the potential benefits and risks of treatment with medical cannabis.

Team goal: Identifying the chief complaint, initial physical exam, gathering history, and safety assessment

Identify problematic substance use, differentiate problematic substance use from substance use disorder, and use a nonjudgmental engagement approach to patients who need intervention.

Working as a team

Patient: Helps the BHP understand what role substances play in his/her life. Works with BHP to develop suicide safety plan, decrease substance-related harm and engage in medically supervised withdrawal, if necessary. Enacts safety plans, begins applying early intervention components in day-to-day life, and identifies self-care techniques as well as supportive relationships to help them during periods of crisis.

PCP: Assumes primary role in initially identifying a possible substance use disorder based on presenting medical or psychiatric issues. Uses short screening instruments and refers to BHP for further evaluation, if necessary. Assesses the need for medically supervised alcohol or opioid withdrawal. Assesses teratogenic risk, as indicated. Assesses for related medical problems. Connects patient to BHP for further psychosocial risk assessment and plan development.

BHP: Screens for substance use disorder, and if necessary, conducts full assessment. Screens for co-occurring psychiatric disorders. Helps identify risky behavior using a compassionate and nonjudgmental style. Begins to develop a strong therapeutic alliance. Assesses high-risk substance-related behavior such as suicidal thoughts, drinking and driving, and acquisition and use of street drugs and risk for overdose. Works with patient to develop safety plan and track use of it.

PC: Assists in identifying a formal diagnosis of a substance use disorder. Works with BHP to develop a substance-use disorder assessment battery. Helps in conceptualizing the most appropriate therapeutic approach tailored to fit patients' needs. Broadens safety plan as indicated. Reviews suicide risk.

Case example

A 44-year-old White/European-American male with no significant medical history presents to his PCP for a chief complaint of "left ankle pain." He states that two days ago he was walking home when he tripped on the curb and twisted his left ankle. He is concerned that it is "broken." His ankle is swollen with ecchymosis and tenderness around the lateral malleolus. This is his fourth fall in the past six months. He has a hard time describing why he is falling more or how he falls. During this time, he has also lost weight, and he appears disheveled. At past appointments, he has endorsed drinking regularly on the weekends.

After further evaluating the patient's left ankle, the PCP asks the patient when he drank last and observes for any current signs of intoxication or withdrawal, of which there are none. The patient is then asked to fill out the AUDIT-C and introduced to the BHP to review the patient's answers to the AUDIT-C. His score is an 11, as he drinks 4 or more times a week, with an average drinking amount of 7 drinks, on a daily or near daily basis. The patient later states he likes to drink to unwind but has been drinking responsibly, and walking home from the bar to avoid drinking and driving. The BHP validates this decision, but also shares that the AUDIT-C results are concerning because they indicate a potential alcohol use disorder that can interfere with his health and general quality of life. The BHP discusses these findings with the PCP, who orders a number of tests and reschedules the patient for a follow-up visit. The BHP discusses the case with the PC who reviews the criteria of an alcohol use disorder with the BHP.

Differential diagnosis and identifying a provisional diagnosis

Substance-induced psychiatric disorders are important to distinguish from primary psychiatric disorders. (Table 6.1, Table 6.2) Providers should take a detailed psychiatric history to assess whether symptoms persist during both periods of substance use and abstinence from substances, whether the

Table 6.1 Screening and assessment for substance-use disorders

Diagnosis	Behavioral health measure/tracking severity
Alcohol use disorder	Audit-C (three-item measure)
Opioid, stimulant, and cannabis use disorders	"How many times in the past year have you used an illegal drug or used a prescription medication for nonmedical reasons?"

Other disorders to consider: Substance-related disorders (intoxication, withdrawal), other substance/medication-induced mood disorders, psychotic disorders, antisocial personality disorder (adults), attention-deficit hyperactivity disorder, conduct disorder (adolescents), anxiety disorders (especially post-traumatic stress disorder), bipolar disorder, depressive disorders.

Table 6.2 Common substance-use disorders in primary care (ICD-10-CM)

Alcohol use disorder	Mild F10.10
	Moderate F10.20
	Severe F10.20
Cannabis use disorder	Mild F12.10
	Moderate F12.20
	Severe F12.20
Opioid use disorder	Mild F11.10
	Moderate F11.20
	Severe F11.20
Stimulant use disorder	Mild, Amphetamine type F15.10
	Moderate, Amphetamine type F15.20
	Severe, Amphetamine type F15.20
	Mild, Cocaine F14.10
	Moderate, Cocaine F14.20
	Severe, Cocaine F14.20

All disorders have mild, moderate, and severe categories.

psychiatric disorder preceded the substance-use disorder, and whether there is family history of psychiatric disorders.

Psychiatric related conditions

Comorbid psychiatric disorders are very common. Of US adults with a past-year substance-use disorder, 42.3 percent had co-occurring mental illness. Additionally, comorbidity with other substance use disorders (i.e., polysubstance use disorders) occurs in 1 percent of the US population. It is important to keep in mind that one substance may be used to reduce symptoms of withdrawal or modulate or enhance the effects of other substances.

Alcohol: psychotic disorders, bipolar disorders, depressive disorders, anxiety disorders, antisocial personality disorder, and PTSD

Opioids: depressive disorders, sleep disorders, sexual dysfunctions, delirium, anxiety disorders, other substance use disorders (especially tobacco, alcohol, cannabis, stimulants, benzodiazepines to moderate/modulate opioid withdrawal and intoxication), antisocial personality disorder, post-traumatic stress disorder

Stimulants: psychotic disorders, bipolar disorders, depressive disorders, anxiety disorders, obsessive-compulsive disorders, sleep disorders, sexual dysfunction disorders, delirium, post-traumatic stress disorder, antisocial personality disorder, attention-deficit/hyperactivity disorder, gambling disorder

Medical related conditions

Cardiovascular: angina, myocardial infarction, essential hypertension, heart failure, arrhythmias, cardiomyopathies, infective endocarditis

Gastrointestinal: viral hepatitis, hepatic carcinoma, peptic ulcer disease, IBD, pancreatitis, gastritis, cirrhosis, cirrhotic varices

Hematologic: anemia, thrombocytopenia, coagulopathies

Endocrine: hypo/hyperthyroidism, diabetes mellitus type II (DMII), hypogonadism

Immunological: HIV, immune suppression leading to opportunistic infections (e.g., TB, pneumonia), necrotizing vasculitis

Metabolic: hypoxia, dehydration, electrolyte abnormalities

Neurological: stroke, encephalopathy, traumatic brain injury, epilepsy, epidural abscess, peripheral neuropathy, Wernicke/Korsakoff syndrome

Respiratory: chronic obstructive pulmonary disease (COPD), asthma, nasal septal perforation

Dermatologic: skin abscesses

Team goal: Differential diagnosis and identifying a provisional diagnosis

Diagnose substance use disorder as well as any psychiatric and medical comorbidity associated with this disorder.

Working as a team

Patient: Helps PCP identify other medical and psychiatric concerns. Begins to develop therapeutic relationship with BHP.

(Continued)

PCP: Identifies the medical and mental health consequences and co-occurring disorders of substance use, including conducting HIV and viral hepatitis screening. Engages patients in discussion of the relationship between their substance use and related medical problems.

BHP: Provides further screening and evaluation for co-occurring psychiatric disorders. Supports patient in following through on medical recommendations such as getting lab work, and returning for follow-up appointments.

PC: Assists in clarifying diagnosis and impact of co-occurring disorders. Broadens search for other associated medical, psychiatric, or substance problems.

Case example

The patient returns to his primary care provider for review of the lab tests. Electrolytes, CBC, and ECG were normal, and an x-ray of his left ankle was negative for a fracture. Due to his concerning AUDIT-C, a comprehensive review of systems was performed but found to be negative. The rest of the patient's physical exam was significant for a slightly less kempt appearance than at previous visits, but his neurological exam and orthostatic vitals were normal. On the single-item screening, the patient denied drug use. He was returned to the BHP for further psychiatric assessment.

During the assessment, the patient admitted to drinking over a longer period of time and in greater amounts than intended during the past six months. He reported this was due to relationship problems. He admitted to almost daily craving, sneaking drinks throughout the day to "take the edge off," and missing deadlines at work, which had almost cost him his job. To screen for anxiety and depression, the BHP conducted the GAD-7, which was negative, and the PHQ-9, which was 8. The patient denied other psychiatric problems. The patient was diagnosed by BHP in consultation with PC with a moderate alcohol use disorder.

Treatment

Initiate treatment

General approaches

Use of a motivational interviewing style is key to approaching discussion of substance use and substance use treatment (Table 6.3). Motivational interviewing allows the provider to build rapport with the patient and elicit change talk from them that may encourage and solidify motivation to make positive behavior changes. Please see Miller & Rollnick's (2013),

Table 6.3 Team-based treatment for substance use in primary care

	PCP approaches	BHP approaches
Biological	**Evidence-Based Medication Treatment:** Medications treatment can be safe and effective for alcohol and opiate use disorders. **Alcohol use disorders:** Oral-form medications, such as naltrexone, acamprosate, and disulfiram, are most useful in highly motivated patients and patients under regular supervision. Extended-release naltrexone is recommended for less compliant patients. **Opioid-use disorders:** There are two primary paths that may be taken: medically supervised withdrawal or longer-term agonist maintenance. It should, however, be noted that the evidence base indicates longer-term agonist maintenance is superior to withdrawal for patients with moderate-to-severe opioid-use disorders.	**Evidence-Based Medication Treatment:** • Assess for potential barriers to engaging in medication treatment if indicated. • Support patients through making medication changes and troubleshoot adherence challenges.
Psychosocial	**Evidence-Based Behavioral Treatment:** • Provide an explanatory model that helps patients understand the biopsychosocial underpinnings of substance use and substance-use disorders as well as the multiple paths to recovery. • Acknowledge different stages in readiness for change and support patients' self-efficacy in achieving their goals.	**Evidence-Based Behavioral Treatment:** • There are a number of evidence-based behavioral interventions for substance use disorders. Assessing for readiness with change regarding use is the first step. • Patients are not currently motivated for abstinence: Motivational interviewing and brief motivational interventions can help engage patients and build rapport.

(Continued)

Table 6.3 (*Continued*)

PCP approaches	BHP approaches
• Assess engagement with and reinforce the behavioral treatment components of their integrated plan during medical visits.	• Harm reduction techniques that are tailored to individuals' risk factors should be suggested. • Patients are motivated for abstinence: • Cognitive-behavioral approaches may be used to continue to support patients' self-efficacy and to teach them ways to cope with high-risk situations, lapses, and relapses • Twelve-step facilitation, which is an evidence-based accompaniment to twelve-step program attendance, may be considered to support patients who are interested in attending twelve-step mutual help groups.

Motivational Interviewing: Helping People Change (3rd edition), for an excellent primer in patient engagement around substance use problems.

- Provide an explanatory model that helps patients understand the biopsychosocial underpinnings of substance use and substance-use disorders as well as the multiple paths to recovery.
- Assess what patients would like to see happen with their substance use.
- Assess patients' readiness for change and to support their self-efficacy in achieving their goals.
- If patients do not want to stop using, providers should discuss ways in which they can minimize their substance-related harm.
- If patients want to stop using, providers should assess the need for and refer to medically supervised withdrawal, as necessary.
  Ways to provide patient-centered treatment for substance-use disorders:
- [Following an assessment of substance-use disorder symptoms and relevant urine toxicology or lab tests:] "You told me you have experienced the following symptoms [name symptoms]. Additionally, lab tests were

conducted using your blood and urine samples. Taken together, these would suggest you are currently experiencing problems with [substance] that are affecting your [name affected areas]."

- "Many people experiment with and use substances, but some people are more likely to develop a substance-use disorder because of environmental, genetic, and other biological reasons."
- "You are not alone. Nearly [20 percent for alcohol/approximately 10 percent for other drugs] of Americans have experienced problems with [alcohol/drugs] in their lifetimes."
- "Fortunately, there are some effective ways to make changes in your substance use—however you might define that."
- "What kinds of things would you like to see happen for yourself? ... I would be happy to work with you toward those goals."
- "If you want, we can talk about some ways to make changes in your substance use."
- "There are some medications and some kinds of talk therapy/counseling that can support the changes you would like to make."

PCP approaches
General principles
Risky substance use is an appropriate target for brief interventions. Patients with substance use disorders require further evaluation to determine disorder severity, need for medically supervised withdrawal, readiness for change, and treatment goals.

- More frequent visits have been linked with more positive outcomes in primary care settings.
- Co-occurring substance use disorders and other psychiatric disorders are most effectively treated concurrently.
- Substance use disorders can often be successfully addressed and treated in primary care settings.

Prescribing principles (Table 6.4)

Alcohol use disorders
- Patients with no signs of alcohol withdrawal after five days from their last use do not need pharmacotherapy for alcohol withdrawal.
- Medically supervised withdrawal from alcohol in an outpatient setting has been well-established for appropriate patients. Such patients include those with a Clinical Institute Withdrawal Assessment for Alcohol Revised Scale (CIWA-Ar) score of < 15 who are medically and psychiatrically stable, have a support person available, are not in need of polysubstance withdrawal, and have no history of delirium tremens or seizures.

Table 6.4 Medications commonly used in the treatment of alcohol, opioid, and stimulant use disorders

Buprenorphine/ naloxone	Must have a waiver to prescribe for opioid use disorder treatment. Induction on medication should occur when patient in active withdrawal. Stabilization dose can take one to two months to establish and often involves ranges between 16 mg/4 mg and 20 mg/5 mg.
Naltrexone	For alcohol use disorder, start 50 mg qday. Range 25 mg–150 mg/d. For opioid use disorder, 50 mg qday is a sufficient dose. Significant interaction with opioids. Avoid in active hepatitis. Otherwise well-tolerated. May be used for use reduction or harm reduction as well as abstinence-based goals. Discontinue opioids for at least five days prior to use.
XR Naltrexone IM	380 mg q4wks. Range: One injection per month. Significant interaction with opioids. Avoid in active hepatitis. Nausea, fatigue, and injection site reactions common. Side effects often improve by five days and can be managed. May be used for use reduction or harm reduction as well as abstinence-based goals. Discontinue opioids for at least five days prior to use.
Naloxone	For treatment of opioid overdose, 10 ml multidose vial 0.4 mg/mL, intranasal syringes. Administer 1 mg per nostril, may repeat in five minutes if respiratory depression persists. Patient will need to instruct family and/or friends regarding indications for use and how to administer. Typically works in 2–5 minutes.
Acamprosate	Start 666 mg tid. Range: 333–666 mg/tid. Alternative for patients taking opioids. Diarrhea most common side effect. SI rare but reported. Renally excreted, reduce dose with CrCl 30–50ml/min, no liver toxicity, no drug interactions. Potential adherence problems.
Disulfiram	Start 250 mg qday. Range: 125–500 mg. Should have abstained from alcohol for at least 24 hours prior to first dose. Most effective for those committed to abstinence with good social support for observed ingestion. Avoid in severe cardiac disease and active hepatitis. Review alcohol disulfiram reaction and less well-recognized uses of alcohol (e.g., cologne, deodorant, cough syrups, vinegars). Several significant drug-drug interactions. Monitor liver functions throughout. Educate patients about symptoms of liver disease.
Gabapentin	Start 300 mg qday and titrate up to 300 mg in am, 300 mg in midday, and 600 mg qhs by day three. Range: 900 mg–1200 mg/day. Useful for ambulatory medically supervised mild to moderate withdrawal and protracted alcohol withdrawal symptoms: depression, anxiety, and insomnia. Doses of 1200 mg/day can be used for cannabis withdrawal and relapse prevention.

Table 6.4 (*Continued*)

Clonidine	Start 0.1 mg q8hours prn for opioid withdrawal symptoms. Hold if blood pressure <90/50, or P<50, excessive sedation, or orthostatic. Increase dosage as tolerated until withdrawal controlled or side effects supervene. Maximum dose 1.2 mg per 24 hours in divided doses. Taper over 2–3 days after withdrawal symptoms subside.
Benzodiazepines	Have the most evidence for management of alcohol withdrawal, including the prevention of seizures. Lorazepam and Chlordiazepoxide are commonly used.

The information provided here is a summary of current clinical practice. For full prescribing details for any of these medications, please consult drugs@fda.gov.

- All patients with alcohol-use disorders who require specialized, medically supervised withdrawal should be prescribed appropriate medication (e.g., chlordiazepoxide, lorazepam, gabapentin) prior to their quit date.
- Both the oral and intramuscular forms of naltrexone, an opioid receptor antagonist, can be used safely in patients who are abstinent or current drinkers and have been shown to reduce alcohol craving, heavy drinking days, and relapse.
- Acamprosate, a synthetic glutamate antagonist, has been shown to reduce return to relapse and increase accumulated days of abstinence. Acamprosate can be useful for patients with contraindications for naltrexone, such as physical dependence on opioids or acute liver disease.
- Disulfiram blocks the metabolism of ethanol leading to a build-up of acetaldehyde and uncomfortable symptoms. This medication can be useful for patients who have already initiated and want to maintain total abstinence. It should not be used in patients who have use reduction or harm reduction goals.
- Oral-form medications, such as naltrexone, acamprosate and disulfiram, are most useful in highly motivated patients or patients under regular supervision. Extended-release formulations improve medication adherence and lower the risk of an excessive dose.

Opioid use disorders
- There are two primary paths that may be taken. First, longer-term agonist maintenance is the most effective treatment. Second, if the patient is fully committed to achieving abstinence, medically supervised withdrawal and follow-up treatment with extended-release naltrexone may be considered. It should, however, be noted that the evidence base indicates

longer-term agonist maintenance is superior to withdrawal for patients with moderate-to-severe opioid use disorders.

- Pharmacotherapies for opioid use disorders target two primary goals: medically supervised withdrawal or longer-term agonist maintenance and include opioid agonists, partial agonists, antagonists and alpha-2-adrenergic agonists. It should be noted that abrupt withdrawal protocols have limited long-term effectiveness. Longer-term agonist therapy such as methadone maintenance or buprenorphine/naloxone are currently recommended over alpha-2-adrenergic agonists (e.g., clonidine) for treatment of withdrawal.
- Agonists and partial agonists:
  - Methadone is an effective opioid agonist used for maintenance. It must be prescribed and administered by specially accredited opioid treatment programs and cannot be used for addiction treatment in primary care.
  - On the other hand, a partial opioid agonist, buprenorphine/naloxone (i.e., Suboxone), is a Schedule III drug. It can be prescribed by primary care physicians who complete an approved 8-hour training course and apply for a federal waiver. Buprenorphine/naloxone is effective in treating withdrawal symptoms and as a maintenance therapy.
  - Opioid maintenance therapy with buprenorphine/naloxone has been shown to be effective in a variety of primary-care settings for moderate to severe disorders.
  - In some clinical settings, considerations for offering treatment for opioid-use disorders with buprenorphine/naloxone could include the following elements:
    - Local administrative and clinical support for developing treatment protocols
    - Screening, assessment, induction, monitoring, psychosocial treatment, termination, and referral policies
    - BHPs trained to support treatment with buprenorphine/naloxone
    - Ability to provide or refer appropriate counseling or nonpharmacological therapies according to DATA 2000
  - Although it is not as effective as buprenorphine/naloxone, clonidine may be used to treat opioid withdrawal as a second-line treatment.
- Antagonists:
  - Naltrexone
    - Oral-form naltrexone, an opioid antagonist, has been shown to be effective in maintaining abstinence among treatment-mandated patients but not in nonmandated patients due to low adherence.

- A single trial of extended-release naltrexone, a 30-day injectable formulation of naltrexone, has shown additional effectiveness because it resolves adherence problems. However, there is still a dearth of convincing evidence for use of naltrexone in opioid-use disorder treatment.
  - After completion of a naloxone challenge test, oral or intramuscular naltrexone may be started after 7–10 days of abstinence.
- Naloxone for overdose prevention is effective in reducing overdose death in patients continuing to use opioids. Prescribing naloxone to someone at risk of overdose is legal, although laws about third-party administration vary by state (see http://www.temple.edu/lawschool/phrhcs/Naloxone/Naloxonepolicy.htm). Naloxone should be prescribed along with psychoeducation regarding:
  - Preventing, identifying, and responding to overdose with naloxone
  - Rescue breathing and calling 911
  - Instructions for patient to educate their peers
  - Community-based programming for additional information (e.g., stopoverdose.org).

Stimulant use disorders

- No medications have strong empirical support in treating withdrawal symptoms or assisting in relapse prevention for methamphetamine/amphetamine use disorders.
- Although antidepressants are often prescribed to treat insomnia and depression experienced during cocaine withdrawal, there is not consistent evidence that they are more effective than placebo in staving off withdrawal or reducing use or relapse.

Cannabis use disorders

- In a small randomized controlled study, gabapentin, a calcium channel/GABA modulating drug, was found to reduce withdrawal symptoms and reduce cannabis use.
- That said, no medications have a strong empirical base to treat cannabis use disorders or withdrawal.

Choice of medication

Alcohol use disorders

- Start with naltrexone for patients desiring to cut back or stop drinking.
  - Check liver function tests prior to initiating medication.
  - Medication does not need to be titrated.

- Consider extended-release IM naltrexone in case of poor adherence with oral formulation.
- Do not use naltrexone if patient is physically dependent on opioids.
- Consider acamprosate if naltrexone is contraindicated, the patient cannot tolerate it, and the patient does not want to stop drinking.
- Disulfiram is most appropriate for highly motivated patients who have a goal of alcohol abstinence, and it works best under supervised conditions. Liver function tests should be checked at baseline and subsequently during treatment, as disulfiram can rarely (1/25,000 patient treatment years) cause liver failure.
- In comorbid conditions, consider the following
  - Physical dependence on opioids: acamprosate or disulfiram
  - Cocaine use disorder: disulfiram if naltrexone is contraindicated and abstinence is the patient's goal
  - Protracted alcohol withdrawal: consider gabapentin in addition to other medications

Opioid use disorders

- Refer to methadone maintenance or buprenorphine/naloxone treatment or develop a primary care-based buprenorphine/naloxone program.
- Consider opioid antagonists in patients with brief history of opioid use disorders or among patients who refuse opioid substitution therapy.
  - Start with naltrexone po for initial trial and consider IM if adherence is an issue.
  - Obtain liver function tests at baseline.
  - Monitor and treat opioid withdrawal symptoms carefully, prior to starting medication, as risk of relapse is high during withdrawal period.

Stimulant use disorder

- Amphetamines
  - Although studies have indicated some preliminary support for disulfiram for cocaine-use disorder and mirtazapine and bupropion for the treatment of methamphetamine-use disorders, there is not yet a sufficient evidence base to ensure their effectiveness.

Cannabis use disorder

- Cannabis
  - Gabapentin can be considered for patients desiring abstinence.
  - Cannabinoid agonists show some promise in reducing withdrawal, but there is not yet sufficient evidence to ensure their effectiveness.

Brief behavioral interventions
- Brief interventions in primary care settings are most effective for risky alcohol use that does not involve physical dependence. Brief interventions for drug use do not have a sufficient evidence base for recommendation.
  - Brief interventions can be delivered in 10–15 minute visits. (For an example, see http://pubs.niaaa.nih.gov/publications/Practitioner/PocketGuide/pocket.pdf)
  - Common components:
    - Provide feedback about diagnosis
    - Discuss safe amounts and offer advice about change
    - Assess readiness for change
    - Discuss goals and strategies for change
    - Arrange for follow-up
- It is important to introduce relapse prevention strategies for individuals who have achieved abstinence.
- For those who are not interested in achieving abstinence, providers may discuss ways to minimize risks of substance use.

BHP approaches
Psychosocial Approaches
It is important to use evidence-based, patient-centered, culturally appropriate approaches that are tailored to the patient's severity level, background, relevant psychosocial factors, and medical comorbidity.

After establishing some rapport, the BHP should elicit patients' treatment goals.
- The BHP can ask: "We will be seeing each other for the next [amount of time]. I am wondering what kinds of things you would like to see happen for yourself during this time? Some people call these treatment goals." It is recommended that treatment goals be patient-driven. This means they are generated by the patient based on their priorities and do not have to be exclusively substance-related.
- Next, the BHP can assess how important each of these goals is and how able a person feels to achieve these goals:
  - "On a scale from zero percent to one hundred percent, where zero percent is not at all important and one hundred percent is the most important thing, how important is [goal] to you?"
  - "On a scale from zero percent to one hundred percent, where zero percent is not at all able and one hundred percent is totally able, how able do you currently feel to work toward this goal?"

- If the patient indicates high levels on these measures, the BHP can provide affirmation by saying, "Wow! What makes you rate this goal so high/what makes you so confident you can achieve this goal?" The patient then has the opportunity to reiterate the importance of the goal and thereby solidify commitment. If this discussion brings up potential barriers, these can be addressed as well.
  - If the patient indicates lower levels, the BHP can ask why it wasn't an even lower number. Discussion of this can provide affirmation that the participant does have some foundation from which they can work to achieve this goal.
- BHPs should be careful not to make assumptions about goals or level of motivation for treatment.
- Such motivational assessment techniques are available in NIAAA's Tip 35.

If patients are not currently motivated for abstinence:
- Motivational interviewing and brief motivational interventions may help initially engage patients and build rapport (see http://pubs.niaaa.nih.gov/publications/ProjectMatch/match02.pdf for an example). It can also be used to help patients develop discrepancy between their current use and their goals and resolve this discrepancy in the direction of positive health behavior change.
- For individuals who are not interested in abstinence-based goals, harm reduction techniques that are tailored to individuals' risk factors should be suggested.

Harm reduction ideas for common substance use disorders
- For alcohol use disorders, suggestions could include supporting drinking moderation and discussing how to stay safer when drinking (e.g., self-monitoring drinks, drinking in a safe place with friends, not drinking and driving, taking B vitamins).
- For opioid-use disorders, this may include avoiding "Krokodil" (i.e., an opioid known for precipitating gangrene), a discussion of naloxone, importance of using clean works and not sharing paraphernalia (i.e., syringes, cookers, cottons, and rinse water), and appropriate vein care.
- With stimulant use disorders, this may include discussions of the potential for levamisole poisoning (cocaine) and avoiding sharing paraphernalia (crack pipes, syringes).

- For adolescents, please see the evidence-based BASICS manual.
- For adults, Denning and Little provide a practical approach for engaging patients around these topics.
- Finally, for cannabis use disorders, a comprehensive discussion of the potential benefits and risks of cannabis use can be helpful to ensure patients have fully considered their personal risk-to-benefit ratio.

If patients are motivated for abstinence
- Cognitive behavioral approaches may be used to continue to support patients' self-efficacy and to teach them ways to cope with high-risk situations, lapses (brief returns to problematic substance use) and relapses (full, sustained return to problematic substance use; see http://pubs .niaaa.nih.gov/publications/ProjectMatch/match03.pdf for an example). 12-step facilitation, which is an evidence-based accompaniment to 12-step program attendance, may be considered to support patients who are interested in attending 12-step programs. For a sample manual, please see: http://pubs.niaaa.nih.gov/publications/ProjectMatch/ match01.pdf.
- Further evidence-based approaches that may be applied in more specialty settings include contingency management, community-reinforcement approaches, or the matrix model. For more information about these interventions' evidence base and relevant tools, please see the SAMHSA National Registry for Evidence-Based Practice (http://www.nrepp .samhsa.gov/).

Working with medications
Because patients may be using various substances in addition to prescribed medications, it is especially important to ask about medications at every session:
- Reconcile medications (and all substances being used) at each appointment,
- Troubleshoot adherence challenges,
- Be responsive to concerns and side effects,
- Support patient through making medication changes,
- Help patient schedule an appointment with PCP to address medications, and
- Help patient write down questions.

Team goal: Initial treatment planning

The team should work together to enhance motivation to engage in treatment and develop a treatment plan appropriate for patient's current motivation to change.

Working as a team

Patient: Develops specific patient-driven treatment goals related to substance use (i.e., harm reduction, use reduction, cessation, relapse prevention) and other aspects of their mental and physical health and well-being. Works toward these goals with support of BHP and PCP. Continues to work on developing coping strategies and a recovery support network. Discusses with BHP barriers to medication adherence, if necessary, or issues around substance use and goals. As necessary/desired, obtains further support such as mutual-help groups or more intensive treatment options.

PCP: Engages patients in a nonjudgmental and compassionate style. Provides patient with information about substance use and treatment options, but allows patient autonomy in making treatment decisions. Uses a motivational interviewing approach to discuss prescribing and monitoring medications. Monitors baseline and follow-up labs and vital signs; health care maintenance and consideration of long-term medication consequences. Makes referrals as needed to treatment or mutual-help groups (e.g., Smart Recovery or 12-step, depending on a participants' goals). Provides brief intervention to at-risk substance users.

BHP: Engages in motivational interviewing to continually assess motivation to change and promote use of patient-selected treatments, including medication. Assists in safety planning. Provides treatment planning and follow-up for patients to engage them in efforts to change their patterns of use. Identifies patients needing extra support for desired behavioral changes.

PC: Supports treatment planning, medication recommendations, and prescribing details. Identifies other behavioral recommendations. Provides recommendations for referral to a higher level of care, when indicated.

Case example

The PCP recommended the PRINCE approach (protection, rest, ice, NSAIDs, compression, elevation) for the patient's ankle pain. The PCP conducted a brief intervention for alcohol use during which the patient expressed ambivalence about changing his drinking. The PCP referred the patient to the BHP. During consultation, the PC recommended the BHP use motivational interviewing to further engage the patient around his alcohol use and to discuss ways he could minimize his risks should he choose to continue drinking. The PC also worked with the BHP to review the patient's suicide risk.

Follow-up and treatment adjustment to achieve treatment to target

When to consider referring

- Inpatient medically supervised withdrawal for alcohol is indicated.
- Opioid substitution treatment is indicated (unless able to provide buprenorphine/naloxone treatment).
- Condition is not responding to treatment in primary-care setting.
- Comorbid conditions exist that require longer term, more intensive, or specialist psychotherapy or medical care.
- Higher level of need is present including the need for long-term case management.
- When patients need employment services. (Especially if people have criminal justice involvement, gaps in employment because of treatment episodes, frequent relapses.)

PCP approaches

Behavioral Approaches

Continued patient engagement is fundamental in the treatment of substance use disorders because patients may experience ups and downs in their substance use trajectories. Patient engagement can be fostered through an equitable partnership that draws on the nonjudgmental and compassionate approach described in the above sections. Such an approach is exemplified through a sense of gentle curiosity about and appreciation of the patient and their social context, as well as an identification and validation of the patient's own knowledge about their substance use. Likewise, it is important to avoid "interrogating" the patient regarding substance use or engaging in authoritarian advice-giving. Finally, as part of the team-based nature of treatment, it is important to inquire about the efficacy of behavioral approaches whether initiated by the PCP or BHP. The PCP can play a powerful role in supporting patients' motivation to engage in behavioral approaches.

Regular monthly follow-up with the PCP, supporting more frequent follow-up with the BHP should be continued until the patient has shown sustained stability. If patients experience difficulty achieving their treatment goals, more regular contact to review medical stability and support positive behavioral changes can be instituted. Consideration for referral for a higher level of care can also be given.

Pharmacotherapy

In assessing a patient in follow-up, it is important to evaluate adherence, efficacy, as well as side effects of a medication. Adherence can be improved through ongoing colearning between the PCP and patient around how the medication works and is working for the patient. Current barriers to medication adherence can be evaluated and discussed. Identification of current side effects and their management should also be addressed. Attention to necessary dosage adjustments is crucial.

BHP approaches

As treatment progresses, the BHP should address any difficulties in team coordination of the overall plan. As the patient becomes more engaged with the BHP, the BHP can often act as an advocate with the medical providers to help mediate therapeutic alliance issues and instruct the patient and medical team about issues the patient may be struggling with due to substance use.

It is also important to note that motivation for treatment and treatment goals shifts and morphs over time. Thus, providers should regularly revisit patient-driven goals, assess progress toward goals, and revisit goals, as indicated. When participants' motivation for treatment seems to wane, it is important for providers to find a positive step the patient has taken and to reflect this back to the participant. For example, "Although you didn't achieve the goal you had set out last time, you made it to this appointment today. That shows real strength and persistence!" This is known as a strengths-based affirmation. Reflecting and affirming patients' strengths help to increase and stabilize motivation for change as well as the therapeutic alliance.

Team goal: Revising treatment planning and stepping up care
Focus on keeping patients engaged during the hard work of changing behaviors and anticipating the need to adjust treatment as needed to achieve patient goals.

Working as a team
Patient: Updates treatment goals and provides ongoing feedback regarding progress made toward treatment goals; fills out behavioral health measures to monitor treatment progress; reports functional changes in daily activities due to medical, psychiatric, or substance-use problems; gives feedback regarding his/her own attempts to manage symptoms; discuss any difficulties with provider interactions; discusses progress on behavioral and medical treatment recommendations to the PCP and BHP and discusses any difficulties with the treatment plan to help trigger further treatment adjustments.

   PCP: Addresses therapeutic alliance issues as needed, consulting with the BHP as needed; follows through on medical treatment goals and outcomes of medical referrals as needed; continues to monitor progress; adjusts prescriptions as needed. Depending on patients' needs, may consider urine toxicology testing to monitor progress or lab monitoring for liver disease in patients with alcohol use disorders or hazardous drinking.

BHP: Continues to address engagement, crisis management, and safety planning as needed; steps up brief behavioral interventions as needed to address comorbid mental health issues; continues to facilitate communication between team members; supports referral follow through and case management as needed (disability, vocational rehab, social services, chemical dependency, additional psychotherapy); monitors measures and advocates for stepping up care as measures and function monitoring indicate poor improvement.

PC: Supports treatment planning; supports safety planning; advocates for stepping up care and altering medication recommendations as needed; and supports and suggests behavioral management recommendations.

Case example

After a few motivational interviewing sessions with the BHP, the patient acknowledged he would like help in cutting back on his drinking. At that point, the PC recommended the PCP begin a course of naltrexone with regular follow-up from the BHP for further motivational interviewing around medication adherence, alcohol consumption, and his functional status. The PC also recommended the PCP review the patient's risk of alcohol withdrawal and discuss with the patient dangers about quitting abruptly on his own. The BHP began moving into the planning phases of motivational interviewing with the patient, weaving in cognitive behavioral strategies for reducing use into their sessions (e.g., setting drinking limits, avoiding high-risk situations, engaging in other pleasurable activities that do not involve substances).

Completing treatment and relapse prevention

Team goal: Relapse prevention

After an acute episode of a substance use disorder resolves, the team must focus on developing a strong plan to continue to support positive treatment gains as well as a reengagement plan should the patient return to baseline levels of harmful drinking or drug use.

(Continued)

Working as a team

Patient: Continues to provide feedback on treatment goals and progress made toward them; fills out measures to monitor treatment progress; reports functional changes in daily activities due to medical, psychiatric, or substance-use problems; gives feedback on own attempts to manage symptoms; discuss any difficulties with provider interactions; discusses progress on behavioral and medical treatment recommendations to the PCP and BHP and discusses any difficulties with the treatment plan to help trigger further treatment adjustments.

PCP: Continues to addresses therapeutic alliance issues as needed, consulting with the BHP as needed; follows through on medical treatment goals and outcomes of medical referrals as needed; continues to monitor progress; adjusts prescriptions as needed. Continues to reinforce therapeutic approach of BHP.

BHP: Continues to address engagement, crisis management, and safety planning as needed; steps up brief behavioral interventions as needed to address comorbid mental health issues; continues to facilitate communication between team members; supports referral follow through and case management as needed (disability, vocational rehab, social services, chemical dependency, additional psychotherapy); monitors measures and advocates for stepping up care as measures and function monitoring indicate poor improvement.

PC: Supports treatment planning; supports safety planning; advocates for stepping up care and altering medication recommendations as needed; and supports and suggests behavioral management recommendations.

Case example

After two months of treatment, the patient's AUDIT-C had dropped to a 5, and his PHQ was 0. The patient's ankle pain resolved with appropriate conservative treatment. He reported no longer drinking at work and noted a noticeable decrease in his desire to drink. He reported feeling much better overall and expressed a desire to stop drinking altogether. The BHP discussed the importance of self-help or mutual-help support (e.g., 12-step programs, Smart Recovery, Harm Reduction, Abstinence from Alcohol, Moderation and Support [HAMS] Network).

Web resources

- National Institutes of Health – National Institute of Alcohol Abuse and Alcoholism: http://www.niaaa.nih.gov/
- National Institutes of Health – National Institute of Drug Abuse: http://www.drugabuse.gov/
- Substance Abuse and Mental Health Services Administration: http://store.samhsa.gov/home
- American Society of Addiction Medicine http://www.asam.org/practice-support
- American Academy of Addiction Psychiatry: http://www.aaap.org
- American Psychological Association Division 50 (Society of Addiction Psychology) website: http://www.apa.org/divisions/div50/
- *SAMHSA/CSAT Treatment Improvement Protocols*: http://www.ncbi.nlm.nih.gov/books/NBK82999/
- Self-help and mutual help:
  - Alcoholics Anonymous: http://www.aa.org/
  - Smart Recovery: http://www.smartrecovery.org/
  - Harm Reduction, Abstinence from Alcohol, Moderation and Support [HAMS] Network: http://www.hamsnetwork.org/

References

Bowman, S., Eiserman, J., Beletsky, L., Stancliff, S., & Bruce, R. D. (2013). Reducing the health consequences of opioid addiction in primary care. *American Journal of Medicine, 126,* 565–571.

Dimeff, L. A., Baer, J. S., Kivlahan, D. R., & Marlatt, G. A. (1999). *Brief alcohol screening and intervention for college students (BASICS): A harm reduction approach.* New York: Guilford Press.

Bush, K., Kivlahan, D. R., McDonnell, M. B., Fihn, S. D., & Bradley, K. A., (ACQUIP) ftACQIP. (1998). The AUDIT alcohol consumption questions (AUDIT-C). *Archives of Internal Medicine, 158,* 1789–95.

Chan, Y. F., Hsiang, H., Sieu, N., & Unützer, J. (2013). Substance screening and referral for substance abuse treatment in an integrated mental health care program. *Psychiatric Services, 64.*

Denning, P. & Little, J. (2012). *Practicing harm reduction psychotherapy: An alternative approach to addictions.* New York: Guilford Press.

Gowing, L., Ali, R., & White, J. M. (2009). Buprenorphine for the management of opioid withdrawal. *Cochrane Database of Systematic Reviews, 3,* 1–70.

Kaner, E. F., Dickinson, H. O., Beyer F., Pienaar, E., Schlesinger, C., Campbell, F., … Heather, N. (2009). The effectiveness of brief alcohol interventions in primary care settings: A systematic review. *Drug and Alcohol Review, 28,* 301–23.

Miller, W. R. (1999). *Enhancing motivation for change in substance abuse treatment, 35.* Rockville, MD: US Department of Health and Human Services.

Miller, W. R. & Rollnick, S. (2012). *Motivational interviewing: Helping people change* (3rd edition). New York: Guilford Press.

Rösner, S., Hackl-Herrwerth, A., Leucht, S., Vecchi, S., Srisurapanont, M., & Soyka, M., (2010). Opioid antagonists for alcohol dependence. *Cochrane Database of Systematic Reviews, 12,* CD001867.

Stotts, A. L., Dodrill, C. L., & Kosten, T. R. (2009). Opioid dependence treatment: Options in pharmacotherapy. *Expert Opinion in Pharmacotherapy, 10,* 1727–40.

Sullivan, J. T., Sykora, K., Schneiderman, J., Naranjo, C. A., & Seller, E. M., (1989). Assessment of alcohol withdrawal: The revised clinical institute withdrawal assessment for alcohol scale (CIWA-Ar). *British Journal of Addiction, 84,* 1353–1357.

TIP 24: A Guide to Substance Abuse Services for Primary Care Clinicians. 24 ed. (2008). Rockville, MD: Substance Abuse and Mental Health Services. http://www.ncbi.nlm.nih.gov/books/NBK64827/.

Chapter 7 **Chronic Pain**

Catherine Q. Howe and Kari A. Stephens

Clinical impact

Chronic pain is very common in patients, particularly adults seen in primary care. Persistent low back pain is the most common, with a prevalence of ~30 percent in the general population, and close to 50 percent in primary care.

Definition of chronic pain: Pain lasting longer than 3–6 months, or alternatively, pain persisting for at least one month beyond the usual course of an acute illness or the time required for an injury to heal.

Chronic pain limits patients' ability to function and can increase the risk for common mental health and substance use disorders. Patients with comorbid mental health disorders have been found to have greater functional impairment and higher rates of health service use and costs along with worse outcomes for surgical interventions, and they are more likely to receive prescription opioids compared to patients without mental health disorders. Pain that interferes with daily activities has been found associated with poor response to depression treatment. Chronic pain can also increase the risk for having serious suicidal ideation.

> **TIP:** Consider mental health and substance abuse problems because they are common in this population, they can complicate treatment, and increase risk for poor outcomes.

Integrated Care: Creating Effective Mental and Primary Health Care Teams, First Edition.
Anna Ratzliff, Jürgen Unützer, Wayne Katon, and Kari A. Stephens.
© 2016 John Wiley & Sons, Inc. Published 2016 by John Wiley & Sons, Inc.

Assessment

Identify chief complaint, associated somatic and psychological symptoms, functional impairment, and safety concerns

General principles
- Chronic painful conditions are systematically characterized based on duration, type, and location of pain
- Commonly presenting chronic pain syndromes are recognized using a structured approach to diagnosis

Key elements in pain-related health history
- PQRST of pain: Provocation, Quality, Region (location), Severity (scale of 0–10), Temporality (onset, course, fluctuation)
- Current and past treatments for pain (e.g., injections, physical therapy, massage, acupuncture, surgery)
- Current pain coping strategies (e.g., relaxation, mindfulness, pacing strategies) and how they are being used
- Medical comorbidities (e.g., diabetes, HIV, obesity, inflammatory bowel disease)
- Psychological comorbidities (e.g., depression, anxiety, posttraumatic stress disorders)
- History or active substance use disorders (e.g., history of illicit drug use, regular use of benzodiazepines or alcohol, receipt of opioids from more than one provider, repeated emergency department visits seeking opioids)
- Surgical history (e.g., spinal surgery)
- Legal history and history of disability claims
- Social history (e.g., financial, housing, and family stressors)
- History of childhood physical or sexual abuse
- Family history

Current physical functioning
- Activities of daily living (how does the patient spend his/her day?)
- Physical activities
- Falls, injuries, accidents
- Eating
- Sleeping
- Side effects of pain medications

Current psychosocial functioning
- Mood and anxiety level
- Enjoyment of life

- Relationships
- Social activities
- Solicitous or illness-reinforcing behavior from family or friends
- Work or employment status
- Hobbies
- Sex

Determine type of pain pathophysiology
- Nociceptive Pain
  - Pain that arises from actual or threatened damage to nonneural tissue and is due to the activation of nociceptors
  - Caused by injuries, infection, inflammation, or intestinal obstruction
- Neuropathic Pain
  - Pain caused by a lesion, disease, or dysfunction of the somatosensory nervous system
  - Can be periphery (e.g., neuroma, nerve entrapment, herpes zoster, diabetic neuropathy), central (e.g., multiple sclerosis, spinal injury), or mixed (e.g., fibromyalgia, trigeminal neuralgia)

Measures
Screen for depression, anxiety, PTSD, pain rating, pain interference in function/life rating. See Figure 7.1 for an example of the pain assessment questionnaire used in an integrated pain care program.

Assessing for safety

Self-Harm
- As many as 50 percent of chronic pain patients report having seriously considered suicide at some point
- Comorbid psychiatric and substance use disorders further increase the risk of suicidality
- Due to this elevated risk, any patient presenting with chronic pain should be screened for suicidality and monitored at follow-up visits. (See Management of Suicidality)

Other Safety Risks
- Serious inability to care for self (grave disability)
- Environmental or social issues posing safety risks: housing/shelter risks, violence (i.e., domestic violence and other dangerous social circumstances)

1. What number best describes your *pain* on average in the past week:

0	1	2	3	4	5	6	7	8	9	10
No Pain										Pain as bad as you can imagine

2. What number best describes how, during the past week, pain has interfered with your *enjoyment* of life?

0	1	2	3	4	5	6	7	8	9	10
Does not interfere										Completely Interferes

3. What number best describes how, during the past week, pain has interfered with your *general activity*.

0	1	2	3	4	5	6	7	8	9	10
Does not interfere										Completely Interferes

4. Chronic pain may limit activities that are very important to you (eg. Caring for children, walking the dog). We hope your pain treatment will make it easier for you to do these important activities. Please list one important activity that is difficult for you to perform so that we can monitor it during your pain treatment.

Activity:

You said that you are having difficulty with _____.

Please rate how able you are to do this activity as of today.

Figure 7.1 Pain assessment questionnaire (PEG three item scale[1] & activity limitation[2]).

[1] Krebs, D. D., Lorenz, K. A., Bair, M. J., et al. (2009). Development and initial validation of the PEG, a three-item scale assessing pain intensity and interference. *J Gen Intern Med, 24*(6), 733–738.
[2] Items from the *Current Pain Tracker* reproduced with permission from Mark Sullivan, MD.

Team goal

Identifying the chief complaint, initial physical exam, gathering history, and safety assessment for pain symptoms. Triage patients with chronic pain to the behavioral health specialist to: (a) evaluate mental health comorbidities and other psychosocial factors needed to determine a behavioral treatment plan for chronic pain including self-management; (b) coordinate the start of the care plan; and (c) begin and solidify treatment engagement. Assess for safety related issues and invoke safety planning practices consistent with clinic policy.

Working as a team

Patient: Describes desired treatment goals, pain, and mood symptoms, and relevant history to the PCP and BHP. Shares symptoms of past and current suicidal ideation with the treatment team, informs the team if symptoms worsen. Shares environmental and risk factors with the treatment team.

PCP: Gathers pain-related health history, conducts physical exam, reviews results from diagnostic studies and specialist consultations to formulate the biological chronic pain assessment. Grows and fosters a therapeutic alliance with the patient, centering on patient driven treatment goals for pain management. Assesses for safety; coordinates with BHP to monitor safety issues and implement safety plan as clinically indicated.

BHP: Completes detailed assessment of psychosocial and substance use history, use of behavioral pain coping strategies, and readiness to move to self-management of chronic pain. Assesses for therapeutic alliance issues with the PCP and specialists, and treatment adherence including the use of medications. Assesses for resource needs addressable via case management. Places pain symptoms in the psychosocial context to provide an integrated perspective on the patient's pain complaints and pain behaviors. Engages patient complete mood and pain rating scales. Assesses safety issues and helps with safety planning; tracks safety plan.

PC: Assists in identifying and evaluating psychiatric comorbidities. Helps place pain symptoms in the psychosocial context to provide an integrated perspective on the patient's pain complaints and pain behaviors. Recommends treatment strategies to address psychosocial contributors to functional impairment/pain syndrome. Assists in safety planning as needed.

Case example

Ms. T is 43-year-old woman who presents to her PCP with history of chronic lower abdominal pain of unclear etiology, asking for help with pain reduction. She reports persistent daily pain, trouble eating, inability to concentrate and focus at work, which has led to her inability to work and related financial and emotional stress. Extensive workup by OB/GYN, including repeated laparoscopies and laparotomies are negative. She has been prescribed

(Continued)

methadone 10mg/day and hydromorphone as needed up to 8mg/day for over a year. Her pain is poorly controlled despite the opioids, and she makes frequent trips to emergency departments for pain crises, nausea, and opioid withdrawal.

Ms. T is told by her PCP that she would like her to be seen by the team's BHP to help with developing a comprehensive plan to address her pain and help her achieve the best quality of life possible. The BHP discovers Ms. T's daily activities are very limited. She has trouble sleeping at night and spends much of the day lying down napping. Her daughter does most of the cooking and household management activities, takes her to all of her doctor appointments, and pushes her around in her wheelchair. In the evenings, she watches TV with her family. She avoids doing many activities because she feels that would make her pain worse and wants a clear diagnosis for her pain and treatment plan that will help stop her pain. Mental health screening using the PHQ-9 and the GAD-7 indicates high levels of depression and anxiety without suicidal ideation. Upon further assessment, she endorses a history of childhood physical abuse and posttraumatic stress symptoms from domestic violence. Ms. T also states she likes her PCP, but does not believe her PCP thinks her pain is real and just wants to take her off her opioid medications, which she believes is the main thing that helps her pain.

Ms. T denied current suicidal ideation and stated she struggled in the past with one suicide attempt in her remote history as a young adult with no associated hospitalization. She also stated her past abusers were no longer in her life and stated she felt safe at this point with her living and social circumstances.

Differential diagnosis and identifying a provisional diagnosis

Working together, the team will develop a differential diagnosis of pain symptoms and assess for comorbid mental health disorders. See Table 7.1 for differential diagnosis of pain and Table 7.2 for common pain diagnoses.

Rule out common contributing medical problems and substance-related conditions

Medical conditions

- Osteoarthritis
- Inflammatory arthritis
- Tumors
- Chronic infection (e.g. incompletely treated septic joint)
- Acute-on-chronic injury
- Poor nutrition, hygiene related issues, sleep disturbance

Table 7.1 Differential for common causes of chronic pain syndromes

Chief complaint	Differentiating history and physical findings	Differential diagnosis
Back Pain	Presence or absence of radicular findings History of spinal surgery	Discogenic pain Degenerative pain Myofascial pain Radiculopathy Failed back surgery syndrome
Musculoskeletal Pain (Non-Spinal)	Trauma or injuries Repetitive motion Structural deformity Inflammatory markers	Osteoarthritis Posttraumatic arthritis Inflammatory arthritis Tendonitis
Headaches	"PQRST" of headaches Cervical range of motion Muscular trigger points	Migraine Tension headache Cervicogenic headache Temporo-Mandibular disorders
Periphery Neuropathic Pain	Metabolic disease (e.g., diabetes, thyroid disease) Infectious history (e.g., HIV, herpes zoster) History of receiving chemotherapy Nutritional deficit Dermatome distribution	Diabetic neuropathy Postherpetic neuralgia HIV neuropathy Nerve entrapment Vitamin B12 deficiency Autoimmune neuropathy
Abdominal and Pelvic Pain	Gastrointestinal symptoms Urinary symptoms Dysmenorrhea History of sexual trauma Abnormal discharge	Irritable bowel syndrome Inflammatory bowel disease Interstitial cystitis Endometriosis Prostatitis Pelvic inflammatory disease
Widespread Pain	Distribution of pain region Tender points	Fibromyalgia Regional myofascial pain Opioid withdrawal

Other disorders to consider: Complex regional pain syndrome, trigeminal neuralgia, spinal cord injury pain, multiple sclerosis, cancer pain

Substance-related conditions
- Opioid diversion: selling medications, supplying family/friends
- Overuse of opioid medications

Assessment of comorbid psychiatric disorders and psychological difficulties
- Chronic pain is highly comorbid with common mental health and substance use disorders. The presence of these comorbid conditions

Table 7.2 Common chronic pain syndromes in primary care (ICD-10)

- Abdominal pain - R10.x
- Chronic pain syndrome - G89.4
- Fibromyalgia - M79.7
- Joint pain - M25.5x
- Low back pain - M54.5
- Migraine - G43.x
- Other idiopathic peripheral autonomic neuropathy - G90.09
- Pain disorders exclusively related to psychological factors - F45.41
- **Pain, unspecified - R52**

makes functional improvement more difficult to achieve. Treatment of these comorbid conditions can significantly improve suffering from pain, support pain self-management and functional improvement.

- Specific comorbidities (see other chapters for more detailed information about specific psychiatric disorders):

  Somatic Symptom Disorder: Patients with chronic pain often have excessive thoughts, feelings, and behaviors associated with their pain experiences that can lead to suffering that can be relieved through addressing pain self-management strategies and cognitive behavioral therapy. These thoughts, feelings, and behaviors can overlap with symptoms from other mental health disorders but often center or exacerbate during the pain experience or pain flare.

  Illness Anxiety Disorder: Some patients with chronic pain may have heightened bodily sensations, be intensely anxious about the possibility of an undiagnosed illness, or devote excessive time and energy to health concerns, often obsessively researching them.

  Major Depression: Chronic pain increases the risk of a depression diagnosis 2–5 times. Patients with both pain and depression have more pain complaints, higher pain intensity and pain chronicity.

  Post-Traumatic Stress Disorder (PTSD): The prevalence of PTSD in chronic pain population is 2–4 times higher than in populations without chronic pain. A history of childhood maltreatment and PTSD increases the risk for developing chronic pain.

  Panic Disorder: Chronic pain increases the likelihood of a panic disorder diagnosis by 6–25 times. Chest pain, irritable bowel syndrome, and chronic recurrent headaches are frequently associated with panic disorder.

  Substance Use Disorders (SUD): The prevalence of both current and lifetime SUD is significantly higher among chronic pain patients than in the general population. Patients with chronic pain and current substance abuse are more likely to be prescribed chronic opioids despite the fact that active SUD is considered a contraindication for long-term opioid therapy by treatment guidelines.

- Common psychological difficulties:

  Fear/avoidance: Patients with chronic pain often avoid physical activities and delay return to work due to erroneous beliefs that physical activities that might make pain worse should be avoided and that pain equals harm.

  Pain catastrophizing: A thought process in which pain is viewed as awful, horrible, and unbearable and the mind goes to the worst-case scenarios. Catastrophizing was found to predict pain, disability, and distress independent of physical findings, age, gender, or duration of pain.

  Secondary gains: Patients can be inadvertently reinforced by family, loved ones, the medical system (and providers), and/or financial systems (i.e., Social Security Disability Insurance, Workers' Compensation, etc.) to stay in a help-seeking, rather than self-management role with chronic pain

  Passive coping: Patients can often come from a frame of externalizing solutions, meaning they expect others (i.e., often providers) to "fix" or "cure" their pain. Sometimes this stems from having their pain medicalized for many years or can be a part of a psychological denial phase for patients as they work toward acceptance of their chronic condition.

Team goal: Differential diagnosis and identifying a provisional diagnosis

Share significant information between team members to ensure treatment planning is patient-centered, appropriate, safe, and effective. Discover the mental health comorbidities that should be addressed as part of a comprehensive and effective treatment plan.

Working as a team

Patient: Works with PCP and BHP and follows through on recommended diagnostic testing; reports patterns of medication use and potential side effects, tracks and reports physical and social activities as recommended by the BHP. Describes appropriate mental health history and their pain "story," to include current views on illness, acceptance of chronic pain, use of current coping strategies, and views on the role of opioid pain medications.

(Continued)

PCP: Evaluates possible treatments and/or medical interventions to alleviate chronic pain; monitors pain medication use, including urine lab tests for substance use and medication adherence as appropriate; obtains additional diagnostic testing and medical consultation as appropriate. Considers comorbidities and refers to BHP for additional assessment as needed. Prescribes medications for common comorbid mental health disorders such as depression as clinically indicated.

BHP: Helps track physical and emotional symptoms, physical and social activities and functioning; connects the patient to PCP for evaluation and adjustment of treatment as needed; supports client in care planning and following through on medical recommendations such as consistently engaging the PCP, getting lab work, and seeing specialists. Conducts a thorough psychosocial assessment. Works with the PCP and PC to work through differential diagnoses to refine mental health treatment targets and plan. Helps the patient learn about how to apply a biopsychosocial model of chronic pain to understand his/her illness and treatments.

PC: Expands medical and psychiatric differential and recommends additional assessment as needed. Considers additional comorbidities for which to screen. Assists BHP in differential diagnosis as needed. Helps provide objectivity to assist BHP in working through potentially complicated countertransference/provider alliance issues that may be confounded by mental health disorders or substance use problems.

Case example

The PCP tells the BHP that Ms. T is persistently asking for more methadone and would like to understand better the context of the request before making a medication change in her treatment plan. Ms. T then tells the BHP that she is not eating regularly, with no appetite and states she wants to "make sure the methadone works the best" so she restricts her eating for hours after taking the medication. The BHP also asks if Ms. T feels she has enough methadone for her pain, and Ms. T states she worries that her brother-in-law is stealing her medication. The BHP tells the PCP about Ms. T's depression, poor eating habits, and drivers for requests for more medication (possible theft and misunderstandings on how to take the medication properly). The PC recommends the BHP assess if appetite loss coincided with depressions onset and Ms. T reports her appetite declined significantly and she had lost 15 lbs in the last six months, which coincided with her latest onset of major depression.

During Ms. T's assessment by the BHP, she reveals a history of persistent dysphoria and anhedonia, and also a history of childhood abuse by her alcoholic father and physical abuse by a prior boyfriend. She has frequent panic attacks, recurrent nightmares, symptoms of avoidance, and emotional numbing. She denies current or past substance abuse but admits to wanting to use more of her prescription opioids than prescribed. She reports a history of treatment for major depression and post-traumatic stress disorder.

Treatment

Initiate treatment

General approaches

Patient Education

- Provide an explanatory model for chronic pain as a pathological process involving a mechanism known as "central sensitization," which is a reduction of the central nervous system's inhibitory function, resulting in amplification of painful signals.

   Examples of patient education about central sensitization include:
   - "Even though your back has healed from the surgery, the parts of your brain that respond to sensory inputs from your back have, over time, become a lot more sensitive, and make you feel pain even when nothing is hurting your back."
   - "For reasons we still don't understand very well, the parts of the brain that respond to pain signals can sometimes 'misfire,' causing people to feel chronic pain even when the injuries are already healed."

- Introduce the biopsychosocial model of chronic pain. Chronic pain usually begins as a biological process and psychological and social factors often play key roles in the development and experience of chronic pain. Therefore, treatment for chronic pain is best done in a multidisciplinary model of care.

   Examples of patient education about the biopsychosocial model of chronic pain include:
   - "Chronic pain is experienced in the brain as your nervous system processes the pain signals. Your brain is also constantly filtering signals it's taking in, including ignoring sounds, sights, even sensations on a regular basis because it's impossible to track everything all the time. We can take advantage of these strengths in the brain by working to train your brain to focus differently, which can help to reduce the pain from interfering in your life. We often work with behavioral specialists, who can figure out the best way to work with you to do this piece."

- "Chronic pain is a very complex experience because it mainly occurs in the brain and therefore we use lots of different methods to treat it. Some might be medications that affect the brain's experience of pain, some might be physical interventions like physical therapy to train the body, and some might be behavioral treatments that help you find ways to manage pain better, and some might be working on reducing stressors in your life that can make pain worse. We've learned that using all these approaches together is what helps people have the best quality of life they can when they have to live with pain."

Setting treatment goals
- Focus on functional improvement, not reduction in pain intensity. Typically effective chronic pain treatment does not necessarily reduce overall physical pain, but does significantly decrease pain interference in the patient's life.
  - Example: "Tell me how you would like your life to be different, without using the word 'pain.'" "What would you be doing if you were not limited by the pain?" "How could you achieve some of these goals even with the pain?"
- Behaviorally defined and measurable: Goals should be concrete and specific and above all, driven by the patient's perspective. Make sure the goals relate to what is of high priority for the patient. Often providers make the mistake of setting goals the patient does not value or feels are impossible to reach.
  - Example: "Be able to walk two miles at a moderate pace, three days a week, starting at walking half a mile a day, three days a week."
- Make sure the patient participates in the development and "owns" or at least co-owns the treatment plan. The BHP can help make sure the treatment team is patient centered and advocate for crafting goals in ways that will be most engaging to the patient. If initial plans do not succeed, the BHP can help explore alternatives that are more likely to help the patient achieve his/her goals. Examples of how the team can work together to provide treatment are listed in Table 7.3.

Early brief behavioral interventions
Biopsychosocial chronic pain model: Promote a multidisciplinary approach to chronic pain treatment. Providers can explain the biopsychosocial model of pain to patients to help them understand pain is not only biological, but made worse and potentially better through psychological and social factors.

Table 7.3 Team-based treatment for chronic pain

	PCP approaches	BHP approaches
Biological	***Evidence-Based Medication Treatment:*** • Long-term opioid therapy (>90 days) is rarely beneficial for chronic noncancer pain, and should be considered treatment of last resort. • Medication treatment approaches that emphasize improving function and quality of life, instead of focusing solely on pain reduction. • Nonopioid analgesics, including acetaminophen and nonsteroidal anti-inflammatory drugs (NSAIDs), are effective in relieving mild to moderate pain. • Antidepressants have analgesic properties independent of antidepressant effect by acting on a number of neurotransmitters, receptors and cytokines. ***Evidence-Based Nonpharmacological Treatments:*** • Physical rehabilitation, through physical therapy and exercise programs involving walking, aquatic exercises, and gentle stretching, is the core treatment for most forms of chronic pain. • Spinal manipulation, massage therapy and acupuncture can be considered.	***Evidence-Based Medication Treatment:*** • Troubleshoot adherence challenges: Patients often do not take medications as prescribed. • It can be helpful to explore the timing and use of medications and other treatments using a treatment diary. • ***Opioid tapering tips:*** helping support opioid tapering plans that allow patients to control pacing of the taper, while maintaining a consistent timeline to carry the taper forward. • Help patients adjust expectations if needed— medications typically do not stop chronic pain, but may provide some relief especially during pain flares.

(Continued)

Table 7.3 (*Continued*)

	PCP approaches	BHP approaches
Psychosocial	*Evidence-Based Behavioral Treatment:* • Providers can explain the biopsychosocial model of pain to patients to help patients understand pain is not only biological, but made worse and potentially better through psychological and social factors. • Cognitive Behavioral Therapy (CBT) has the strongest evidence base for helping patients improve quality of life with chronic pain. Providers can make referrals to CBT therapists or encourage patients to work with BHPs using a CBT approach.	*Evidence-Based Behavioral Treatment:* Common areas to address with CBT include: • Helping patients with a mourning process around losses they have experienced due to chronic pain can often help with moving patients toward acceptance and effective self-management habits for their chronic pain. • Mood issues related to depression and anxiety using CBT should be addressed simultaneously. • BHPs working on the primary care team have opportunities to address some common pitfalls many patients with chronic pain face. • Addressing poor engagement • Set patient-centered goals • Opioid tapering support/adherence • Measurement based care

Therapeutic alliance: Listen to the patient's pain story, create a strong therapeutic alliance. Many patients have experienced negative judgments from providers (i.e., being treated as an addict, providers feeling burned out or judgmental of patients who don't seem to take initiative to manage their pain, providers frustrated with feeling accused of not helping or caring) and are sometime struggling to trust or open up to their providers. Patients can lash out in anger at providers, feeling defensive about perceived judgments (that may or may not have basis) and/or because of skills that may be lacking from the patient to communicate effectively. PCPs can use the BHPs as a resource to work through poor alliance issues and move to a patient centered care plan.

Safety planning
- For patients presenting with chronic pain, treatment of comorbid psychiatric disorders contributing to suicidality can reduce the patient's risk of suicide.

PCP approaches
General principles
- Chronic pain can respond well to treatment approaches that emphasize improving function and quality of life, instead of focusing solely on pain reduction.
- Avoid treatments that cause oversedation or reduce energy and motivation.
- Help patients overcome fear of pain, avoidance of activity, and deconditioning.

Prescribing principles
- Long-term opioid therapy (>90 days) is rarely beneficial for chronic non-cancer pain, and should be considered treatment of last resort.
- Nonopioid analgesics, including acetaminophen and nonsteroidal anti-inflammatory drugs (NSAIDs), are effective in relieving mild to moderate pain. NSAIDs are particularly helpful in relieving pain from osteoarthritis and inflammatory arthritis. Adequate trials of such nonopioid drugs should be considered as first for medication management.
- Antidepressants have analgesic properties independent of antidepressant effect by acting on a number of neurotransmitters, receptors, and cytokines.
- Antidepressants with both serotonin and norepinephrine reuptake inhibition, such as serotonin-norepinephrine reuptake inhibitors (SNRIs) and tricyclic antidepressants (TCAs) are first-line options for neuropathic pain.
- Certain antiepileptic drugs, including gabapentin and pregabalin, reduce neuronal hyperexcitability and are considered first-line drugs for neuropathic pain and fibromyalgia.
- Muscle relaxants only have evidence of efficacy in *acute* back pain and *acute* exacerbations of chronic muscle pain. Avoid using benzodiazepines and carisoprodol (Soma), which metabolizes into meprobamate, a barbiturate-like tranquilizer, due to their addiction potential and respiratory depression effect.

Choice of medication (see Tables 7.4 and 7.5)

- Patients should have adequate trials of nonopioid analgesics (e.g., acetaminophen or NSAIDs) as clinically appropriate.

Table 7.4 Medications commonly used in the treatment of chronic pain

Nonopioid analgesics		
Acetaminophen	**Start:** 325–500 mg tid-qid. **Max:** 4 g/d.	Lower dose or avoidance for patients with liver disease.
Celecoxib (Celebrex)	**Start:** 100 mg bid or 200 mg qday. **Range:** 200–400 mg/d	COX-2 selective NSAID.$
Diclofenac (Voltaren)	**Start:** 50 mg bid-tid. Range: 150–200 mg/d.	Acute and chronic pain of osteoarthritis, rheumatoid arthritis, ankylosing spondylitis.
Ibuprofen (Advil, Motrin)	**Start:** 200–400 mg q4–6 hr. **Max:** 3200 mg/d.	Mild to moderate musculoskeletal pain, dysmenorrhea.
Meloxicam (Mobic)	**Start:** 7.5 mg/d. Max: 15 mg/d	Pain associated with osteoarthritis, rheumatoid arthritis.
Nabumetone (Relafen)	**Start:** 1000–2000 mg/d divided qd-bid. **Max:** 2000 mg/d.	Pain associated with osteoarthritis, rheumatoid arthritis.
Naproxen (Naprosyn)	**Start:** 250–500 mg q12h. **Max:** 1500 mg/d x 6 mo. **Strength Clarification:** 200, 250, 500 mg naproxen = 220, 275, 550 mg naproxen sodium	Acute and chronic pain of osteoarthritis, rheumatoid disorders, dysmenorrhea.
Naproxen Sodium (Aleve)	**Start:** 220–550 mg q12h. **Max:** 1650 mg/d x 6 mo. **Strength Clarification:** 220, 275, 550 mg naproxen sodium = 200, 250, 500 mg naproxen	Acute and chronic pain of osteoarthritis, rheumatoid disorders, dysmenorrhea. More rapid onset than naproxen.
Antiepileptic Drugs (AEDs)		
Gabapentin (Neurontin)	**Start:** 300mg QHS then ↑ by 300mg/d every 3–7d. **Range:** 300–1200mg TID.	Weight gain, edema, cognitive slowing, and dizziness are common side effects. ¢
Pregabalin (Lyrica)	**Start:** 50mg TID; may ↑ to 100mg TID in 1 week. **Range:** 50–100mg TID.	Similar side effect profile as gabapentin, but much more expensive. $

Table 7.5 Antidepressants commonly used in the treatment of chronic pain

Selective Serotonin Reuptake Inhibitors (SSRIs)	Citalopram (Celexa)
	Escitalopram (Lexapro)
	Fluoxetine (Prozac)
	Sertraline (Zoloft)
Serotonin-Norepinephrine Reuptake Inhibitors (SNRIs)	Duloxetine (Cymbalta)
	Venlafaxine (Effexor)
Mixed Receptor Antidepressants	Bupropion (Wellbutrin)
	Mirtazapine (Remeron)
Tricyclic Antidepressants (TCAs)	Desipramine (Norpramin)
	Nortriptyline (Pamelor)

For prescribing details and protocols, please see Chapter 11, "Evidence Based Psychopharmacology for the Collaborative Care Team."

- For patients with comorbid pain and unipolar depression, start with an SNRI or a TCA.
- If there is a high level of comorbid anxiety, start with a serotonin reuptake inhibitor (SSRI) such as citalopram or sertraline, which may be better tolerated than SNRIs or TCAs.
- Start gabapentin or pregabalin for neuropathic pain. These medications may also be beneficial for certain anxiety disorders. Other medications that can help with neuropathic pain include noradrenergic antidepressants such as venlafaxine, duloxetine, or tricyclic antidepressants such as nortriptyline.
- Do not start an antidepressant without input from a psychiatric consultant if the patient has been diagnosed with bipolar disorder.
- For patients with comorbid PTSD, in addition to the use of an antidepressant for anxiety, consider use of low dose prazosin for nightmares and symptoms of hyperarousal.

Nonpharmacological approaches
- Physical rehabilitation is the core treatment for most forms of chronic pain. Consider physical therapy referral to a therapist familiar with chronic pain issues if the patient is physically inactive, deconditioned and not currently engaging in an exercise program.
- Encourage the patient to establish an exercise routine that can include moderately paced walking, aquatic exercises, yoga, and tai chi.
- Spinal manipulation, massage therapy, and acupuncture can be considered if the relevant resources are available.
- Cognitive behavioral therapy (CBT) has the strongest evidence base for helping patients improve quality of life with chronic pain. Encourage the

patient to work with the BHP using a CBT approach, or refer the patient to a CBT therapist if such specialty resource is available.

BHP approaches

Common areas to address with CBT include:

- Helping patients with a mourning process around losses they have experienced due to chronic pain can often help with moving patients toward acceptance of their chronic pain. Addressing poor acceptance is often necessary before gains can be made to help patients establish effective self-management habits for their chronic pain.
- Mood issues related to depression and anxiety using CBT should be addressed simultaneously, given often mood issues stifle patients' success with pain self-management strategies.
- Patients may have anxiety about causing more pain by becoming more active. Checking in with the medical provider to reassure patients they are medically cleared for increases in activity can help patients engage in physical activity. Addressing anxiety management and exposure issues can be helpful.

BHPs working on the primary care team have opportunities to address some common pitfalls many patients with chronic pain face.

Addressing poor engagement: Patients with chronic pain often have difficulty establishing trust with providers, often based on a history of negative medical experiences. Patients with comorbid anxiety issues, histories of trauma and/or childhood abuse, which are common in patients with chronic pain, also can have difficulty with provider alliances. BHPs can assess for poor alliance issues with the PCP and potentially other medical specialist providers and help the team be more effective in care by providing: a safe place for patients to process frustrations, skills, and guidance for patients to effectively communicate with their PCP, and advocacy for the patient with providers to help improve engagement and the patient's perspective in the overall care plan.

Setting patient-centered goals: BHPs have more time to hear and elicit the patient's pain story and desired treatment goals. This can help clarify key points that drive motivations for patients to get more active and engaged in chronic pain self-management. The BHP can help convey patient centered goals for treatment.

Opioid tapering adherence: Patients often struggle with tapering opioid medications. BHPs can help assess adherence issues and address ambivalence with tapering, while teaching pain coping strategies. Having a clear and consistent plan that the patient feels invested in, as well as a clear line of communication with the clinical team members can help patients stay compliant and address concerns as they arise. Tapering opioid medications is often quite a complicated process that often needs to incorporate addressing psychosocial factors to avoid adherence issues. As nonprescribers, BHPs can often educate patients about risks of chronic opioid therapy, including: habituation (i.e., need for higher doses over time), hyperalgesia (i.e., opioids can increase sensitivity to pain over time), and the dangers of high doses (i.e., risks of stopping breathing) in ways that can be less threatening and more acceptable to patients. The BHP can often play a crucial role in helping the team be successful at tapering.

Measurement based care: Measuring improvements is key to making sure treatment is working. Measuring chronic pain interference in life is doable by asking a single item like "How much has your pain interfered in your life over the past week (0–10)?" or by using scales like Cleeland's Brief Pain Inventory or its brief 3-item version in the PEG.

BHPs can provide key psychoeducation for chronic pain to help patients understand, accept, and manage their chronic condition. Several key points of psychoeducation include:

Gate control theory: Chronic pain often requires a multidisciplinary approach that includes addressing multiple factors to help achieve the best quality of life. Helping patients understand that their actions can both decrease (i.e., getting proper sleep, exercise, and food, good mood, massage, relaxation, distraction, etc.) or increase (i.e., overdoing activities, becoming more inactive overall, muscle tension, depression, anger, focus on the pain) pain can help patients understand how self-management of chronic pain can reduce pain interference. These ideas are part of Gate Control Theory, which explains how patients can control the "opening" or "closing" of the neurological gate on pain via the Gate Control Mechanism, a bundle of nerve cells that extend along the spinal cord.

Depression and pain: Chronic pain increases the risk of depression and often treating depression can help with chronic pain management. Patients who have not experienced depression until they began experiencing chronic pain often find it helpful to hear about the physical overlap in brain circuitry between chronic pain and depression, as well as becoming more open to trying serotonin based medications for both depression and pain.

Suffering vs. pain: Separating the physical sensation of pain from the idea of suffering can help patients set achievable goals for treatment. While reducing physical pain might not always be possible, reducing suffering often is. Suffering is based on interpretations of physical pain and shifting these negative interpretations can lead directly to reducing suffering.

Pain medications: Many patients can have high expectations for pain relief from medications. However, pain medications in general are expected to help only 0–30 percent with pain control.

Team goal: Initial treatment planning
Create an initial treatment plan that is in line with the patient's goals for treatment and appropriate to the biopsychosocial assessment of the patient's unique chronic pain syndrome. The patient should have an initial understanding of the role of each provider in the plan, a sense that all of the providers are working together and with him/her to help achieve the patient's goals, and a clear sense of how the plan addresses his/her pain and goals.

Working as a team
Patient: Actively participates in exploring treatment options and formulating an initial treatment plan. Voices concerns about the plan's safety and effectiveness. Follows through on initial treatment recommendations, speaks up about issues and concerns as treatment progresses.

   PCP: Establishes and maintains therapeutic alliance; educates the patient about components of the treatment plan, in particular the use of medications and other medical treatments; emphasizes the importance of also addressing psychosocial contributors to pain and working closely with the BHP; sets and reviews medical treatment goals and monitors progress; prescribes and monitors medications; makes medical referrals as needed.

   BHP: Establishes and maintains therapeutic alliance; addresses crisis management and safety planning strategies; reviews the full treatment plan with the patient and addresses questions and concerns; provides brief behavioral interventions addressing comorbid mental health issues and promoting chronic pain self-management; facilitates communication between team members; makes and supports referrals (e.g., disability, vocational rehab, social services, chemical dependency, additional psychotherapy).

   PC: Resource for diagnosing and treating psychiatric comorbidities; supports treatment planning; supports safety planning; medication and behavioral management recommendations.

Case example
A medication and behavioral plan were determined to initially address Ms. T's presenting problems and initial diagnoses. The BHP, PC, and PCP communicated about the joint assessment and the BHP coordinated an initial care plan that was communicated to the Ms. T at her next appointments with the PCP and with the BHP. Ms. T was mainly concerned about her having her stomach pain addressed. A trial of methadone dose reduction to 5mg/day was initiated due to the lack of evidence for benefit. She signed an opioid agreement

stipulating no rescue opioids outside of the methadone and hydromorphone she was receiving from the clinic. She was provided as needed ondansetron for nausea. The BHP discussed Ms. T's case with the PC, who recommended starting citalopram and to later consider adding low dose nortriptyline and prazosin to address persistent depressive and anxiety symptoms, as well as nightmares related to PTSD. The BHP conveyed these medication recommendations to the PCP and initiated biweekly visits to track on the patient's progress, treatment adherence, and complications, and to provide brief cognitive behavioral therapy, specifically with plans to address improving her nutrition intake and behavioral activation for depressive symptoms and to further assess and address anxiety related issues as she initiated her opioid taper, as well as to work on readiness for self-management of chronic pain. Treatment with the BHP was initially focused on maintaining and growing a therapeutic alliance to increase engagement and adherence with the treatment plan and later moved more to behavioral treatments as engagement solidified.

Follow-up and treatment adjustment to achieve treatment to target

General approaches

As patients become more engaged in treatment and move toward acceptance of chronic pain, self-management strategies can begin to move and comorbid psychiatric disorders can continue to be treated. Adjust medications and behavioral treatments as appropriate to step up care.

Track patient goals and use care plan: Work with the BHP to stick to a consistent care plan for the patient, making sure to help set patient centered goals for treatment. It is important to track functional outcomes with treatment (using a measure such as Figure 7.1: Pain Assessment Questionnaire). It is important to stay consistent with the plan as well, to not inadvertently add chaos and intermittent reinforcement to behaviors from the patient that are problematic (i.e., increasing opioid doses in response to a spontaneous presentation of crisis when the plan was to hold the dose steady or taper). This can undermine the care plan and treatment effectiveness.

Tapering opioids: It can be helpful to allow the patient some control in tapering opioid medications by allowing the patient to set the tapering schedule to some degree (i.e., reduce their dose whenever they want in the next two weeks, knowing the overall prescription will be reduced at the next visit) and to allow for a small surplus of medications particularly for highly anxious patients (i.e., allowing for a few extra tablets in between prescriptions in case a pain flare were to occur, with a strict plan to count tablets at the next visit to monitor the surplus), when medically appropriate. This can help patients manage their anxiety and adhere with an opioid taper by feeling more in control of the process, but also balance setting boundaries as the provider to ensure the prescribed dose continues to decrease. Collaborate with the BHP to keep tabs on the patient's willingness and ambivalence to taper and communicate the tapering plan to the BHP so s/he can assist with supporting adherence.

When to refer
- Condition not responding to treatment
- Conditions that may benefit from interventional procedures or surgery
- Conditions requiring longer-term, more intensive, or specialist psychotherapy
- Higher level of need including long-term case management
- Employment Services: Especially if people have developed avoidance patterns
- Occupational Therapy: To help translate treatment gains into the capacity to accomplish goals at home or at work
- Disability: More severe cases, especially if anticipate inability to work for greater than a year

PCP approaches
Ongoing medication management
- Initial response to antidepressants usually occurs within four to eight weeks
- Partial responders after four weeks should be titrated to higher doses, if tolerated
- If *no response* after four to six weeks at therapeutic dose, consider switching or augmenting treatment in consultation with psychiatric consultant

Working with opioids
- When to consider:
  - The principal reason for prescribing opioids is to provide sufficient pain relief such that the patient is able to participate in physical rehabilitation (such as exercise therapy) in order to improve functional status.
  - Opioids have been increasingly used to treat chronic noncancer pain in the last two decades, but the practice is controversial due to a parallel increase in opioid death. Long-term opioid effectiveness for chronic pain has *not* been demonstrated.
- Specific concerns regarding long-term opioid therapy:

  Hyperalgesia: Long-term opioid use may lead to increased sensitivity to pain through opioid hyperalgesia.

Iatrogenic addiction: The risk of inducing addiction in patients without previous history substance abuse is low. However, there is a risk of worsening or reactivating addiction in patients with a current or previous substance use disorder.

Hormonal and immune effects: Chronic opioid treatment has been associated with suppression of testosterone, estrogen, cortisol, LH and FSH levels. It may also suppress immune function.

Respiratory depression and accidental overdose: Deaths from accidental opioid overdose have exceeded motor vehicle deaths in 30 states in the United States. Respiratory suppression is a particular concern when patient is receiving high dose opioids or using alcohol or sedative and hypnotic medication concurrently.

- How to initiate treatment:
  - Informed consent and opioid agreement: Opioid therapy should be a conscientious decision made jointly by the prescriber and the patient based on informed consent about the potential risks and benefits of opioid use.
  - A formal opioid risk assessment can be made using a screening questionnaire.
  - Start with a short-acting opioid at the lowest PRN dose necessary to achieve sufficient pain relief. Avoid further dose escalation once a therapeutic dose is established.
- How to monitor treatment response:
  - Continued opioid prescription needs to be contingent on the patient showing functional improvement with opioid use
  - Check with your state's opioid prescription tracking system if you have one to check what other providers might be prescribing opioids to the patient.
  - Periodic urine toxicology screens in patients receiving opioid therapy can help detect aberrant opioid behaviors such as the use of street drugs (e.g., cocaine) or nonprescribed opioids, and diversion (when no opioid is detected in urine).
- When to discontinue treatment:
  - Aberrant opioid use behavior: early refills; aberrant urine toxicology findings; receipt of opioids from more than one provider; repeated ED visits seeking opioids
  - Lack of demonstrated functional improvement
  - Epidemiological data have shown that once 90 days of continuous therapy is received, opioid use often persists for years. Therefore, a decision regarding whether to continue opioid therapy is ideally made before reaching the three-month mark.

BHP approaches

Working with medications

- Be able to recognize the names of opioid and nonopioid medications commonly used in treating chronic pain and be familiar with the medical team's expected use and expected outcome of the medication for the patient. Often patients' expectations, understanding, and experiences with the medications are not in line what is understood by the prescribing providers. It is often useful to ask the provider directly about prescriptions and track doses prescribed and used by the patient.
  - Troubleshoot adherence challenges
    - Patients often do not take medications as prescribed. They may take too little or too much. They may take the medications at the wrong times (e.g., after pain has become so severe that the patient is not able to be physically active as planned). It can be helpful to explore the timing and use of medications and other treatments using a "treatment diary."
    - **Opioid tapering tips:** helping support opioid tapering plans that allow patients to control pacing of the taper, while maintaining a consistent timeline to carry the taper forward (i.e., give the patient the choice of when to drop the dose within a set window of time); support patients with significant anxiety issues in negotiating a small surplus of extra medication be allowed who are at low risk for aberrant use; monitor specific behavioral function during the taper to keep close track of tapering tolerance and mediate misattributions of withdrawal and other stressors.
  - Offer psychoeducation for benefits of medication use, particularly for psychotropic medications
  - Be responsive to concerns and side effects
  - Support the patient through making medication changes
  - Help patient schedule an appointment with PCP to address medications
  - Help patient write down questions

Team goal

Be prepared to adjust the treatment plan until treatment targets are achieved.

As patients become more engaged in treatment and move toward acceptance of chronic pain, self-management strategies can begin to move and comorbid psychiatric disorders can continue to be treated. Adjust medications and behavioral treatments as appropriate to step up care.

Working as a team

Patient: Is an active partner in trying treatment strategies and communicates concerns with treatment, potential side effects, and misalignment of treatment goals if they arise; fills out measures to monitor treatment progress; reports functional changes in activities related to pain interference; gives feedback on attempts with self-management strategies for pain; discuss any difficulties with provider interactions; discusses progress on behavioral and medical treatment recommendations to the PCP and BHP and discusses any difficulties with the treatment plan to help trigger further treatment adjustments.

   PCP: Addresses therapeutic alliance issues as needed, consults with the BHP as needed; follows through on medical treatment goals and outcomes of medical referrals as needed; continues to monitor progress; adjusts prescriptions as needed.

   BHP: Continues to address engagement, crisis management, and safety planning as needed; steps up brief behavioral interventions as needed to address comorbid mental health issues and promoting chronic pain self-management; continues to facilitate communication between team members; gives the patient hope even if initial treatments are not successful; works closely with the patient to explore why treatments may not be effective; supports referral follow through and case management as needed (disability, vocational rehab, social services, chemical dependency, additional psychotherapy); monitors, measures, and advocates for stepping up care as measures and function monitoring indicate poor improvement.

   PC: Supports treatment planning; supports safety planning; advocates for stepping up care and altering medication recommendations as needed; supports and suggests behavioral management recommendations.

Case example

Ms. T complied with the opioid taper and reported the initial reduction led to severe exacerbation of pain and more difficulty with daily functioning. She also had more emergency department (ED) visits where she received antiemetics and hydromorphone. She was asked to sign an opioid agreement to limit outside prescriptions of medication, her taper was halted, and her 10mg dose of methadone was resumed. After she signed the opioid agreement, her ED visits ceased. Concurrently, she did well with prazosin, increasing her dose gradually to 6mg nightly and her nightmares ceased and sleep improved significantly. She also tolerated the citalopram and nortriptyline well, titrating to effective

(Continued)

therapeutic doses. In her sessions with the BHP, she worked on addressing financial applications, and discussed struggles with adjusting to not working and losses she had experienced from developing chronic pain to help her move toward readiness for self-management of chronic pain. Ms. T conveyed appreciation to the team for being responsive and caring and reported on her measures that her anxiety had not decreased. The BHP began discussing addressing anxiety issues and reassessing anxiety as primary target for treatment, which Ms. T was not willing to address as she continued to work on pain issues. The treatment team with Ms. T's consent reprioritized her anxiety issues as a primary target and the team agreed to work on addressing anxiety management and further pain coping strategies before returning to an opioid taper. The BHP helped her set functional goals related to her anxiety and avoidance of physical and social activities, including a walking and water exercise program with appropriate pacing, and a plan for increasing her social interactions outside of her immediate family.

Completing treatment and relapse prevention

- In most cases, chronic pain does not resolve or significantly improve over time; expectations for medication management of pain typically improves pain control 0–30 percent; therefore, the treatment targets for chronic pain treatment are significantly improving function and quality of life and shifting patients to a maintainable routine of effective self-management of chronic pain
- Comorbid depression and anxiety issues will often improve, noted by clinically significant drops in standard measures of depression and anxiety

Team goal
Reinforce a clear ongoing care plan for the patient to maintain an optimal level of functioning and reduce the risk of setbacks such as exacerbations in pain or psychiatric symptoms; clarify and reinforce self-management strategies, medication use; review early warning signs of worsening medical or psychiatric problems and develop strategies for what to do if symptoms worsen and when to return for further treatment.

Working as a team
Patient: Participates in establishing a relapse prevention plan with the BHP and the PCP; tracks the ongoing plan and reengages in additional care if pain or functional impairment significantly worsen

PCP: Provides plan for ongoing medication management appropriate for pain management and comorbid psychiatric disorders and clear instructions to the patient to request reevaluation

BHP: Reviews successes and gains in treatment, as well as the ongoing behavioral changes and treatment plan; clarifies team roles and who to reengage should function decline or mood and anxiety worsen

PC: Clarifies to the team recommendations for long-term use of medications and supports the BHP in creating a treatment summary and relapse prevention plan as needed

---

Case example

Ms. T at the end of treatment reported the following gains: measures of depression (PHQ-9) and post-traumatic stress (PCL-C) were in the mild range and her pain interference rating had dropped; her pain levels remained stable and her methadone dose remained stable at 10mg; her ED visits had stopped; she was eating regularly and overall well-being was stated as much improved; her sleep remained improved with an absence of nightmares, and she avoided staying in bed and stopped taking naps during the day; she was actively using relaxation techniques for anxiety; she took a 30-minute, moderately paced walk almost every day, and went to a local pool for aquatic exercises two to three times per week; and she was gradually increasing her social activities by using anxiety management and exposure strategies. The PCP planned to continue prescribing her methadone, to continue citalopram, low-dose nortriptyline, and prazosin, and Ms. T was asked to report any exacerbations in her abdominal pain, physical function, depression, or anxiety. Ms. T was pleased with her progress and stated that she was functioning better than she had in years.

Self-help books and web resources

- The Pain Survival Guide, by Dennis Turk & Frits Winter
- Managing Pain Before It Manages You, by Margaret Caudill
- Video "Understanding Pain: What to do about it in less than five minutes?" http://www.youtube.com/watch?v=4b8oB757DKc
- Brief Pain Inventory's 3-item PEG version, designed for quick use in primary care http://openi.nlm.nih.gov/detailedresult.php?img=2686775_11606_2009_981_Fig1_HTML&req=4
- Activity pacing handouts from the Veteran's Administration http://www.mentalhealth.va.gov/coe/cesamh/docs/Activity_Pacing-patients.pdf
- Free brochure on chronic pain and depression offered via NIMH http://www.nimh.nih.gov/health/publications/depression-and-chronic-pain/index.shtml

References

American Pain Society. (2006). *Pain control in the primary care setting*. Glenview, IL.

Arnow, B. A., Blasey, C. M., Lee, J., Fireman, B., Hunkeler, E. M., Dea, R., Robinson, R., & Hayward, C. (2009). Relationships among depression, chronic pain, chronic disabling pain, and medical costs. *Psychiatric Services, 60*(3), 344–50.

Bruns, D. & Disorbio, J. M. (2013). *The psychological assessment of patients with chronic pain* In: Deer, T. R., Leong, M. S., Buvanendran, A, et al. (eds). *Comprehensive treatment of chronic pain by medical, interventional, and integrative approaches: The American Academy Of Pain Medicine textbook on patient management:* 1st edition. New York, NY: Springer, 805–26.

Chou, R. & Huffman, L. H. (2007). Nonpharmacologic treatments for acute and chronic low back pain: A review of the evidence for an American Pain Society/American College of Physicians clinical practice guideline. *Annals of Internal Medicine, 147*, 492–504.

Edlund, M. J., Fan, M. Y., DeVries, A., Braden, J. B., Martin, B. C., Sullivan, M. D. (2010). Trends in use of opioids for chronic non-cancer pain among individuals with mental health and substance use disorders: the TROUP study. *Clinical Journal of Pain, 26*, 1–8.

Gatchel, R. J., Peng, Y. B., Peters, M. L., & Turk, D. C. (2007). The biopsychosocial approach to chronic pain: Scientific advances and future directions. *Psychological Bulletin, 133*, 581–624.

Morlion, B. (2011). Pharmacotherapy of low back pain: targeting nociceptive and neuropathic pain components. *Current Medical Research and Opinion (Opi 27)*, 11–33.

Saarto, T. & Wiffen, P. J. (2007). Antidepressants for neuropathic pain. *Cochrane Database of Systematic Reviews 2007*, (4) Art. No.:CD005454, 2007.

Sullivan, M. D., Edlund, M. J., Fan, M. Y., DeVries, A., Braden, J. B., Martin, B. C. (2008). Trends in use of opioids for non-cancer pain conditions in commercial and Medicaid insurance plans, 2000–2005: The TROUP Study. *Pain. 138*, 440–449.

Turk, D. C., Swanson, K. S., & Tunks, E. R. (2008). Psychological approaches in the treatment of chronic pain patients – when pills, scalpels, and needles are not enough. *Canadian Journal of Psychiatry, 54*(3), 213–223.

Turk, D. C. & Winters, F. (2006). *The pain survival guide: How to reclaim your life*. American Psychological Association. Washington, DC.

Chapter 8 **Attention Deficit Hyperactivity Disorder (ADHD)**

Jennifer Sexton, Ryan Kimmel, William French, David A. Harrison, and Kim Kensington

Clinical impact

Attention-deficit hyperactivity disorder (ADHD) is a neuro-developmental disorder with childhood onset characterized by hyperactivity, impulsivity, and inattention, which often persist into adulthood and can lead to chronic and pervasive impairment in academic, social, and vocational functioning. In patients diagnosed with ADHD as children, studies show continuation into adulthood of the full syndrome in up to 50 percent of patients, resulting in an adult prevalence rate between 4 and 5 percent. The majority of adults diagnosed with ADHD have at least one additional psychiatric disorder, and adults with ADHD often complain of severe psychosocial difficulties that result in a lower sense of self-efficacy and self-esteem.

Special considerations for children and adolescents

ADHD is the most common neuro-developmental disorder in children and adolescents with an estimated prevalence of 8 percent. The majority of children with ADHD have one or more comorbid disorders (e.g., oppositional defiant disorder, learning disorder) and academic and social impairment. ADHD is highly treatable and treatment may minimize later impairment and development of psychiatric comorbidity.

Integrated Care: Creating Effective Mental and Primary Health Care Teams, First Edition.
Anna Ratzliff, Jürgen Unützer, Wayne Katon, and Kari A. Stephens.
© 2016 John Wiley & Sons, Inc. Published 2016 by John Wiley & Sons, Inc.

Assessment

Identify chief complaint, associated somatic and psychological symptoms, functional impairment, and safety concerns

Diagnosis is primarily based on a detailed patient history, assessment of current behavior and symptoms, level of functioning and impairment, collateral history, and childhood history.

Special considerations for children and adolescents
- Correctly diagnosing ADHD in preschool children (4–5 years old) can be challenging due to lack of nonparent informants, ongoing family dysfunction, or difficulty distinguishing the behaviors from developmentally normal overactivity and inherent instability of preschool behavior.
- Adolescents (13–18 years old) may present with inattention without hyperactivity/impulsivity and may not have a single "best" teacher to serve as an informant; the lack of an ADHD diagnosis being made at an earlier age raises concern for alternative diagnoses (e.g., substance abuse or anxiety) and should lead to an inquiry about earlier childhood symptoms that were possibly missed.

Common psychological symptoms
- Easily distracted
- Difficulty sustaining attention
- Impulsive decision-making
- Trouble organizing tasks or activities with poor multitasking
- Procrastination
- Difficulty stopping activities
- Starting projects without reading or listening to directions
- Failing to follow through on commitments to others
- Feeling paralyzed or unable to get in gear
- Difficulty doing things in their proper order
- Spending disproportionate amounts of time trying to "catch up" at the expense of other activities
- Quickness to anger and rapidly changing emotions
- Poor stress tolerance
- Inability to slow down during leisure time
- Internalized shame for the extra effort needed to keep up with peers
- Compensation strategies (seen in higher functioning patients):
  - excessive caffeine or other substance use
  - all-night cram sessions
  - staying late at work or going in on weekends
  - compulsive stacks of notes

- rigid organizational systems or multiple systems
- multiple alarms
- hiring help or excessive delegation

Common physical/Somatic symptoms
- Hyperactivity
- Restlessness
- Fidgeting
- Fatigue (common with the inattentive subtype)

Common functional impairments
Relationships: much higher rate of separation and divorce

Education/Work: lower socioeconomic status, higher occurrence of prior academic problems, more job changes, chronic dissatisfaction with jobs

Health behavior: increased risk of sleep deprivation, poor nutrition, overeating, smoking, lack of exercise, and automobile accidents

Medical environment behavior: often late to or missing medical appointments, falling behind on prescription renewals or frantic calls for refills and lost prescriptions, unpaid medical bills, forgetting needed items for appointments

---

Special considerations for children and adolescents

Common functional impairments include poor self-esteem and difficulty in family functioning and social relationships; academic underachievement; school suspension, expulsion, and dropout, and high risk behaviors such as substance abuse, reckless driving, and unprotected sex.

Team goal

Identifying the chief complaint, initial physical exam, gathering history, and safety assessment:

Use the initial visit with the PCP and BHP to understand the functional impairment related to hyperactivity, impulsivity, and inattention. The whole team will also need to gather information to inform the differential diagnosis. A good assessment of functional impairment will also shape the goals for treatment.

Working as a team

Patient: Describes symptoms and functional impairment; brings in documentation of outside ADHD assessment and/or treatment, presents childhood history; asks friends/family to give collateral history

(Continued)

PCP: Primary role in identifying possible ADHD and assessing current physical and psychological symptoms

BHP: Completes detailed assessment, gathers childhood history as well as collateral history to confirm adult symptoms; often develops a more complete understanding of the functional impairment and treatment goals

PC: Helps interpret results from measures; considers whether the patient meets DSM criteria; helps make sense of symptom set and functional impairment

Case example

A 26-year-old Caucasian male presents to his PCP with a chief complaint of poor focus that has made it difficult for him to keep jobs, and he is now unemployed. He states that he had a difficult time in school and dropped out of high school after 10th grade. He also endorses feeling restless with difficulty sitting through a movie or reading more than one to two pages from his book at a time. His girlfriend accompanied him to his appointment and states that he does not listen well, loses things often, and leaves projects around the house unfinished. The patient was able to give some details around his difficulty focusing in school as a child, though he was never formally diagnosed. His girlfriend was able to confirm the patient's difficulty with attention, organization, and task completion during previous employment as well as in the home.

Differential diagnosis and identifying a provisional diagnosis

Rule out common medical diagnoses and substance/drug-related conditions

Medical conditions to consider when evaluating ADHD

Endocrine: thyroid disease, low testosterone levels

Gastrointestinal: hepatic disease

Neurological: petit mal or complex partial seizure disorders, lead toxicity, traumatic brain injury, encephalopathy, hearing deficits

Respiratory: obstructive sleep apnea

Other: medication interactions, anemia, chronic fatigue

Substance-related conditions to consider when evaluating ADHD (impacting attentiveness)

Recreational: nicotine, caffeine, marijuana, and alcohol

Prescribed: anticholinergics, antihistamines, steroids, pain medications, chemotherapy agents, and anticonvulsants

Special considerations for children and adolescents
- Most children with ADHD have an unremarkable medical history, but possible conditions that cause ADHD-like symptoms include head injury; fetal alcohol syndrome (FAS); lead exposure; sleep apnea (or other cause of poor sleep); hearing, speech, language, or vision impairments; and thyroid disease.
- Antidepressants can be associated with "activation," especially in younger children, and may mimic or worsen ADHD symptoms.

Develop and refine differential diagnosis

From the chief complaint and core presenting symptoms, generate a broad differential to generate a list of diagnoses to consider (see Table 8.1, Table 8.2 for Children and Adolescents). Use the key questions and differentiating symptoms listed to narrow the differential. ADHD diagnoses are listed in Table 8.3. Many rating scales are available and can be helpful for clarifying the diagnosis, assessing severity, and tracking symptoms over time. For children and adolescents, teacher, parent, and self-report forms are available.

Here are some of the most commonly used rating scales:
- Adult ADHD Self-Report Scale Symptom Checklist (ASRS v1.1)
- Brown Attention-Deficit Disorder Rating Scale and Diagnostic Form
- Connors Adult ADHD Rating Scales
- Wender Utah Rating Scale
- For children and adolescents: Connors Early Childhood (ages 2–6) and Connors 3 (ages 6–18); Vanderbilt (nonproprietary, ages 6–12)

Psychological or neuropsychological testing, when available, can be helpful in identifying comorbid learning disorders or cognitive impairment, finding individual strengths and weaknesses, and documenting disabilities for appropriate academic accommodations.

Assessment of comorbid psychiatric disorders and psychological difficulties

The majority of patients with ADHD meet criteria for an additional psychiatric diagnosis. It can be very difficult to differentiate ADHD from other psychiatric conditions given the overlap of symptoms.
- There is a relatively high incidence of lifetime diagnoses of anxiety disorders, major depressive disorder, antisocial personality disorder, and alcohol or drug dependencies in adults with ADHD
- Learning disorders are particularly difficult to differentiate from ADHD given the common outcome of poor academic functioning
- It is generally recommended that substance use be addressed prior to beginning ADHD treatment, followed by reassessment for ADHD symptoms after abstinence is achieved

Table 8.1 Generating the differential for ADHD in adults

Diagnosis	Key questions	Differentiating symptom	Behavioral heath measure
ADHD	Do you struggle with impulsivity, hyperactivity, or problems with attention?	Poor focus	ASRS v1.1
Major Depressive Disorder	Have you been feeling depressed or having difficulty enjoying things in your life?	Low mood or anhedonia	PHQ-9
Bipolar Disorder: Hypomania or Mania	Do you have periods of time with much less sleep than usual and not really missing it the next day?	Decreased need for sleep	MDQ CIDI-3
Generalized Anxiety Disorder	Have you been worrying excessively for greater than six months? Are you a worrier?	Worry	GAD-7
Obsessive-Compulsive Disorder	Do you have any repetitive thoughts or behaviors that bother you?	Repetitive thoughts or behaviors	Yale Obsessive Compulsive Checklist (Y-BOC)
Learning Disabilities	Do you have a history of poor academic performance in any specific domain?	Failure to acquire reading, writing, or math skills at age expected levels	No measure available (consider psychometric or neuropsycho-logical testing)
Antisocial Personality Disorder	Do you have a history of frequent fights, stealing, vandalism or other legal problems?	General disregard for and violation of the rights of others	No measure available
Trauma and PTSD	Do you have a history of trauma or abuse with nightmares and flashbacks?	Recurring traumatic memories, hyperarousal, and avoidance behaviors	PCL-C

Other disorders to consider: Mental retardation, Traumatic Brain Injury, Delirium, Dementia, Malingering

Table 8.2 Generating the differential for ADHD in children

Diagnosis	Key questions	Differentiating symptom	Behavioral Health measure
ADHD	Does your child struggle with impulsivity, hyperactivity, or problems with attention compared to their classroom peers or in structured activities, like sports?	Poor focus	Connors Early Childhood (ages 2–6) Connors 3 (ages 6–18); Vanderbilt (nonproprietary, ages 6–12)
Oppositional Defiant Disorder	Does your child often lose his or her temper, argue or behave defiantly with adults, or become resentful or vindictive when things do not go his or her way?	Context dependent emotional and behavioral reactivity	Child Behavior Check List (CBCL)
Conduct Disorder	Does your child have problems with fighting, destructive behavior, lying or stealing?	General disregard for and violation of the rights of others	CBCL
Trauma and PTSD	Does your child have a history of severe neglect, maltreatment, trauma or prolonged exposure to psycho-social adversity?	Recurring traumatic memories, hyperarousal, and avoidance behaviors	UCLA PTSD Index Trauma Screen, PCL-C
Autism Spectrum Disorders	Does your child seem uninterested in people or display repetitive behaviors or a narrow range of interests?	Impaired social communication along with restricted interests and repetitive behaviors	Social Communication Questionnaire (SCQ)

Other disorders to consider: Mental retardation, Traumatic Brain Injury

Table 8.3 Common ADHD disorders in primary care (ICD-10)

- Attention-deficit hyperactivity disorder, predominantly hyperactive type - F90.1
- Attention-deficit hyperactivity disorder, predominantly inattentive type - F90.0
- Attention-deficit hyperactivity disorder, combined type - F90.2
- Attention-deficit hyperactivity disorder, other type - F90.8
- Attention-deficit hyperactivity disorder, unspecified type - F90.9

Special considerations for children and adolescents
Inattention and/or poor impulse control problems that develop *de novo* in the context of an anxiety, depressive, or bipolar disorder do not justify a separate ADHD diagnosis.

- More than 50 percent of children with ADHD also meet criteria for Oppositional Defiant Disorder and many of these children later develop Conduct Disorder.
- Anxiety often occurs concurrently with ADHD while depression is likely to present several years after the onset of ADHD.
- As with adults, it is generally recommended in adolescents with recently diagnosed ADHD and co-occurring substance abuse that substance abuse be addressed prior to beginning ADHD treatment.

Team goal: Differential diagnosis and identifying a provisional diagnosis
Once the PCP has evaluated for medical causes for symptoms of hyperactivity, impulsivity, and inattention, the team will work together to complete screening for common mental health conditions, to identify any comorbid diagnoses, and to make a provisional anxiety diagnosis of ADHD if appropriate.

Working as a team
Patient: Monitors symptoms; reports to PCP and/or BHP; and follows through on medical recommendations or consultations. Presents all relevant information related to the expanded differential and completes needed measures. Presents all relevant information for comorbid illness; follows through on any additional assessment or treatment recommended.

PCP: Primary role in evaluating possible medical etiology for presenting complaints starting with a review of medications and complete physical exam;

screening labs should be based on physical exam abnormalities (no labs indicated in context of normal exam); send for additional tests and medical consultation as appropriate. Coordinates with BHP to refine differential and often starts initial screening for comorbidities (e.g., PHQ-9 and GAD-7). Considers comorbidities (such as anxiety and depressive disorders), gathers basic history around the other suspected disorders, and refers to BHP for additional assessment.

BHP: Important role in noting any concerning physical symptoms and connecting patient to PCP for evaluation; gathers detailed substance use history; supports the patient in following through on medical recommendations (which can be particularly difficult for patients with ADHD). Chooses and follows through on necessary measures; asks appropriate follow-up questions for any positive screens and refers for neuropsychological testing when learning disorders or cognitive impairment are suspected; discusses screening results with PC as needed; offers provisional diagnoses and clarifies the diagnoses with the help of the PC. Considers and screens for anxiety, depression, antisocial personality disorder, and substance use; refers for substance use treatment as necessary and follows up on reassessment after abstinence is achieved.

PC: Expands medical differential as needed, with close attention to cognitive disorders and substance use; recommends additional assessment, such as cognitive assessments, when needed. Refines and/or expands differential; confirms the BHP's provisional diagnoses. Considers additional comorbidities, helps differentiate between comorbidities by considering key differences; reviews any neuropsychological testing completed; helps determine when substance use treatment should be pursued and reassesses for ADHD symptoms after abstinence is achieved.

Case example

The patient was further assessed by his PCP and no medical comorbidities were found by review of systems and exam, no labs were indicated. He was also screened for substance use and endorsed a history of four years of amphetamine abuse from which he was now clean, though not in treatment.

(Continued)

An ASRS was completed and he was found to have symptoms highly consistent with ADHD. The patient's girlfriend also expressed concern for anxiety. He was given a PHQ-9 and scored a 3/27, with minimal symptoms. GAD-7 was also given and he scored a 7/21, symptoms were consistent with mild generalized anxiety.

The PCP referred the patient to the BHP for further assessment of ADHD, anxiety and past amphetamine abuse. The BHP screened him for PTSD, OCD, panic disorder, and bipolar disorder, and all were negative. He denied suicidal thoughts but did endorse chronic, low self-esteem and a belief that he was "not smart enough" to keep a job.

Treatment

Initiate treatment

General approaches

Psychoeducation provides an explanatory model in a specific way that might be helpful for the primary care team when working with patients with ADHD to develop a treatment plan (Table 8.4). Psychoeducation about the effects of ADHD and its response to treatment is almost universally agreed upon as the starting point for psychosocial treatment. Examples of psychoeducation around ADHD include:

- "Adults with ADHD are often trying extremely hard and have the best of intentions, but because their brains have trouble keeping track of time, or remembering what they were in the middle of doing, the result is often failure and disappointment."
- "A lifetime of ADHD behaviors and problems can lower self-esteem and affect your relationships. Individual counseling, medications, and support groups can help."
- "There are small, strategic changes we can help you make in your daily routine to compensate for these difficulties and help you become more successful at work and at home."
- "Believing that you can 'do it right this time' by sheer force of will is a myth. External aids are often essential as some of the issues are out of conscious control."
- "People with ADHD have an increased risk for drug and alcohol abuse, thus drinking only in moderation or abstinence is recommended."

Table 8.4 Team-based treatment for ADHD

	PCP approaches	BHP approaches
Biological	***Evidence-Based Medication Treatment:*** • Adult ADHD responds to medication treatment at rates higher than almost any other psychiatric disorder. • Long-acting stimulants, such as Adderall XR and Concerta, are the first-line medication intervention when there is no history of substance abuse, cardiac disease, significant hypertension, or certain psychiatric disorders (such as bipolar disorder).	***Evidence-Based Medication Treatment:*** • Help patients adhere to their ADHD as adherence can be limited by the patient's disorganization. • Additional monitoring of stimulant use should be provided by the BHP given the risk for abuse, diversion, and nonadherence: • Consider regular pill counts and a stimulant contract for at-risk patients • Recommend urine toxicology to the PCP when diversion or concurrent substance abuse suspected.
Psychosocial	***Evidence-Based Behavioral Treatment:*** • Start by providing psychoeducation about the effects of ADHD, including common symptoms and outcomes, as well as the effectiveness of treatment. • Promote cognitive behavioral therapy (CBT) as an adjunct to medication as it can improve daily life skills affected by ADHD.	***Evidence-Based Behavioral Treatment:*** • Evidence-based behavioral interventions include psycho-education, cognitive-behavioral treatment (CBT), self-management skills training, vocational counseling, neuro-feedback, and ADHD coaching. • Focus on helping the patient lay out specific functional treatment goals and return to these goals to strengthen commitment to treatment when it becomes difficult.

Special considerations for children and adolescents
Psychoeducation for children and adolescents needs to take into account family and patient concerns and treatment preferences and should provide guidance in terms of anticipated developmental changes and challenges, which may occur in the course of treatment. Providers should help parents access community supports and advocate for their child's educational needs (e.g., assisting with a referral for an Individualized Education Program).

Safety issues
Serious side effects to monitor with stimulant use include anger, agitation, mania, even psychosis.

Misuse of "study drugs" is common on college campuses with a 12-month prevalence of 4 percent. Stimulants are also used for recreation, often intranasally and in combination with alcohol.

Red flags for stimulant diversion or abuse include:
- escalating dose
- lost script
- early refills
- specific requests for short-acting formulations
- new-onset psychosis
- new-onset cardiac symptoms

Special considerations for children and adolescents
- The risk of stimulant diversion generally increases with patient's age; however, it is also possible that a parent of a child may be engaged in stimulant diversion.
- Blood pressure, pulse, height, and weight are typically monitored parameters in youth; long-term use of stimulants, especially at higher doses, may be associated with a diminished growth in the range of 1–2 cm.
- Risk of significant cardiac complications, including sudden cardiac death due to cardiac arrhythmias, is extremely low in children without a personal or family history of cardiac disease.

PCP approaches
General principles
In patients with mild ADHD or children under six years old, psychosocial approaches are preferred choice. Combination therapy with both medications and psychotherapy is recommended for individuals (six years and older) with moderate to severe ADHD.

Special considerations for children and adolescents

For preschool children, the American Academy of Pediatrics (AAP) recommends parent behavioral training and/or school-based interventions be tried prior to a medication trial. If moderate to severe symptoms persist following an adequate trial of behavioral interventions, methylphenidate may be prescribed. For elementary school children (6–11 years of age), the AAP recommends combined medication and parent behavioral training and/or school-based interventions when possible. For adolescents, the AAP recommends combined medication and behavioral therapy when possible.

Prescribing principles

Adult ADHD responds to medication treatment at rates higher than almost any other psychiatric disorder. Studies show greater effect sizes for stimulants than nonstimulants in adults with ADHD, but no significant difference in effect between short- and long-acting stimulants. See Table 8.5 for details on medications used in treatment of ADHD.

- Drawbacks of short-acting stimulants include rebound, need for multiple dosing, decreased efficacy in the evening, and greater risk for abuse.
- Long-acting stimulants, such as dextroamphetamine/amphetamine ER (Adderall XR), lisdexamfetamine (Vyvanse), and methylphenidate ER (Concerta), are the first-line medication intervention when there is moderate to severe ADHD and no history of substance abuse, cardiac

Table 8.5 Medications commonly used in the treatment of ADHD

First Line (Stimulants)
dextroamphetamine/amphetamine (Adderall)
dextroamphetamine/amphetamine ER (Adderall XR)
lisdexamfetamine (Vyvanse)
methylphenidate (Ritalin)
methylphenidate ER (Concerta)

Second Line
atomoxetine (Strattera)

Third Line (not FDA approved for ADHD but some evidence for use)
bupropion (Wellbutrin)
venlafaxine (Effexor)
duloxetine (Cymbalta)

For prescribing details and protocols, please see Chapter 11, "Evidence Based Psychopharmacology for the Collaborative Care Team."

disease (if not well controlled), significant hypertension, or certain psychiatric disorders (such as bipolar disorder).

- After long-acting stimulants, atomoxetine is the usual second-line medication (or first line for patients with a history of cocaine or amphetamine use disorders).
- Bupropion and SNRIs have demonstrated treatment response, if not always full symptom remission, in limited placebo-controlled trials.
- Many clinics use stimulant contracts as part of clinic prescribing protocols.

Special considerations for children and adolescents

Finding the optimal medication and dose with the fewest side effects may take several months; initially, frequent (i.e., twice monthly) follow-up may be necessary until treatment is optimized; once optimized, follow-up every 3–4 months is recommended. In general, long-acting stimulants are preferred as first-line agents in children > 16 kg in weight; in smaller children, short-acting agents are typically used initially and then traded for long-acting formulations as tolerated. (See Tables 8.5 and 8.6 for details.)

- Preschool children (3–5 years of age) are less likely to benefit from stimulant use and are more sensitive to side effects compared to school-age children; mean optimal dosing for methylphenidate is approximately 0.7 mg/kg/day for preschoolers versus 1 mg/kg/day for school-age children, though there can be substantial individual variability.
- Common side effects in children of all ages include appetite suppression, insomnia, abdominal discomfort, affective flattening, and weight loss; preschoolers are more likely to experience irritability and mood lability, especially if developmentally delayed.
- Low doses of short-acting stimulants can be administered in the late afternoon or early evening to help with medication rebound (worsening behavior and irritability after daytime medication wears off) in children of all ages, for older children with heavy homework assignments, and for safety reasons, such as automobile driving.
- Failure to respond to one stimulant class (e.g., amphetamine) does not predict failure to the alternative class (e.g., methylphenidate), so switching stimulant classes is recommended prior to trying second-line agents (e.g., atomoxetine).

Table 8.6 Other medications commonly use in pediatric populations

clonidine (Catapres)	**Start:** for children < 45 kg, 0.05mg qhs × 3–7d, then↑ by 0.05 mg/day q3–7 d; for children > 45 kg, 0.1 mg qhs × 3–7d, then↑ by 0.1 mg/day q3–7 d. **Range:** 27–40.5 kg, 0.05–0.2 mg tid-qid; 40.5–45 kg, 0.05–0.3 mg tid-qid; >45 kg, 0.1–0.4 mg tid-qid	Second line treatment. *Not* FDA-approved for ADHD. Often used in conjunction with stimulants or atomoxetine for persistent ADHD symptoms and/or to help with sleep, anxiety, irritability, tics, and aggression. To discontinue, taper slowly over 4–14 days to avoid rebound hypertension. ¢
clonidine ER (Kapvay)	**Start:** for children > 6 yo, 0.1 mg qhs × 7d, then ↑ by 0.1 mg/day qweek. **Range:** 0.1–0.4 mg qd-bid	Second line treatment. FDA-approved for ADHD in children 6–17 years old. Often used in conjunction with stimulants or atomoxetine for persistent ADHD symptoms and/or to help with sleep, anxiety, irritability, tics, and aggression. To discontinue, taper slowly over 4–14 days to avoid rebound hypertension. $
guanfacine (Tenex)	**Start:** for children < 45 kg, 0.5mg qhs × 3–7d, then↑ by 0.5 mg/day q3–7 d; for children > 45 kg, 1 mg qhs × 3–7d, then↑ by 1 mg/day q3–7 d. **Range:** 27–40.5 kg, 0.5–2 mg bid-qid; 40.5–45 kg, 0.5–3 mg bid-qid; >45 kg, 1–4 mg bid-qid	Second line treatment. *Not* FDA-approved for ADHD. Often used in conjunction with stimulants or atomoxetine for persistent ADHD symptoms and/or to help with sleep, anxiety, irritability, tics, and aggression. To discontinue, taper slowly over 4–14 days to avoid rebound hypertension. ¢
guanfacine ER (Intuniv)	**Start:** for children > 6 yo, 1 mg qd × 7d, then ↑ by 1 mg/day qweek. **Range:** 1–4 mg/d	Second line treatment. FDA-approved for ADHD in children 6–17 years old. Often used in conjunction with stimulants or atomoxetine for persistent ADHD symptoms and/or to help with sleep, anxiety, irritability, tics, and aggression. $

Table Key: ¢: Generic $: More expensive

Brief behavioral interventions

Cognitive behavioral therapy (CBT) is helpful as an adjunct to medication as it can improve daily life skills affected by ADHD. Help the patient identify at least three specific impairments due to ADHD and track how they change over time with treatment. Support the work of the BHP by:

- Communicating closely with the BHP
- Ask the patient about behavioral changes discussed in therapy sessions and how s/he has followed through with those recommendations
- Review any symptom tracking or logging the patient has recorded as part of therapy with the BHP

Special considerations for children and adolescents

Parent behavior training is recommended before a trial of medication for preschool children and is recommended to be used in conjunction with medications for all children, especially in children with comorbid ODD, aggression, and internalizing symptoms such as anxiety. Close collaboration with schools is important to insure appropriate educational and behavioral interventions are in place. Adolescents, like adults, may benefit from CBT.

BHP approaches

General principles

Evidence-based behavioral interventions include psychoeducation, cognitive behavioral treatment (CBT), self-management skills training, vocational counseling, neurofeedback, and ADHD coaching. Start by providing psychoeducation about the effects of ADHD, including common symptoms and outcomes, as well as the effectiveness of treatment.

cBT principles for adult ADHD

cBT emphasizes the interactive role of automatic thoughts, images and belief systems as well as behaviors in perpetuating symptoms of ADHD (small c, capital B to emphasize the behavioral component). Focus on helping the patient lay out specific functional treatment goals and return to these goals to strengthen commitment to treatment when it becomes difficult. Help the patient improve organizational, time-management, and problem-solving skills by:

- Chunking large tasks into smaller steps
- Introducing a daily planner and emphasizing use of one planner or notebook only
- Manage to-do's using assistive devices, such as mobile phones
- Starting tasks well in advance of their deadline

- Reducing distraction (i.e., clutter-free desktop, windowless and quiet space to work)
- List making and task prioritization
- Self-monitoring with regular completion of behavioral checklists and logging
- Target behaviors as they come up in session, such as arriving late for appointments or losing homework

Facing these longstanding difficulties may trigger self-criticism, negative self-thoughts, and frustration, so much of the treatment is about reducing shame:

- Target the negative cognitions and beliefs as they come up to prevent worsening comorbidities such as anxiety and depression
- Relate back to initial treatment goals to help push through barriers

---

Special considerations for children and adolescents

Parent Behavioral Training (PBT)

PBT is a psychosocial intervention designed to help parents acquire skills in behavioral techniques they can use with their children to target associated behavioral problems; in addition to psychoeducation regarding ADHD, components include:

- Helping parents establish realistic and observable behavioral expectations for their child
- Discussing and modeling clear and specific caregiver communication skills
- Helping parents understand and implement changes in the home environment which promote increased structure, predictability, and consistency
- Helping parents improve relationships and behavior by encouraging them to: 1. Increase their focus on rewarding desirable behaviors ("catch them being good"); 2. Ignore annoying or attention-seeking behaviors; and 3. Apply appropriate discipline (e.g., loss of privileges) in a consistent, predictable, and immediate fashion
- Helping promote improvement of parent-child relationships by "prescribing" daily child-directed play time
- Reviewing child's daily schedule with parents to screen for inappropriate activities or inadequate levels of supervision; provide recommendations if necessary (e.g., supervised day camps during the summer)
- Ideally, behavioral plans and interventions can be coordinated between home and school so that expectations and consequences for behavior are consistently applied across these domains.

Working with medications

Helping patients adhere to their medications is especially important when treating ADHD as adherence can be limited by the patient's disorganization. Additional monitoring of stimulant use should be provided by the BHP given the risk for abuse, diversion, and nonadherence:

- Consider regular pill counts and a stimulant contract for at-risk patients
- Recommend urine toxicology to the PCP when diversion or concurrent substance abuse suspected

---

Team goal: Initial treatment planning

Using the provisional diagnosis of ADHD and patient preference, the team must work together to make sure medication and behavioral treatments are initiated and that the patient is engaged in the overall plan.

Working as a team

Patient: Engages in recommended therapy and follows through on homework (may need to set alarms to check in or have regularly scheduled appointments), starts medications as prescribed

   PCP: Engages the patient in treatment with basic psychoeducation on ADHD and brief behavioral interventions; prescribes and monitors medications (patients on stimulants should initially be monitored monthly); checks baseline labs as well as vital signs (particular attention to HR and BP in patients on stimulants)

   BHP: Engages patient in treatment by helping him/her lay out specific treatment goals, follows up psychoeducation on ADHD started with the PCP; develops full treatment plan and shares it with the patient; initiates cBT

   PC: Reviews treatment planning; gives medication recommendations and prescribing details; guides BHP through laying out treatment goals and providing psycho-education around ADHD

Case example

In order to engage the patient in treatment, the BHP first helped him lay out goals. His primary functional goals were to be able to read 20 pages without being distracted, keep better track of medical appointments, show up on time for things, and contribute to grocery shopping and meal planning in the home. The patient was discussed with the PC who recommended starting atomoxetine 40mg daily with reevaluation and titration after 4–6 weeks. Stimulants were not recommended due to past amphetamine abuse and bupropion was avoided due to concern for worsening anxiety. The medication was initiated at the patient's next PCP appointment. The PC also recommended the BHP provide psychoeducation on adult ADHD and begin cBT to target both ADHD symptoms and anxiety symptoms. The BHP also referred the patient to 12-step meetings for more support around maintaining abstinence from amphetamines.

Follow-up and treatment adjustment to achieve treatment to target

When to refer

- ADHD is not responding to treatment or the patient is not able to tolerate treatment
- Conditions requiring longer-term, more intensive, or specialist psychotherapy
- Employment Services: Especially important in adults with ADHD given vocational difficulties identified in outcome studies
- Disability: More severe cases, especially if anticipate inability to work for greater than a year

Ongoing medication management

The same behavioral measures that are used for diagnosis can also be used to assess ongoing care, but it is also helpful to identify functional goals (e.g., patient's ability to read for a longer length of time, attend to conversations, and finish specific projects) and use these to judge efficacy of treatment over time.

- Patients not responding to initial dosing may benefit from an increased dose; see Chapter 11 for dosing details
- There are no known factors that correlate with prescribing dose (e.g. age, sex, body weight, or symptom severity). Medications should be titrated based on effect and max dosage limitations.
- Patients who do not respond to an adequate dose and duration of treatment or who have significant side effects to the initial treatment choice should be switched to second-line treatment
- Patients on stimulants not following treatment recommendations or showing concerning signs or symptoms for abuse or diversion should be switched to nonstimulant treatment (atomoxetine, bupropion, or an SNRI)

It is recommended that the BHP ask the patient about their ADHD medications at each contact:

- Troubleshoot adherence challenges
- Be responsive to concerns and side effects

- Support patient through medication changes
- Help patient schedule an appointment with PCP to address medications
- Help patient write down questions for their PCP

Special considerations for children and adolescents
Children and adolescents generally should not be allowed to self-administer their medications due to safety concerns, potential for diversion, and high rates of nonadherence. Developmental changes (such as increased weight) or an increase in developmental demands (such as academic expectations) may require higher doses of medications. Intermittent medication holidays, such as during summer vacations, may benefit youth with evidence of diminished growth and weight loss.

Team goal: Revising treatment planning and stepping up care
Monitor progress on the identified behavioral targets related to ADHD, and adjust treatment to until target and goals achieved.

Working as a team
Patient: Reliably reports back to team regarding all treatment concerns and attends recommended referrals

PCP: Monitors for medication adherence, response, and tolerance and follows through on related PC recommendations; watches for signs of abuse or diversion of stimulants, considers long-term medication consequences and health maintenance issues; monitors any relevant labs and continues to follow vital signs (for patients on stimulants); places medical referrals as needed

BHP: Helps patient track refills and medical appointments (encouraging patient to schedule next appointment before leaving), sends appointment reminders the day prior if possible; facilitates communication between team members (particularly if substance abuse issues are present); makes and supports referrals (disability, vocational rehab, social services, substance use treatment, additional psychotherapy); monitors improvement in functional goals over time

PC: Monitors for medication adherence, response, and tolerance and makes specific medication recommendations to for the PCP; watches for signs of abuse or diversion of stimulants; supports BHP delivery of cBT by trouble-shooting stuck points in therapy

Case example

After one month of treatment, the patient had made some progress in his functional goals. He was reading about five pages at a time without distraction, attending most medical appointments though often late, helping his girlfriend with groceries, and planning one meal per week. The BHP was helping him use task lists, a daily planner, and reminders on his phone with some success. The BHP also flagged the patient for reconsultation with the PC and helped him follow through with PCP appointments. The patient told his PCP the atomoxetine at 40mg was improving his level of restlessness and he had no significant side effects from it. The PCP increased the dose to 80mg daily, upon recommendation by the PC.

Completing treatment and relapse prevention

ADHD is a life-long disorder and often requires chronic treatment. Treatment goals should be rooted in functioning, as described above, thus the "target" varies from patient to patient. Once a therapeutic dose of a medication with minimal side effects is found, treatment is indefinite. Stimulants (with the exception of growing children) should not require escalating doses over time to achieve the same effect. If a patient continues to require increased dosages, it may be a warning sign for abuse or diversion. Relapse preventions requires monitoring for:

- Treatment adherence (particularly important with ADHD given forgetfulness and disorganization)
- Abuse, diversion, or side effects when stimulants are prescribed (recommend regular visits with PCP and/or BHP throughout treatment period)
- Early warning signs of relapse
- Follow through on referrals

Team goal: Relapse prevention

Coordinate across all team members to determine agreement that an ADHD treatment plan is optimized with patient goals adequately met, develop a relapse prevention plan (especially plan of any stimulant prescriptions) and support patient transition to ongoing management as part of the PCP general panel.

(Continued)

Working as a team

Patient: Continues to adhere to medications and attends all medical and BHP appointments; monitors for early warning signs of worsening inattention or hyperactivity and reports to either PCP or BHP

   PCP: Continues to prescribe medications at therapeutic dosages and monitors for side effects or loss of efficacy; encourages patients to follow through on all BHP recommendations and therapy homework; communicates with BHP as needed

   BHP: Continues regular screening for anxiety, depression, and ADHD symptoms; continues cBT but at decreased frequency once goals are reached with a focus on relapse prevention; monitors for early signs of relapse and flags patient for psychiatric consultation when needed; encourages adherence to all medications

   PC: Continues to track results of behavioral health measures on the electronic registry and offers consultation with BHP and/or PCP if symptoms increase

Case example

After 12 weeks of combination treatment (medication plus psychotherapy), the patient's repeat GAD-7 decreased to a 2/21. He was engaging in therapy with the BHP and tracking changes with weekly behavioral logs. He was also making progress in his functional goals—reading for 15–20 pages at a time, showing up for medical appointments, and planning one meal per week. His feelings of self-efficacy were improving and he held a new goal of attending vocational rehab to find part-time work. He spaced out his appointments with his BHP to monthly with a focus on relapse prevention and continued to see his PCP regularly for ongoing medication treatment.

Resources

- NAMI http://www.nami.org/
- NIH http://www.nimh.nih.gov/health/publications/adhd-listing.shtml
- CDC http://www.cdc.gov/ncbddd/adhd/
- CHADD http://www.chadd.org/
- AACAP http://www.aacap.org
- AAP http://www.aap.org

References

A 14-month randomized clinical trial of treatment strategies for attention-deficit/hyperactivity disorder. The MTA Cooperative Group. Multimodal Treatment Study of Children with ADHD. (1999). *Archives of General Psychiatry, 56*(12), 1073–86.

Barkley, R. A. (2010). *Taking Charge of Adult ADHD*. New York: Guilford.

Davidson, M. A. (2008). ADHD in adults: A review of the literature. *Journal of Attention Disorders, 11*(6), 628–641.

Faraone, S. V. & Glatt, S. J. (2010). A comparison of the efficacy of medications for adult attention-deficit/hyperactivity disorder using meta-analysis of effect sizes. *Journal of Clinical Psychiatry, 71*(6), 754–63.

Kessler, R. C., Adler, L., Barkley, R., Biederman, J., Conners, C. K., Demler, O., Zaslavsky, A. M. (2006). The prevalence and correlates of adult ADHD in the United States: results from the National Comorbidity Survey Replication. *American Journal of Psychiatry, 163*(4), 716–23.

Kooji, S. J., Bejerot, S., Blackwell, A., Caci, H., Casas-Brugué, M., Carpentier, P. J., Asherson, P. (2010). European consensus statement on diagnosis and treatment of adult ADHD: The European Network Adult ADHD. *BMC Psychiatry, 10*(67).

Montano, B. (2004). Diagnosis and treatment of ADHD in adults in primary care. *Journal of Clinical Psychiatry, 65*(Suppl. 3), 18–21.

Pliszka, S. (2007). AACAP Work Group on Quality Issues. Practice parameter for the assessment and treatment of children and adolescents with attention-deficit/hyperactivity disorder. *Journal of American Academy of Child and Adolescent Psychiatry, 46*(7), 894–921. Review.

Ramsay, R. J. (2007). Current status of cognitive-behavioral therapy as a psychosocial treatment for adult attention-deficit/hyperactivity disorder. *Current Psychiatry Reports, 9*, 427–33.

Subcommittee on Attention-Deficit/Hyperactivity Disorder; Steering Committee on Quality Improvement and Management: Wolraich, M., Brown, L., Brown, R. T., DuPaul, G., Earls, M., Feldman, H. M., Ganiats T. G. ... Visser, S. (2011). ADHD: clinical practice guideline for the diagnosis, evaluation, and treatment of attention-deficit/hyperactivity disorder in children and adolescents. *Pediatrics, 128*(5), 1007–22.

Part 2

Collaborative Care Interventions

Chapter 9 **Challenging Clinical Situations**

Kyl Dinsio, Anna Ratzliff, and Kari A. Stephens

Case example

A 50-year-old Caucasian woman is followed in primary care with recurrent major depressive disorder, chronic pain, pain disorder with high anxiety and depression, and ADHD. Her treatment is focused on a Suboxone taper and mental health (focusing on depression and pain self-management). She has regularly scheduled appointments in the clinic but is regularly late—often arriving more than halfway through the allotted appointment time. She has also been observed to be frequently in distress and highly emotional during her appointments. As a result, the limited time available is usually focused on helping her cope in the moment rather than working on other treatment goals about her depression and self-care.

Clinical impact

Difficult and challenging patient-doctor situations (Table 9.1) are common in clinical practice. An estimated 15 to 30 percent of primary care visits are described as being difficult. Primary care practitioners can regularly expect to have three to four challenging encounters daily. These difficult encounters are stressful for providers as well as patients. Physicians endorsing frequent difficult encounters have been found to have lower job satisfaction and higher rates of burnout and to report suboptimal care performance and expectation of future errors.

Integrated Care: Creating Effective Mental and Primary Health Care Teams, First Edition.
Anna Ratzliff, Jürgen Unützer, Wayne Katon, and Kari A. Stephens.
© 2016 John Wiley & Sons, Inc. Published 2016 by John Wiley & Sons, Inc.

Table 9.1 Common difficult situations in primary care

- Thinking about the patient invokes dread ("heartsick" or "head in hands" patient)
- Secretly wishing the patient will fire you or not return to the clinic
- The patient who verbally abuses providers and staff
- The patient who asks for help but ignores medical advice ("help-rejecting patient")
- Patient frequently shows dissatisfaction with care
- Frequent team discussion or debates about treatment approach or plan
- Care expectations that are unrealistic
- Ongoing conflict over treatment plan or medications, repeated requests for unnecessary tests
- Poor alliance, mistrust (suspected malingering)
- Team members blaming each other for difficulties

Historically, writings around difficult situations centered on characteristics of the "difficult patient." Modern perspectives have shifted to appreciating that all clinical interactions are complex interplays between patient, provider/team, illness, and environmental factors. When clinical encounters are stressful, unsatisfying, or conflict-laden, there are typically multiple factors contributing to the situation.

The good news is that "targets" for improving the patient-provider relationship exist. Although patient characteristics are one factor to consider, the provider and team have the most influence and opportunity to improve the situation for everyone involved. A brief, structured, team-based intervention can have a significant positive impact. These interventions provide an opportunity for team building since team members can problem solve together to improve the experience for the patient and the providers. This chapter outlines a five-step process to help Collaborative Care team members better cope with difficult clinical situations.

- Difficult clinical situations are common in daily practice.
- The provider/team has the most influence and opportunity to make positive changes in the treatment relationship.
- Addressing difficult patient-doctor situations requires a tailored and individualized approach based on the particular challenges presented by an individual patient situation.
- A five-step approach can help the team better cope with common difficult situations.

Assessment

Step 1: Name the emotions that working with the patient evokes in you.

General principles
Difficult provider-patient interactions generate strong emotions in everyone involved. The first step to improving these clinical situations is to acknowledge the emotional reaction that *you* are experiencing.

Answer the questions
- How do I feel when this patient shows up on my schedule?
- How do I feel when this patient leaves my office?

While it might seem counterintuitive, the emotion that you are presently feeling is often the most accessible and easily identifiable way to start the process of improving these challenging situations. Eventually, the goal will be to identify the behavioral causes of the problem, but first providers need to take stock of how they are feeling about the situation.

Emotions exist on a continuum from very mild to extreme, and emotions generated by clinical situations are no different. Negative emotions fall into five primary categories.

Scared: (examples include: blamed, hopelessness, avoidant, panicked, overwhelmed)

Disgusted: (examples include: contemptuous, exasperated, dismissive)

Bad: (examples include: exhausted, unappreciated)

Ashamed: (examples include: doubtful, bored, uncertain, inept)

Angry: (examples include: frustrated, impatient, bitter, defensive, irritated)

Occasionally team members will blame each other (privately or even in public) for difficult clinical situations. This is a **red flag** that the entire team needs to discuss the situation. Blaming one of our colleagues breaks down team unity and can affect much more than just this one patient's care. Even if the team unity is not in question, if just one team member is struggling with a patient interaction, then it is worth the team's time to help problem-solve the interaction.

Frequently, team members have similar emotional reactions to a particular patient situation. However, it is also common for different providers to vary in their emotional responses. This doesn't indicate that some providers are "wrong" or "right" regarding their feelings in working with a particular patient, just that everyone has individual responses. Some common pitfalls in team members naming their emotions in challenging clinical situations are listed in Table 9.2.

Table 9.2 Potential pitfalls in naming the emotions that working with the patient evokes in you

Potential pitfalls of step 1	How to recognize it	How to mediate it
Defensiveness	A provider may respond with suspicion and feel that their professionalism or competence is being questioned. A provider may feel pestered and not want to participate in the team process of solving the problem ("shutting down").	Validate and normalize the negative emotions associated with working with this patient. Elicit the provider's concern about engaging in the process. Disclose that other members of the team are struggling and would appreciate the provider's wisdom in helping to solve the problem. Educate the provider about the stepped process outlined in this chapter. Explain how a discussion starting with emotions leads to making a plan to improve the situation later in the process.
Blaming the patient	A provider may insist that the problem lies solely with the patient or the patient's demands. A provider may want to "fire" the patient or transfer care to another clinic.	Acknowledge that the provider is having strong feelings toward the patient. Encourage the provider to describe the feelings and why they are so strong for this particular patient. Agree that firing the patient or transferring care are always "last resort" options, but that first it may help to see if the situation can be improved before taking such a drastic step.
Denial	A provider may insist that there are no problems in working with a particular patient. A provider may dismiss others' concerns about their ability to work with the patient. A provider may blame team members for the difficult situation, aligning with the patient against the rest of the team.	Acknowledge that although the provider is not feeling burdened, other team members are and are asking for the team's help. Encourage the provider to engage in the process, possibly by describing or offering guidance or "tips" for how s/he is able to work effectively with the patient. Gently address the issue of how blaming our colleague has a negative impact on team unity, esprit de corps, and job satisfaction.

Step 2: Define the patient's problematic behaviors in a concrete, specific, and observable way.

General principle

When providers feel frustrated, hopeless, or angry with patients, there is usually some problematic patient *behavior* that is eliciting the negative response. Focusing on the *specific problematic behaviors* is key to solving the problem as it creates a *target* for intervention (Table 9.3).

Table 9.3 Common problematic patient behaviors

- Showing up late
- Help seeking/help rejecting
- Patient is emotional during appointments
- Patient is always in suicidal crisis ("chronic SI")
- The patient who won't talk
- The patient who always agrees, but never follows through
- The patient who yells and is verbally aggressive
- The patient who wants something you can't offer (tests, medications, answers to unanswerable questions)
- The patient who shows up to appointments intoxicated
- The patient who idealizes some member of the team and devalues others ("splitting")

Answer the question

- What exactly is this patient doing that is getting in the way of care?
- What happened during our last encounter that prevented effective engagement?

To be effective at problem solving, we need to be concrete and specific. A statement such as "that patient is just manipulative" is vague; it is unclear what the actual behavior is that needs to be addressed. There are likely many complex things going on, none of which are explained by the word "manipulative." Rephrasing it as "patient cries through the entire appointment without being able to be redirected" is a statement of the particular behavior that is causing a problem in the treatment relationship.

An additional reason for focusing on behavior is that it can be tracked and measured over time so that you can see if the interventions are working. The patient in the case example was chronically late to appointments and the team chose to focus on trying to get her to appointments on time. How often the patient was late and by how many minutes could then easily be tracked over time. This data can be then shared with the team and with the patient for future strategizing and treatment planning.

Lastly, focusing on behaviors (i.e., what the patient is *doing*) helps align the team with the patient, helps align the team with each other, and promotes patient-centric care.

Examples of concrete and specific problematic behaviors:

- "The patient calls frequently and frantically in crisis several times a week."
- "The patient agrees to the plan but does not complete homework."
- "The patient asks for a stimulant prescription at every appointment and becomes angry when it is declined."
- "The patient does not answer important assessment questions or data points that the provider needs."

Examples of vague and poorly formulated problematic behaviors:

- "Patient disagrees with everything."
- "Patient blames the provider for his/her problems."
- "Patient is just personality disordered."

Step 3: Identify provider problematic behaviors (your own and your team).

General principle

Often without realizing it, providers contribute to difficult interactions with their own problematic behaviors.

Answer the questions

- What am I doing that supports this patient's problematic behavior or worsening the situation for everyone involved?

  Hint: Some of these behaviors may have started out as engagement strategies.

- What are other team members doing that support this patient's problematic behavior or worsening the situation for everyone involved?

A common example of this is a provider who extends the appointment past the scheduled time for a patient who is frequently late. Another example is a provider who responds to a patient who frequently presents in crisis with long, thorough, warm, and emphatic interactions. Common problematic provider behaviors are listed in Table 9.4.

It is additionally important to address how team members *differ* in their response to the patient's behavior and how this can contribute the perpetuation of problematic behaviors. Is everyone consistent in abiding by the scheduled appointment time? Who fields phone calls and how are those handled? Are providers involved in a "splitting" situation whereby some providers are viewed as "good" and others as "bad"?

Table 9.4 Common problematic provider behaviors

- Extending appointment times
- Always responding in a warm and empathetic way when a patient frequently presents in crisis
- Responding in a cold, matter-of-fact way when patient presents in a noncrisis (often because you are mad from the last crisis)
- Not praising patient for things he/she *are* doing to help themselves
- Provider cancels patient appointments without rescheduling
- Provider appears impatient or distracted during appointments (watching the clock; taking other phone calls or pages during appointment)
- Failing to return the patient's phone calls or delay in calling back
- Making negative/derogatory statements about the patient to other team members; aligning with another team member against the patient
- Joining with the patient to make negative statements against another team member ("splitting")
- Being inconsistent with regard to the patient's treatment plan between providers ("not being on the same page")
- Arbitrarily changing policies with the patient without explaining why
- Not providing the patient clear expectations for acceptable behavior
- Not being transparent about reasoning for declining patient requests (e.g., why aren't benzos, opiates, or stimulants being prescribed? why isn't a referral to neurology indicated?)
- Dismissing patient concerns without thorough investigation or assessment
- Over attributing physical symptoms to mental health problems (e.g., not doing standard work-up)

The treatment environment can also play a role in perpetuating difficult situations. Do all team members have a private and quiet area to meet with the patient? Are treatment rooms free of distractions and interruptions? Is front desk staff pleasant and professional toward the patient at check-in? Is the patient able to park easily at the clinic? Is there a bus stop nearby? While some of the treatment environmental conditions may not be easily modifiable (clinic location, bus stop, etc.), working with the patient to problem-solve the difficulty these challenges present may be a key part of addressing the problematic behavior (see Step 4).

Step 3 is most effective when team members take a moment to thoughtfully step back and look at the overall patterns of behavior (both patient and provider) that have developed over time. Table 9.5 (below) lists many common problematic provider behaviors and details the negative effects on both patients and the providers. In a particularly difficult situation, it may be worth the team's time to review the entire list to generate ideas. Ultimately the consequences for all the behaviors are the same: the patient doesn't get better and the team burns out.

Table 9.5 Effects of common problematic provider behaviors

Common problematic provider behaviors	Negative effect on patient behavior	Negative effect on provider/team
Extending appointment times to accommodate patient lateness or crisis	The patient got his/her needs met despite not being on time. So there is no incentive for being on time. In fact, some patients may have an *even longer* appointment if they show up late, making it *even more* reinforcing to never be on time. The patient will expect the same longer appointment in the future.	Provider's schedule is disrupted; provider gets behind and feels annoyed. Sets up team discord when one provider will spend extra time with a patient but another provider will not. Sets up a scenario where team splitting may happen.
Always responding in a warm and empathetic way when a patient presents in crisis frequently	A patient who receives a warm response from a provider when in crisis will be more likely to come to clinic in crisis every time. It makes it more likely that the patient will continue to use all the available appointment time for crisis management.	Providers feel exhausted and burned out by each crisis appointment and managing negative patient affect. Spending appointment time doing crisis management doesn't leave time to further assess underlying issues.
Responding in a cold, matter-of-fact way when patient presents in a noncrisis	Patient learns that the way they receive warm treatment from provider is by being in crisis. Patient may feel that their provider only cares about them when they are in crisis.	Providers miss the opportunity to encourage desirable patient behaviors! It should be most rewarding for a patient to come to clinic NOT in crisis.
Not praising patient for things they *are* doing to help themselves	Patient feels invalidated. Patient feels discouraged when trying hard to follow provider's recommendations.	Similar to the parenting concept of "catch them being good," providers need to be their most warm and fuzzy when patients show even the smallest improvement in behavior.

Table 9.5 (*Continued*)

Common problematic provider behaviors	Negative effect on patient behavior	Negative effect on provider/team
Canceling patient appointments without rescheduling	Patient feels disrespected, particularly if cancellation is not standard clinic policy.	Worsens patient behavior when the appointment finally does happen.
Failing to return the patient's phone calls or delay in calling back	Patient gets the message that his/her concerns are not important. Patient may escalate to crisis behavior in an effort to gain more of provider's focused attention.	Passive aggressively damages alliance.
Appearing impatient or distracted during patient appointments (watching the clock, taking other phone calls or pages during appointment time)	Patient feels disrespected and unimportant to provider. Patient may escalate to crisis behavior in an effort to gain more of provider's focused attention.	Provider may overlook or not recognize important aspects of patient's presentation ("miss something"). Passive aggressively damages alliance.
Making negative/ derogatory statements about the patient to other team members	Patients easily detect staff negative attitudes about them, which can lead to poor alliance.	Places the burden of a difficult situation on the patient exclusively ("blaming the patient").
Aligning with another team member against the patient	Ultimately results in ineffective engagement of the patient in the treatment process.	Can lead to team discord. Sets up a scenario where team splitting may happen.
Joining with the patient to make negative statements against another team member ("splitting")	The patient is aware that the team is not unified, which can cause uncertainty about their care.	Team is pulled into splitting between providers. Can lead to team discord and job dissatisfaction.
Being inconsistent with regard to the patient's treatment plan between providers ("not being on the same page")	Patient gets conflicting messages and ends up confused about treatment plan. Patient may stop or start treatment abruptly due to confusion about plan. Patient may lose faith in providers and fear that providers are not competent.	Team members can become frustrated by different approaches to challenging patient situations between providers. Can lead to team discord and job dissatisfaction. Sets up a scenario where team splitting may happen.

(Continued)

Table 9.5 (*Continued*)

Common problematic provider behaviors	Negative effect on patient behavior	Negative effect on provider/team
Arbitrarily changes policies with the patient without explaining why	Patient feels punished. Patient may retaliate with escalating crisis behaviors.	Team members may be confused as to why policies are being arbitrarily changed and won't be able to present a "united front."
Not providing the patient clear expectations for acceptable behavior	Patient feels confused, unsure of how s/he is supposed to behave. Patient may be unsure what they are doing to offend providers.	Providers may feel frustrated with patient behavior and feel powerless to intervene, or that they have to "just take it."
Not being transparent about your reasoning around declining patient requests	Patient feels punished. Patient may retaliate with escalating crisis behaviors. Patient may feel judged and feel s/he has been labeled unfairly (e.g., "drug-seeker").	Provider feels ongoing pressure to relent to patient request. Provider needs to discuss the request at every visit, leaving less time for addressing other issues.
Dismissing patient concerns without thorough investigation or assessment	Patient feels his/her concerns are not taken seriously. Patient loses confidence in provider. Patient not referred to mental health services.	Provider may overlook significant comorbidities such as mental health problem, substance abuse problem, or violence.
Overattributing physical symptoms to mental health problems (e.g., not doing standard work-ups)	Patient feels concerns are not taken seriously. Patient loses confidence in provider.	Provider may overlook true medical illness, causing delay in diagnosis or treatment. Provider is vulnerable to malpractice allegations.

- A key component of this step is nondefensiveness in viewing your own contribution and open flexibility to changing your approach when needed.
- Environmental factors also contribute to difficult situations.
- The ultimate result of all problematic provider behaviors is that the patient doesn't get better and the provider burns out.

Working as a team

Patient: Shares how s/he feels about treatment; discusses conflict with providers openly, particularly focusing on patient's feelings about it; clarify patient's goals for seeking care.

PCP: Identifies feelings generated by difficult situations; discusses conflict with patients and team members openly; defines problematic patient presentation in behavioral terms and identify contributing problematic provider behaviors, including their own.

BHP: Identifies feelings generated by difficult situations; discusses conflict with patients and team members openly; alert to brewing conflicts; tracks and catalogs an inventory of the emotions present across all team players; checks in with how everyone is feeling about the situation; educates team about the five-step process to improving difficult situations; defines problematic patient presentation in behavioral terms and identifies contributing problematic provider behaviors, including their own.

PC: Observes and provides outside perspective; point out patterns in describing the patient that may indicate negative feelings or conflict; checks validity test (does the affect fit the situation?); helps team to define problematic patient presentation in behavioral terms. Partners with BHP or other team members to catalog emotions present across all team players; asks specifically about team players that are "silent" on the issue; alert to what is being "left out" in the description of the situation; validates; a part of team decisions or discussions around particularly challenging cases and educates team about the five-step process to improving difficult situations.

Back to the case

Following the five-step process outlined in this chapter, the treatment team met to discuss their challenges in working with this patient during a morning huddle.

Step 1. Providers described emotions of *frustration, anger, and blame* generated in their work with the patient

(Continued)

Step 2. Providers described the patient's problematic behaviors as: *help-seeking/help-rejecting—constantly late, leaving less than half the appointment time, always comes in distressed initially and requires a great deal of soothing*

Step 3. Providers described their own problematic behaviors as: *team members would reward late behavior by allowing the patient to go over allotted time, providers were scheduling patient at the last minute and staying late past normal clinic hours.*

Treatment

Step 4: Develop a team-based behavioral approach to addressing the difficult situation.

General principle

The frequency of a behavior is determined by the *consequences* or response to the behavior. If the response to the behavior is desirable, then the behavior will increase. If the response is not desirable or aversive, then the behavior will decrease. Different responses are needed for behaviors to reward and behaviors to limit. In other words, to change the patient's behavior, providers need to adjust their *response* to the behavior.

Ask the questions
- What positive behaviors do we want to reward?
- What problematic behaviors do we want to limit?

A behavioral approach to a patient who is chronically late might include strategies to limit the problematic behavior, such as no longer seeing the patient the same day if s/he is more than 10 minutes late, strictly observing scheduled appointment time and not extending appointments, and keeping interactions during business hours only. Strategies to reward the positive behavior (being on time) might include scheduling more frequent appointments in order to avoid crisis-driven appointments, praising small improvements such as being 5 minutes late instead of 15, and encouraging the patient's ability to succeed.

Behavioral plans should be tailored to the particular patient as well as the particular behavior that is a problem. What is rewarding for one patient may be aversive to another. For example, a patient who is frequently late because they do not like engaging with the medical system may respond well to having brief, focused appointments rather than extended interactions with providers.

It is critically important that the patient is aware of the new approach and of the team's expectations. Similarly, the patient should know how the team will respond when expectations are not met. Documentation of the plan should be developed. This plan should be agreed to by the patient and they should be given their own copy along with a copy being kept in the chart for all team members to refer to. Strategies for potential difficult situations are listed in Table 9.6.

- In developing a behavioral plan, it is important to include both ways to *reward* positive patient behavior and also ways to *limit* problematic behavior.
- The success of a behavioral strategy depends on all team members being consistent in their approach to the patient. Patients should be educated about the plan and have a chance to contribute to its development. They should receive a written copy of the finalized plan.

Potential pitfalls to developing a team-based behavioral approach to addressing the difficult situation are listed in Table 9.7.

- The most successful plans target specific behaviors to reward and specific behaviors to limit and are tailored to each individual patient.

Working as a team

Patient: Reviews plan with BHP, offers suggestions for what might work better for him/her, follows through with plan, and communicates openly with the team when having difficulties following the plan

PCP: Works with team members to develop plan; adds particular treatment planning around medication issues and referrals; stays consistent with the plan during patient visits; educates nursing staff on the plan

BHP: Leads the team in designing and implementing plan; communicate plan to patient; reassess if the plan is working, make adjustments as necessary and communicate adjustments to team members; checks in with team members about how patient is responding to the plan

PC: Provides guidance and suggestions in the development of the plan; validates the difficulty of the situation; partner with BHP to make adjustments to the plan over time.

Table 9.6 Strategies for typical difficult situations

Patient presentation	Behavioral strategies
Help/rejecting patient *Ex. Comes in late to appointments; asks for help then gets angry at providers*	Validate Be consistent Practice good boundaries Promote use of skills
Emotionally dysregulated patient *Ex. Calling frequently and frantically; crying entire session without being able to be redirected; overstays sessions*	De-escalation Ground patient in the moment Triage (safety planning, problem solve, crisis manage) Assess their current use of skills Move to treatment—either problem solving or use distress tolerance/crisis management skills
Chronically suicidal patients *Ex. Every other visit patient presents with active SI; regularly threatens to harm self*	Triage (safety planning, problem solve, crisis manage) Develop a crisis plan Assess patient's current use of skills Move to treatment—either problem solving or use distress tolerance/crisis management skills
The splitting patient (I hate my doctor, they hate me; the stories don't match) *Ex. Spends the whole session complaining about PCP; PCP has a story different from patient's*	Validate patient's perspective Support and problem-solve engagement with treating providers Promote use of skills in working with treatment team Create consistent schedule and consolidate care with treating providers
Multiple medical complaints *Ex. Presents many new problems at each visit and never seems satisfied with care*	Perform appropriate and indicated medical work-ups or obtain records from prior treatment Evaluate for comorbid anxiety, mood, or substance use disorders Ask patient to prioritize concerns for each visit. Say, "We have time today to talk about two of these items; which two seem most pressing to you?" Schedule regular appointments Encourage patient decision-making Validate the emotion, if not necessarily the symptoms. Say, "I can see how worried you are about this." Move to treatment—either problem solving or use distress tolerance/crisis management skills

Table 9.6 (*Continued*)

Patient presentation	Behavioral strategies
Suspected malingering Ex. *Patient's symptoms or complaints do not match objective data; suspicion of external motivation such as litigation or disability claim*	Perform appropriate and indicated medical work-ups or obtain records from prior treatment Assess for comorbid substance abuse, anxiety, depression Reassure patient there is no "serious" illness and that improvement is expected. Allow patient to "save face" Enhance engagement in other positive health behaviors
The Non-Engaged Patient **The disappearing patient, who only comes in crisis** Ex. *Presents in crisis, then no shows for several visits, then re-presents in crisis*	Triage (safety planning, problem solve, crisis manage) Assess their current use of skills Move to treatment—either problem solving or use distress tolerance/crisis management skills Create consistent schedule and consolidate care with treating providers Reinforce any noncrisis driven interactions
The patient who won't talk Ex. *Silent; Provider generates all ideas/goals*	Focus solely on engagement (defer treatment) Try to identify motivations for coming in and THEIR treatment goals (not your own)—ask "If our time was spent well, how would you know?"
The patient who always agrees, but never follows through Ex. *Does not complete homework; makes many "great" excuses; says "likes" the idea but does not follow through*	Do more assessment to understand function of "agreeing" behavior • Is it a trust issue and lack of engagement (i.e., pushing for treatment before you have good credibility)? • Is it a cultural issue (i.e., agreeing out of respect)? • Is it a goal issue (i.e., the goal is too overwhelming or the goal is not aligned well with the patient's goals) • Is it a lack of understanding or lack of skill?

(Continued)

Table 9.6 (*Continued*)

Patient presentation	Behavioral strategies
The patient who wants something you can't offer (medication seeking, services, "cures") Ex: *Makes many demands or voices high expectations (housing fix, time, medications)*	Do more assessment to understand function of the request • Is it a problem you can actually address? • Do they have distress tolerance skills to handle having a problem they can't solve? Focus on engagement Better align treatment with patient goals Acknowledge limitations (yours and theirs) Be honest with yourself and with patient about what you will and won't do (e.g., if benzos aren't indicated, explain to the patient that you won't be prescribing them and why) Don't be ambiguous. Don't overpromise.

Back to the case

Step 4: The team decided that the problematic behavior they were going to try to limit was erratic attendance and always in crisis. The positive behavior that they would reward would be arriving consistently and not always in crisis. The team developed the following plan:

• Patient would no longer be seen in the same day if more than 10 minutes late
• All providers were to keep to scheduled appointment times (do not go over allotted time)
• All providers were to keep interactions during business hours only (no extending appointments after clinic hours)
• All providers were to praise and encourage patient during each session and encourage patient's ability to succeed

Although the patient had other problematic behaviors such as always being in distress and frequently crying through the entire appointment, the team decided to address the lateness first. The theory was that if they had more time in their appointments, then they would have more time to assess and address the tearfulness.

Table 9.7 Potential pitfalls to developing a team-based behavioral approach to addressing the difficult situation

Potential pitfalls of step 4	How to mediate it
Patient is running late and they really have a critical issue	If you anticipate this may be a problem, set a policy ahead of time. For example, the policy may be that the patient can call if they are running late and see if they can be rescheduled for later in the day if there are openings (although with the understanding that the answer may be no).
	Alternatively, providers could agree ahead of time that the patient can have "one free pass" or a "one time exception" to be used at the patient's discretion. However, once the "free pass" has been used, then no more exceptions will be made.
Team members are reluctant to change their approach	Elicit the provider's specific concerns about following the plan.
	Educate the provider on the revised approach. For example, say, "We have the best chance of success if everyone agrees to be consistent in our approach to this patient."
	Or, "In order to effectively help this patient, we need to have a plan in place."
	Or, "It may be difficult at the beginning, but ultimately this is in the patient's best interest."
The patient is reluctant to follow the plan	Do more assessment of the patient's concerns. Try to problem-solve concerns.
	• Are they feeling punished by the plan?
	• Is the patient's real problem/motivation for being there being addressed?
	• Are there extenuating psychosocial contributions (domestic violence? immigration issues? financial or transportation difficulties? childcare?)
	• Are there comorbid disorders that contribute to the patient's behavior? Is there active substance abuse?
	• Are there tweaks that could be made that would be more agreeable to the patient but would still accomplish the team's goals?
	Validate the patient's concerns. Try to link the patient's goals for treatment with the team's goals. For example, say, "In order for our team to help you with your chronic pain, we need to be able to see you for the full appointment time each time."
	Or, "We want to get you the best care and in order to do that, we need to have these policies in place."
	Or, "We get upset when you yell at us and that makes it difficult for us to try to address your specific health concerns."
	Or, "It is hard for us to know how to best help you when you come to clinic intoxicated."

Step 5: Address your needs for support in working with this patient.

General principle

Providers need support and validation to manage the stress of working with challenging situations.

Ask the question

- What kind of support do I need to work effectively in difficult situations?
- What kind of support does the team need to work effectively in difficult situations?

The burden of difficult clinical situations is profound and can be damaging over time. When providers feel ill-equipped to manage a difficult situation, their identity as helper and healer is threatened. By using the steps outlined in this chapter, it is hoped that providers in primary care settings will feel more empowered and competent in coming up with practical, targeted plans to improve these difficult encounters. A final, and equally important step, is to make a plan to support yourself and your team.

Practical strategies for support include:

- Acknowledge your own and the system's limitations—maintain perspective on what you can and can't affect.
- Practice good self-care for the emotional distress from your job (and life).
- Validate your efforts and the efforts of other members of your team.
- Seek team and peer support. Don't "go it alone."
- Get good consultation if needed.

Back to the case

Step 5. The team developed the following plan for self-care:

- Congratulate and encourage each other for sticking to the plan
- Being thoughtful about the appointment time (scheduling her at a time of day that works for both patient and provider)
- Providers would take a few minutes before and after appointments with her to prepare, soothe, breathe, and so on.
- Acknowledge that improvement was going to be slow, but hanging in there was progress
- Providers would periodically check in to discuss how the plan is going, make adjustments, and support each other's efforts
- Providers would look to each other for support
- Validate each other's success at keeping boundaries

Summary

Five steps to improve difficult clinical situations

Step 1: Name the emotions that working with the patient evokes in you.

Step 2: Define the patient's problematic behaviors in a concrete, specific, and observable way.

Step 3: Identify provider problematic behaviors (your own and your team's).

Step 4: Develop a team-based behavioral approach to addressing the difficult situation.

Step 5: Address your needs for support in working with this patient

References

Baum, N. H. (2002). 12 tips for dealing with difficult patients. *Geriatrics, 57*(11), 55–7.

Cannarella Lorenzetti, R., Jacques, C. H., Donovan, C., Cottrell, S., & Buck, J. (2013). Managing difficult encounters: understanding physician, patient, and situational factors. *American Family Physician, 87*(6), 419–25.

Grooves, J. (1978). Taking care of the hateful patient. *New England Journal of Medicine, 293*(16), 883–887.

Haas, L. J., Leiser, J. P., Magill, M. K., & Sanyer, O. N. (2005). Management of the difficult patient. *American Family Physician, 72*(10), 2063–8.

Platt, F. W., & Gordon, G. H. (1999). *Field guide to the difficult patient interview.* Philadelphia, Pennsylvania: Lippincott Williams & Wilkins.

Chapter 10 Evidence-Based Behavioral Interventions for the Collaborative Care Team

Kari A. Stephens and Stacy Shaw Welch

How can each member of the team use this chapter?

Patient: The overview of how evidence-based behavioral interventions are included in treatment will be helpful in understanding what to include and how to work best with the team to make treatment most effective and relevant to the patient.

PCP: Understanding the steps involved in using evidence-based behavioral interventions will help the PCP refer patients to this type of treatment and help facilitate the success of treatment. Some clinical skills, such as engagement building by the PCP and BHP, may also be helpful.

BHP: BHPs deliver the bulk of evidence-based interventions, and it is important to understand the overall therapeutic process in the context of a team. Understanding the different stages of the therapeutic process and how behavioral interventions are incorporated in Collaborative Care teams will help the BHPs use these interventions most effectively.

PC: Facilitating and consulting with the BHPs and PCPs about the overall therapeutic process and implementation of evidence-based behavioral interventions can improve care by supporting evidence-based and accountable care with a patient-centered approach. PCs can support the team in problem-solving poor engagement or treatment response.

Integrated Care: Creating Effective Mental and Primary Health Care Teams, First Edition.
Anna Ratzliff, Jürgen Unützer, Wayne Katon, and Kari A. Stephens.

Overview

Evidence-based behavioral interventions are well-established as effective treatments for improving mental and physical health in primary care settings. Many mental health issues that present in primary care can be treated with behavioral counseling techniques, including depression, anxiety, substance abuse, and somatization issues. Behavioral interventions can also support changes needed to improve chronic disease management (e.g., diabetes) and substantially improve health outcomes and decrease medical costs. Many of the previous chapters describe specific behavioral interventions that the team can use in the context of various mental health related issues. This chapter provides an overview of how behavioral interventions play a key role in Collaborative Care teams. We also provide a toolkit to help assess teams' behavioral intervention skills and identify any critical gaps needed to deliver these treatments in primary care settings.

Continuum of care

Engaging patients in psychological/behavioral interventions includes good engagement, followed by assessment, management of crises as needed, and treatment. **Engagement** occurs when both the clinician and patient agree on what the problems are and how they should be treated, and the patient is actively participating in the treatment process. A common pitfall for providers can be to jump too quickly into treatment before engagement exists or a proper assessment has been done to guide appropriate treatment planning. Crises often arise that derail treatment and should be considered the rule, not the exception. It is important that all stages of the continuum be addressed throughout care to ensure treatment is successful.

Figure 10.1 shows relationships among these stages. Notably engagement is needed throughout the psychotherapeutic process, and that stages are connected. Assessment guides treatment planning. Crises must be adequately managed. Assessment, crisis management, and treatment can only occur if engagement is sufficient. Once treatment has begun, clinicians may need to return again and again to engagement, assessment, and crisis planning as needed. This could occur in any order, and sometimes all within one session. Flexibility is encouraged for the purpose of ensuring that treatment occurs and fosters real, measurable change in patients' lives.

Core skills

Every BHP should have a set of core skills for offering foundational behavioral interventions (see Table 10.1). These skills include a nonjudgmental stance

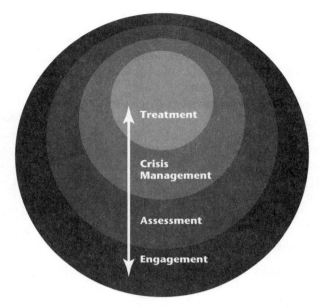

Figure 10.1 The psychotherapeutic process can move between stages over the course of treatment, but each stage must be addressed for treatment to be effective both at the team and individual provider levels.

Table 10.1 Core skills BHPs should have as an effective Collaborative Care team provider

Core Skills for Behavioral Interventions	<ul><li>Nonjudgmental stance of acceptance and understanding</li><li>Active listening skills</li><li>Competency in assessing and applying stages of change, supported by some modality of treatment such as Motivational Interviewing</li><li>Competency in several evidence-based behavioral treatments, to include cognitive behavioral therapies and/or solution-oriented therapies</li></ul>

and active listening skills that allow the BHP to create good engagement with patients. These skills also help them assess for ambivalence about treatment engagement and/or the kinds of behavioral changes that might be required.

Stages of change involve a continuum of readiness to change spanning from *precontemplation* (when patients may be most defensive and spending the least amount of time considering change) to *contemplation, preparation, action,* and finally *maintenance* of change. BHPs and PCPs should be familiar with these stages and able to assess which stage a patient may be in when working with that patient to make changes. For example, when a PCP refers a patient to a BHP, many patients will be ambivalent about engaging. PCPs will need to be prepared to understand why and continue to work with patients to help them engage over time with the BHP. Without a good understanding of stages of change, providers experience common pitfalls such as pushing patients for change before they are ready. One example pitfall includes encouraging action such as giving behavioral homework when there is little buy-in because the patient is still in precontemplation and does not yet think this behavioral homework is something that warrants investment. Ideally the whole team will assess for the stage of change and help each other target the appropriate level of intervention.

Engagement strategies

Engagement, and ultimately good treatment outcomes, rely on a strong alliance between the patient and provider. Strong alliances require an interpersonal connection or bond between the provider and patient, shared goals, and shared tasks (see Table 10.2). In Collaborative Care teams, patients form alliances with both the individual providers and the team. Providers working on Collaborative Care teams must monitor and nurture strong alliances with patients not just individually, but also with the entire team. This means weak alliances with individual providers and lack of agreement or consistency on team treatment goals and tasks can weaken the team alliance and lead to poor engagement and treatment outcome.

Providers sometimes assume that patients are in agreement on goals and tasks, but this should be something that is openly discussed on a regular basis with patients to make sure these assumptions are correct. If providers work to create and maintain a strong alliance, patient-centered goals can be set and

Table 10.2 Engagement strategies for Collaborative Care

Engagement Strategies	**Bond:** A bond between patient and provider is fostered by patients both feeling listened to and feeling accepted by a provider.
	Shared Goals: The patient and provider must have agreed-upon goals for treatment that both parties endorse as meaningful.
	Shared Tasks: The patient and provider must have agreed-upon tasks that must be done to achieve the goals.

maintained throughout treatment (see Chapter 1 for more information on specifics for goal setting).

Therapeutic alliance

Bond: A bond between patient and provider is fostered by patients both feeling listened to and feeling accepted by a provider; providers must demonstrate listening skills to patients through reflective listening skills so patients can determine whether providers have heard what they are trying to message; providers can also demonstrate acceptance by conveying a nonjudgmental stance even in difficult situations, such as when patients do not show up for appointments, are highly emotional in and outside of appointments with providers, or fail to complete agreed upon tasks—patients need to feel they can "fail" without being judged or quickly abandoned by a provider.

Team bond: When patient alliances with providers are poor, providers with strong alliances can often help patients problem solve issues with other providers. For example, the BHP can support patients around frustrations with medical providers when they feel they aren't listened to, feel the overall care plan is unclear, or disagree with the approach. BHPs often have more time to listen and engage patients and can help patients stay engaged in crucial medical care. Alternatively, PCPs can encourage engagement with a BHP even though the changes in behavior being worked on are difficult.

Shared goals: The patient and provider must have agreed-upon goals for treatment that both parties endorse as meaningful; setting goals (e.g., behavioral intervention treatment, medication treatment) that patients are not bought into will not be patient-centric or effective; the patient must help determine the goals for treatment.

Shared team goals: The team must have some agreement and cohesiveness to their treatment goals to make sure they stay patient-centered and not overwhelm the patients with disjointed care plans (i.e., the BHP can help clarify the overall team plan by facilitating communication between providers and the patient, help the team negotiate goals so they remain realistic and in line with what the patient wants).

Shared tasks: The patient and provider must have agreed-upon tasks that must be completed to achieve the goals. Patients must see the direct connection between tasks they are being asked to complete (e.g., activity tracking, physical exercise, exposure exercises) and their goals (e.g., better mood) or they are not likely to complete the tasks, leading to disengaged patients and frustrated providers.

Shared team tasks: The team can work together to track on tasks and give the patient support in making what are often difficult behavioral changes needed to reach their treatment goals.

Patient goals often shift during treatment. Checking in among the team to make sure the patient feels that the most important goals are being addressed in care is very important to maintaining good engagement and reaching good outcomes. Many patients in primary care are somatically focused and wish to address physical ailments. They are often unaware or reluctant to address mental health issues. Strong alliances between providers on the care team can help move patients into readiness to address mental health issues by helping make clear connections for patients between physical issues and mental health issues. For example, chronic pain, insomnia, or poor management of diabetes are common reasons patients seek care. Mood or anxiety issues both exacerbate these issues and can complicate treatment. A strong alliance that includes setting clear patient-centered goals can often help bridge the gap between the relevance of mental health care with their care for physical ailments for many patients. Creating a strong alliance can take patience and skill to avoid jumping too quickly into mental health treatment before goals are mutually set.

Crisis management

Some patients can present in crisis, even before engagement has solidified. If a patient presents in crisis, the team must first assess for safety to address any imminent risk of self-harm or harm to others (see Chapter 1 and the appendix for an example of a safety protocol). Assuming minimal imminent risk, which is true in the majority of cases, providers should focus on engagement before focusing on crisis management skill building. If engagement is strong, providers can triage patients into either problem solving or, if the problem cannot be solved immediately, working on skills to develop better crisis management (e.g., distress tolerance—see Table 10.3). A common

Table 10.3 Distress tolerance strategies BHPs should have as an effective Collaborative Care team provider

Distress Tolerance Strategies	• Self-soothe
	• Distraction
	• Imagery
	• Meditation and affirmation
	• Relaxation
	• Take some time out of the situation
	• Positive self-talk
	• Be creative
	• Physical strategies to weather intense emotions

pitfall for providers is to continue to push for treatment (e.g., behavioral activation, reducing alcohol/drug use) without centering on addressing a crisis for the patient, which can lead to poor engagement and treatment dropout or failure.

In Collaborative Care teams, BHPs can often help the team create behavioral plans to help the patients make shifts to improve crisis management. Sometimes ongoing crises that create chronic high stress and frustration for patients and providers alike can create challenging clinical issues for teams (e.g., high provider frustration, high utilization, frequent no-shows or cancellations). Having a BHP as a resource for safety assessments and difficult clinical situations that involve problematic behavioral patterns can improve the clinic team's overall ability to respond effectively and support providers who often feel overwhelmed by these situations. Left unaddressed, these situations can burn out teams and, in a vicious cycle, lower patient engagement even further. BHPs can lead the creation of behavioral plans in consultation with the PCP and PC to address these situations, which can lead to teams being more effective and avoiding burnout (see Chapter 9).

Treatment

Numerous behavioral interventions have been found to be effective in primary care settings (see Table 10.4). Behavioral interventions should be directly tied to case formulations after initial assessments are completed and should be adjusted over time as formulations change, engagement increases or wavers, and as goals progress. BHPs should have competency in several behavioral interventions that have been shown to be effective as brief treatments and/or adapted for primary care settings (consistent with the principle of evidence based care). PCs should have familiarity of these common evidence-based behavioral treatments so they can support their use among the team. The most common evidence based interventions in primary care settings have typically included cognitive behavioral treatments, solution-oriented therapies, and Motivational Interviewing. Specific evidence based treatments mentioned in the disorder specific chapters are summarized below (see Table 10.4). In addition to the evidence based treatments listed below, the chapters discuss many behavioral strategies individual providers and teams can use to enhance effectiveness of treatment delivery specific to each category of disorder.

Offering behavioral interventions in Collaborative Care teams differs from specialty care settings in that patients can lack motivation to engage in mental health treatment, often have low understanding of the relevance of these treatments, and may be in the process of being diagnosed with a mental health

Table 10.4 Specific evidence-based behavioral interventions for primary care Collaborative Care teams

Mental health disorder	Evidence based behavioral treatments
Mood Disorders— Major Depression (Chapter 2)	• Cognitive behavioral therapy (CBT) for depression • Problem solving therapy (PST) • Behavioral activation (BA) • Interpersonal therapy for primary care (IPT)
Mood Disorders— Bipolar Disorders	• CBT • Family-focused therapy • Social rhythm therapy • Daily routine and activity planning • Sleep hygiene • Depression treatments • Interpersonal therapy • Motivational Interviewing for treatment adherence
Anxiety and Trauma Disorders (Chapter 4)	• CBT treatments for anxiety • Modular Anxiety Therapy—CBT components of exposure and anxiety management behavioral strategies adapted for primary care
Psychotic Disorders (Chapter 5)	• CBT for psychosis • Coping strategies to improve distress from delusions • Medication adherence behavioral support
Substance Use Disorders (Chapter 6)	• Motivational Interviewing • Cognitive behavioral coping skills therapy • Relapse Prevention • 12-Step Facilitation • Others: contingency management, community-reinforcement approaches, matrix model
Chronic Pain (Chapter 7)	• CBT targeting: Negative thoughts about pain Pain interference Acceptance of chronic pain Self-management strategies (i.e., relaxation, pacing) Behavioral change/routine development
Attention-Deficit Hyperactivity Disorder (ADHD) (Chapter 8)	• Psychoeducation • CBT targeting daily life skills • Self-management skills training • Vocational counseling • Neurofeedback • ADHD coaching • Parent behavioral training for adolescents and children

disorder for the first time. Engagement must be strong at the provider and team level because lacking engagement in either realm can weaken the overall treatment effectiveness (i.e., if treatment goals conflict across providers or an alliance is weak with an individual provider, patients' engagement in care may suffer). Given these challenges, the following tips may help improve treatment engagement.

Box 1: Successful behavioral treatment tips in primary care

Engagement: Make sure the patient is engaged in working with the BHP. If the patient is not engaged, take time to create and grow a strong alliance before moving too quickly to behavioral interventions

Time limited care: Patients should be told early in the engagement process that the behavioral interventions will be brief; many patients like hearing treatment will be brief and it can help break stereotypes that "therapy" is a long involved process with no potential for short-term gains.

Target one problem at a time: Many patients present with complex formulations, multiple comorbidities, crises, and very difficult life problems, and sometimes all of the above; while thorough assessments are important, starting simply by targeting one top problem to treat can often lead to better outcomes and lower the risk of trying to do too much at once, which can lead to little to no improvement.

Psychoeducation: Offering psychoeducation about mental health disorders, symptoms, care processes, and complications of comorbid mental and physical illness in a way that is consistent across the team can make for a good experience for the patient and foster engagement. Disjointed or contradicting information from the PCP and BHP can do the opposite and lead to confusion and poor engagement by the patient. It is not uncommon for patients to hear very divergent explanations of mental heath conditions and treatments within the same system.

Make the pitch! Making a pitch for treatment means giving a compelling case as early as possible to patients for the benefits of a behavioral intervention. The pitch should be deliberate, compelling, and concise so that they give direct information on the relevance of behavioral interventions to the patient's goals. Many patients in primary care are naïve to the utility and use of behavioral treatments and even the importance of mental health. They may need time to move toward readiness to engage in behavioral interventions; spending time on engagement and gaining buy-in to treatment is not wasted time, but rather a much more efficient path to good care than pushing treatment when patients either do not understand the rationale or are not ready to engage.

Offer many treatment options: Offer patients as many options for care as possible so they can drive choice to help with keeping treatment patient-centric; try to be as unbiased as possible when offering treatment choices and discuss the pros and cons of all treatment options; be eclectic in treatment, given that one size does not fit all (i.e., some people prefer medication, some people prefer psychotherapy, some prefer both).

Continuous goal setting: Check in frequently to make sure goals are in alignment with treatment efforts and that patients have good buy-in to the treatment plan; make sure the team goals reflect one reasonable plan that the patient agrees with.

Measure progress on goals and symptoms: Keep metrics of goal tracking and symptom severity front and center in the dialogue with patients so useful feedback is given, engagement is motivated, and changes in care can be applied when progress is stalled. Keep in mind the best treatment is the one that works, so measurement-based care is key to determining whether the treatment is worth continuing and when care needs to be increased. At times, the level of care needed may be more appropriate for a mental health specialist in a community mental health center if available and measuring progress can help speed this type of triage.

Help with poor alliance issues: Patients may feel comfortable discussing frustrations with medical care and with medical providers with their BHP; helping patients navigate poor alliances with other providers by coaching them with communication, providing safe harbor for these frustrations, and advocating for patient-centered goals with the entire treatment team can help patients engage more effective medical interventions.

Workforce development/on-going training: Make sure skills for emerging evidence-based brief behavioral interventions are kept up to date; health care reform is driving adoption and adaptation of behavioral treatments and the workforce is often behind in acquiring knowledge and skills needed to offer these treatments; these innovations can include mobile and online technologies that both augment treatment directly for patients and trainings for providers.

Relapse prevention

Behavioral interventions in primary care are typically brief and should be terminated with a clear relapse prevention plan that offers a summary of appropriate behavioral planning that the patient should continue after treatment ends (See Table 10.5). It is helpful to communicate this before

Table 10.5 Relapse prevention planning

Relapse Prevention	<ul><li>Complete at the end of an episode of care</li><li>Communicate to all team members</li><li>Include all interventions that helped the patient improve (both medication and behavioral treatments)</li><li>Include early warning signs and how to return to care</li></ul>

and during termination of treatment, and also to ensure that the relapse prevention plan is communicated to the PCP. The PC consults as needed to the content. Emphasizing progress and gains to the patient and to the team are key to both helping patients maintain gains and helping the team buy-in to BHP roles in the care of patients. It is important for providers and patients to constantly have reminders that if problems arise in the future, it may not be because the treatment failed, but because the patient stopped doing the treatment. Constant encouragement to recall gains and reengage the use of skills gained during treatment is needed from all team members.

Summary

Evidence-based behavioral interventions are an important resource for teams to deliver Collaborative Care. The case example presented below illustrates how behavioral interventions support the delivery of the five principles of Collaborative Care in the context of a typical patient seen in primary care.

Case example

Mr. A, a 31-year-old male, presents to his primary care doctor asking for "sleeping pills." His PCP takes a history and finds out he has not been sleeping for the last month, he has been struggling to get work and missed a few days, he has difficulty concentrating, and his wife is frustrated because he has "just checked out." His PCP suspects he may be experiencing depression.

Patient centered team care: Mr. A's main concern is sleep, and the team has also recognized he is suffering from depression. The BHP works to develop engagement by centering on sleep issues and offering education about depression. The BHP recognizes engagement must be established before treatment adherence can be expected and makes sure Mr. A is in agreement with the treatment goals.

Population-based care: The BHP tracks Mr. A's care in a registry. When Mr. A misses his first follow-up appointment, the BHP proactively reaches out to the patient to reengage him. As engagement develops, the care plan shifts from behavioral interventions for sleep to additionally address depression.

Measurement-based treatment to target: The BHP works in regular assessments on progress toward goals, including measures of depression, linking behavioral interventions to the measures. Depression symptoms continue at first with the main focus on sleep, and the BHP is able to adjust treatment to both begin behavioral interventions for depression, in addition to addressing conflicts with his wife and issues with sleep, while working with the team to support medication adjustments.

Evidence-based care: Mr. A is given information by the PCP and the BHP that both sleep and depression can be most effectively treated with a combination of medication and behavioral interventions. The BHP uses behavioral activation as Mr. A becomes more engaged in treatment for depression to help him reach his goals.

Accountable care: The team works to assess both Mr. A's individual treatment trajectory and the population of patients being treated. The team looks at how efficiently and appropriately behavioral interventions were applied to make sure this mode of treatment is able to be offered systematically across the population when appropriate.

Mr. A's depression goes into remission with his sleep much improved, and he is able to continue working and improve his relationship with his wife. Mr. A has a plan for relapse prevention, including maintaining behavioral changes gained during treatment.

Resources

General:

- Evidence-Based Behavioral Practice (EBBP) offers an online resources for behavioral therapies http://www.ebbp.org/skillsBasedResources.html
- National Institute for Health and Care Excellence (NICE) offers information and guidance for treatment of common mental health conditions in primary care https://www.nice.org.uk/guidancemenu/conditions-and-diseases/mental-health-and-behavioural-conditions
- The Association for Behavioral and Cognitive Therapies offers online clinical resources for evidence based practices http://www.abct.org/Resources/?m=mResources&fa=ClinicalResources

Engagement and Motivational Interviewing:

- Rollnick, S., Miller, W. R., & Butler, C. C. (2007). *Motivational Interviewing in Health Care: Helping Patients Change Behavior (Applications of Motivational Interviewing)*. New York, NY: Guilford Press.

Chapter 11 **Evidence-Based Psychopharmacology for the Collaborative Care Team**

David A. Harrison and Anna Ratzliff

How can each member of the team use this chapter?

Patient: Using the concise summaries of common medications as a guide, it may be helpful to review common side effects as well as compare medications when working with the team to choose treatments. Additionally, cautions and other risks are reviewed to aid in informed consent. Cost information is provided to help guide medication choice.

PCP: The concise prescribing protocols will be helpful for initiating treatment, titrating to target dose, and monitoring appropriately. Safety information and drug-drug interactions are also available for quick reference.

BHP: These protocols will add in taking accurate history of medications (classes, both generic and brand name, typical doses) as well as being able to provide psychoeducation to patient about medications. For most BHP, it would be in the scope of practice to assess for concerns about medications and side effects and connect patient to team as needed to address these.

PC: These concise prescribing directions can be included in notes to help PCP prescribe medications more easily and accurately. This will facilitate evidence-based recommendations.

Overview

Psychiatric consultants recognized early on that PCPs and BHPs would benefit from standardized medication instructions for use in primary care. Based on this need a quick reference guide (Table 11.1) and" after,

Integrated Care: Creating Effective Mental and Primary Health Care Teams, First Edition.
Anna Ratzliff, Jürgen Unützer, Wayne Katon, and Kari A. Stephens.

a collection of succinct prescribing protocols (see below) for commonly prescribed psychotropic medications were developed and tailored to the outpatient setting. These prescribing protocols integrated the drug's FDA label information and information gathered from the published literature, including practice guidelines, together with the clinical prescribing experience of the psychiatric prescribers participating in the Collaborative Care setting. To maximize usability, the prescribing protocols were organized into three sections: dosing information, monitoring, and general information.

The section on **dosing information** is designed to make the prescribing process more straightforward by listing prescribing instructions—including requirements for baseline lab work, if needed—on a week-by-week basis. The dosing protocol includes a **starting dose**, an **initial target dose**, a **typical dosage range**, and a **maximum dose,** where appropriate. As a general rule, doses in elderly and medically debilitated patients should be lower both initially and as target dosages. When specified in the FDA label information, this information will be provided. Where appropriate, dosing instructions are listed for multiple indications and for off-label use. With some medications, e.g., Lamictal, an FDA-recommended tapering protocol is listed. In most cases, general tapering recommendations are provided.

A **monitoring** section was included due to the increasingly recognized importance of tracking metabolic parameters, QTc prolongation, and drug levels when available.

The **general information** section is the longest of the three and includes information about medications thought to be clinically relevant to the prescribers. The information in this section includes:

Mechanism of action: describes the commonly accepted mechanism of action of a drug, recognizing that our understanding of how a psychotropic medication works is often quite incomplete.

FDA indications: delineates the FDA indications for a medication.

Off-label indications: describes well-accepted and often evidence-based off-label uses for a medication.

Pharmacokinetics: lists the $T\frac{1}{2}$ for a medication from the FDA label information, when available. Primarily includes information about the parent compound, but where appropriate (e.g., fluoxetine) includes information about metabolites.

Common side effects: lists common side effects by percentage, when available, from label information on the FDA website. As a general rule the side effect is listed if it occurs at a frequency above 5 percent, is twice placebo, or is clinically relevant. In medications with multiple indications, side effects are listed for more than one indication for the most common uses of the medication.

Black-box warning: summarizes the black-box information for a medication.

Contraindications: summarizes the contraindications for a medication.

Warning and precautions: lists the *specific* medication-related warnings and precautions found in the FDA label information together with clinically significant medication concerns where appropriate. For example, suicidality is not listed as a side effect of antipsychotics when used to treat schizophrenia, as the warning in this case is related to the illness as opposed to the medication. On the other hand, suicidality is mentioned as a warning in an antipsychotic that used for treatment of unipolar or bipolar depression.

Metabolism/Pharmacogenomics: lists information about metabolism and significant pharmacogenomics concerns as mentioned in the FDA label or in the research literature, e.g., the use of fluoxetine in CYP2D6 poor metabolizers.

Significant drug-drug interactions: lists significant drug-drug interactions. Given the complexity of drug-drug interactions with some medications, it may be appropriate to consult with a pharmacist before prescribing a medication.

Pregnancy: Reports pregnancy safety category information based on the FDA label information.

Lactation: Describes safety during lactation on the basis of FDA label information and published reports. Safety is categorized as: "Compatible," "Excreted/Use Caution," "Excreted/Not Recommended," "Contraindicated," and "No data/Not recommended."

Dosage information: lists the available medication forms, e.g., tablet vs. capsule.

Generic available: reports whether a generic form of a medication is available.

Cost: categorizes the cost of medications based on information from GoodRx.com in four categories: inexpensive (¢) < $20, moderately expensive ($) $20–100, expensive ($$) $101–250, and very expensive ($$$) > $250.

Currently the quick reference guide and prescribing protocols are in broad and daily use in the Mental Health Integration Program in Washington State. That being said, it is important to consider the pros and cons of these protocols. These prescribing protocols are intended to facilitate the best possible prescribing practices in the outpatient setting. They should always be used with discrimination and where questions arise, e.g., as new prescribing information comes out about a medication, in consultation with a pharmacist and with current FDA drug label guidelines (available at http://www.accessdata.fda.gov/scripts/cder/drugsatfda/).

Table 11.1 Quick reference guide: Commonly prescribed psychotropic medications

Name generic (trade)	Dosage	Key clinical information
	Antidepressant medications*	
Bupropion (Well-butrin)	Start: IR-100 mg bid X 7d, then ↑ to 100 mg tid; SR-150 mg qam X 7d then ↑ to 150 mg bid; XL-150 mg qam X 7d, then ↑ to 300 mg qam. Range: 300–450 mg/day.	Novel mechanism; Contraindicated in seizure disorder and history of TBI because it decreases seizure threshold; stimulating; not good for treating anxiety disorders; 2nd line TX for ADHD; abuse potential. P: C; L: Excreted/Use Caution. ¢ IR/SR/XL.
Citalopram (Celexa)	Start: 20 mg qday X 7d, then ↑ to 40 mg. MAX: 40 mg qday (MAX: 20 mg qday if ≥60 y/o, hepatically impaired, a CYP2C19 poor metabolizer, or taking a CYP2C19 inhibitor).	Well-tolerated SSRI; minimal CYP450 interactions; good choice for anxious pt. Caution: QTc prolongation. P: C; L: Excreted/Use caution. ¢
Duloxetine (Cymbalta)	Start: 30 mg qday X 7d, then ↑ to 60 mg qday. Range: 60–120 mg/day.	SNRI; TX for neuropathic pain; need to monitor BP; 2nd line TX for ADHD. P: C; L: Excreted/Not recommended. $
Escitalopram (Lexapro)	Start: 5 mg qday X 7d, then ↑ to 10 mg qday. Range 10–20 mg/d (~3X potent vs. Celexa).	Best-tolerated SSRIs; minimal CYP450 interactions. Good choice for anxious pt. P: C; L: Excreted/Use caution. ¢
Fluoxetine (Prozac)	Start: 10 mg qam X 7d, then ↑ to 20 mg qday. Range: 20–60 mg/day.	More activating than other SSRIs; long half-life reduces withdrawal (t $^1/_2$ = 4–6 d). P: C; L: Excreted/Not recommended. ¢
Mirtazapine (Remeron)	Start: 15 mg qhs. X 7d, then ↑ to 30 mg qhs. Range: 30–60 mg/qhs.	Novel mechanism; Sedating and appetite promoting; Neutropenia risk so avoid in the immunosupressed. P: C; L: Excreted/Use caution. ¢
Nortriptyline (Pamelor)	Start: 25 mg qhs X 7d, then ↑ 25 mg qhs - q weekly to 75 mg qhs. Range: 75–150 mg/day.	TCA; Sedating; TX for neuropathic pain; Baseline EKG; Max dosing in the elderly: 100 mg; Lethal in overdose. P: D; L: Excreted/Use caution. ¢

(Continued)

Table 11.1 (*Continued*)

Name generic (trade)	Dosage	Key clinical information
*Antidepressant medications**		
Paroxetine (Paxil)	Start: 10 mg qhs X 7d, then ↑ to 20 mg qday. Range: 20–60 mg/day.	SSRI; Anticholinergic; sedating; Significant withdrawal syndrome. P: D; L: Excreted/Use caution. ¢
Sertraline (Zoloft)	Start: 25 mg qam X 7d, then ↑ to 50 mg qday. Range: 50–200 mg/day.	SSRI; limited CYP 450 interactions; mildly activating. P: C; L: Compatible. ¢
Venlafaxine (Effexor)	Start: IR-37.5 mg bid X 7d, then ↑ to 75 mg bid; ER-75 mg qam X 7d, then ↑ to 150 qAM. Range: 150–375 mg/day.	SNRI. More agitation & GI side effects than SSRIs; TX for neuropathic pain at 225 mg and above; need to monitor BP; Significant withdrawal syndrome. P: C; L: Excreted/Not recommended. ¢ IR $ ER.
Antianxiety and sleep (hypnotic) medications		
Alprazolam (Xanax)	Start: IR-0.25-0.5 mg tid. Usual MAX: 4 mg/d. ER-0.5–1mg qAM Usual MAX: 3–6 mg/d	Equiv. dose: 0.50 mg. Onset: intermediate (1–2 hrs). T$\frac{1}{2}$: 11 hrs. More addictive than other benzos and has uniquely problematic withdrawal syndrome. Try to avoid as 1st line tx. Significant withdrawal syndrome. P: D; L: Excreted/Not recommended. ¢
Amitriptyline (Elavil)	Start: 10 mg qhs X 7d, then consider ↑ 25 mg qhs Range: 10–50 mg/qhs	TCA; Sedating; Helpful in neuropathic pain; Lethal in overdose. P: C; L: Excreted/Use caution. ¢
Clonazepam (Klonopin)	Start: 0.25 mg bid Usual MAX: 4 mg/day.	Equiv. dose: 0.25 mg. Onset: intermediate (1–4 hrs). T$\frac{1}{2}$: 30–40 hrs. Helpful in TX mania. P: D; L: Excreted/Not recommended. ¢
Diazepam (Valium)	Start: 5 mg bid. Usual MAX: 40 mg/day.	Equiv. dose: 5 mg. Onset: immediate. T$\frac{1}{2}$: 50–100 hrs. Caution with liver disease P: D; L: Excreted/Not recommended. ¢

Table 11.1 (*Continued*)

Name generic (trade)	Dosage	Key clinical information
	Antianxiety and sleep (hypnotic) medications	
Lorazepam (Ativan)	Start: 0.5–1 mg bid to tid. Usual MAX: 6 mg/day. Insomnia: 0.5–2 mg qhs.	Equiv. dose: 1 mg. Onset: intermediate. T½: 12 hrs. No active metabolites, so safer in liver dz. P: D; L: Excreted/Not recommended. ¢
Buspirone (BuSpar)	Start: 7.5 mg bid. Range: 10–30 mg bid.	Nonbenzo SSRI-like drug FDA approved for anxiety. May take 4–6 weeks to become fully effective. P: B; L: Not recommended. ¢
Hydroxyzine (Vistaril)	Start: 25–100 mg 3–4 X per day. Usual MAX: 400 mg/day.	Nonbenzo antihistamine FDA approved for anxiety. P: C (Not recommended in 1st trimester); L: Excreted/Not recommended. ¢
Prazosin (Minipress)	Start: 1 mg qhs. Increase q 2–3 d until symptoms abate. Usual MAX: 10 mg qhs.	BP med used to TX nightmares. Warn about orthostasis in AM after 1st dose & after each new dosage change. P: C; L: Not recommended. ¢
Trazodone (Desyrel)	Start: 25–50 mg qhs. Range: 50–150 mg qhs.	Commonly used as sleep aid; inform about priapism risk in men. P: C; L: Excreted/Not recommended. ¢
Temazepam (Restoril)	Start: 15 mg at bedtime. MAX: 45 mg qhs.	T½: 8.8 hrs. Older benzo hypnotic. No P450 metabolism. More potential for physical dependence. P: X; L: Excreted/Not recommended. ¢
Zolpidem (Ambien)	Start: 5–10 mg qhs. MAX: 20 mg qhs.	T½: 2.6 hrs. Potential for sleep-eating and sleep-driving. P: C; L: Excreted/Use caution. ¢ Available in longer acting form (CR $)

(*Continued*)

Table 11.1 (*Continued*)

Name generic (trade)	Dosage	Key clinical information
	Mood stabilizers	
Lithium	Start: 300 mg bid or 600 mg qhs. Target plasma level: acute mania & bipolar depression: 0.8–1.0 meq/L; Maintenance: 0.6–0.8 meq/L. Available in ER form dosed once daily (usually at HS, Lithobid & Eskalith). Plasma levels related to renal clearance.	Black box warning for toxicity. Teratogenic (cardiac malform.) and will need to inform women of childbearing age of this risk. Check Ca^{2+}, TSH and BMP before starting and q6–12 months thereafter. Advise pt about concurrent use of NSAIDS and HTN meds acting on the kidney as can decrease renal clearance. Lithium strongly antisuicidal. P: D (Not recommended in 1st trimester); L: Contraindicated. ¢
Divalproex (Depakote)	Start: 500 mg/day (bid, DR; qday, ER); increase dose as quickly as tolerated to clinical effect. Target plasma level: 75–100 mcg/mL (DR) & 85–125 mcg/ml (ER).	Multiple black box warnings including for hepatotoxicity, pancreatitis, and terato-genicity (need to inform women of childbearing age of this risk). Need to monitor LFTs, platelet counts, and coags initially and q3–6 mo. Weight gain common. P: D/X; L: Excreted/Use caution. $
Lamotrigine (Lamictal)	Start: 25 mg qday for wks 1 & 2; then 50 mg qday for wks 3 & 4; then 100 mg qday for wk 5; and finally 200 mg qday for wk 6+ (usual target dose). Dosage adjustment required when taken w/ drugs that ↓ (e.g., Tegretol, estrogens) or ↑ (Depakote) Lamictal concentration.	Black box warning for serious, life-threatening rashes requiring hospitalization and d/c of TX (Stevens-Johnson syndrome @ approx. 1:1–2000). No drug level monitoring typically required. Need to strictly follow published titration schedule. Fewer cognitive and appetite stimulating side effects. No evidence that doses above 200 mg more effective for mood. P: C; L: Excreted/Not recommended. ¢

Table 11.1 (*Continued*)

Name generic (trade)	Dosage	Key clinical information
	Antipsychotic/mood stabilizers**	
Aripiprazole (Abilify)	Mania. Start: 15 mg qday; Range: 15–30 mg/day. MDD adj tx. Start: 2–5 mg/day; adjust dose q1+ weeks by 2–5 mg. Range: 5–10 mg/day. MAX: 15 mg qday. Schizophrenia. Start: 10–15 mg/day; ↑ at 2 week intervals; Range: 10–15 mg/day; MAX: 30 mg/day.	EPS: Mild; TD Risk: Mild; Sedation: Mild; Metabolic Effects: Mild. Very long half-life: 75 hrs. Least amount of sexual side effects. FDA indication for adjunctive treatment of MDD. Potential increased suicidality in first few months. Need to screen glucose and lipids regularly. P: C; L: Excreted/Not recommended. $$$
Lurasidone (Latuda)	Bipolar Dep: Start: 20 mg qday; Initial target: 20 mg qday Range: 20–60 mg/day. MAX: 120 mg/day. Schizophrenia: Start/Initial Target: 40 mg qday Range: 40–160 mg qday. MAX: 160 mg/day.	EPS: Mild to Moderate; TD Risk: Unknown; Sedation: Moderate; Metabolic Effects: Mild. It is critical to take Latuda with food (at least 350 calories) for optimal absorption (increased by up to three fold). Also, grapefruit juice should be avoided. P: B; L: Excreted/Not recommended. $$$
Olanzapine (Zyprexa)	Mania. Start: 10 mg qhs; Range: 10–20 mg/qhs. MAX: 20 mg/day. Schizophrenia. Start: 5 mg qhs; ↑ by 5 mg qhs per week; Range: 10–15 mg qhs: MAX: 20 mg/day.	EPS: Mild; TD Risk: Mild; Sedation: Moderate; Metabolic Effects: Severe. Do not prescribe to diabetics. Need to screen glucose and lipids regularly. P: C; L: Excreted/Not recommended. ¢

(*Continued*)

Table 11.1 (*Continued*)

Name generic (trade)	Dosage	Key clinical information
	Antipsychotic/mood stabilizers**	
Quetiapine (Seroquel)	Bipolar Dep: Start: 50 mg qhs; Initial target: 300 mg qhs; Range: 300–600 mg/d. Mania. Start: 50 mg bid; Initial target: 200 mg bid. Range: 400–800 mg/d. MDD adj tx. Start: 50 mg qhs; Initial target: 150 mg qhs. Range: 150–300 mg/day. Schizophrenia. Start: 25 mg bid and increase by 50–100 mg/d (bid/tid). Initial target: 400 mg/d. Range: 400–800 mg/d.	EPS: Mild; TD Risk: Mild; Sedation: Moderate; Metabolic Effects: Moderate to severe. FDA indication for bipolar depression and adjunctive treatment of MDD. Potential increased suicidality in first few months. Need to screen glucose and lipids regularly. Abuse potential. Available in an extended release form: Seroquel XR. Avoid or use alternative in combination with methadone due to QTc prolongation. P: C; L: Excreted/Not recommended. IR $/XR $$$
Risperidone (Risperdal)	Mania. Start: 1–2 mg qhs;↑ by 1–2 mg/day per week. Range: 3–4 mg/day. MAX: 6 mg/day. Schizophrenia. Start: 1 mg qhs;↑ by 1 mg/day per week; Range: 3–4 mg/day: MAX: 6 mg/day.	EPS: Moderate; TD Risk: Moderate; Sedation: Moderate; Metabolic Effects: Moderate. Hyperprolactinemia and sexual side effects common. Need to screen glucose and lipids regularly. P: C; L: Excreted/Not recommended. ¢

*Antidepressant Medications warnings/precautions: 1) Potential increased suicidality in first few months, 2) Long term weight gain likely (except venlafaxine & bupropion), 3) Sexual side effects common (except bupropion & mirtazapine), 4) Withdrawal syndrome frequently occurs with abrupt cessation (especially with SSRIs and SNRIs), Increased risk of bleeding with SSRIs and SNRIs (especially in combo with NSAIDs), 5) Risk for Serotonin Syndrome (except bupropion), especially with combination of drugs effecting serotonin metabolism, 6) Hyponatremia sometimes seen with SSRIs and SNRIs especially in elderly.

**Antipsychotic/mood stabilizer warnings/precautions: 1) Increased risk of death related to psychosis and behavioral problems in elderly patients with dementia, 2) Increased risk of QTc prolongation and risk of sudden death (especially in combination with other drugs that are known to prolong the QTc).

ABBREVIATIONS: po = by mouth; prn = as needed; qday = 1x/day; bid = 2x/day; tid = 3x/day; qid = 4x/day; qod = every other day; qam = morning; qhs = at bedtime; qac = before meals. P= pregnancy risk category L= lactation. ¢ = <$20, $ = $20–$100, $$ = $101–250, $$$ = >$250. SSRI = Selective Serotonin Reuptake Inhibitor. SNRI = Serotonin Norepinephrine Reuptake Inhibitor.

Brief medication prescribing protocols

Antidepressant medications

Bupropion (Wellbutrin, Wellbutrin SR, Wellbutrin XL, Forfivo XL, Aplenzin, Zyban)

DOSING INFORMATION: **Wellbutrin (IR):** *Week 1:* Baseline blood pressure. Consider BMP for baseline sodium in older adults. **Start IR:** 100 mg bid. *Week 2:* Increase to 100 mg tid, if tolerated (single dose should not exceed 150 mg). **Wellbutrin SR:** *Week 1:* Baseline blood pressure: **Start SR:** 150 mg qAM. *Week 2:* Increase to an **Initial Target Dose** of 150 mg bid, if tolerated. **Wellbutrin XL:** *Week 1:* Baseline blood pressure. **Start XL:** 150 mg qAM. *Week 2:* Increase to 300 mg qAM, if tolerated. **Note:** Aplenzin has a different titration. **Typical Dosage Range (IR/SR/XL):** 300–450 mg/day. **Max Dose (IR/SR/XL):** 400–450 mg qday. **Discontinuation:** 25 percent per week to 25 percent per month depending on length of treatment in order to minimize risk of relapse.

MONITORING: Blood pressure. Consider posttreatment BMP to rule out hyponatremia in older adults. Reports of false-positive urine immunoassay screening tests for amphetamines have been reported in patients taking bupropion, consult lab if needed.

GENERAL INFORMATION: Wellbutrin has a novel mechanism of action (weak dopamine and NE reuptake inhibitor; stimulant like effect). **FDA Indications:** Major depressive disorder, season affective disorder (prophylaxis), and smoking cessation. **Off-Label Indications:** Second line RX for ADHD. **Pharmacokinetics:** T½ = 21 hr. **Common Side effects (XL-MDD):** Headache (34 percent), dry mouth (26 percent), >5 lb. weight loss (23 percent), insomnia (20 percent), nausea (13 percent), constipation (9 percent), anxiety (7 percent), flatulence (6 percent). **Black-box warning:** Increased SI in patients <25 y/o. Increased risk of neuropsychiatric symptoms and suicidality in patients taking bupropion for smoking cessation. **Contraindications:** Known hypersensitivity reaction to the product, seizure disorder, current or prior diagnosis of bulimia or anorexia nervosa, abrupt discontinuation of alcohol or benzodiazepines, use of a MAOI within 14 days of stopping Wellbutrin, concurrent use of a MAOI including drugs with significant MAOI activity (e.g., linezolid), or use of Wellbutrin within 14 days of stopping a MAOI. **Warnings and precautions:** Clinical worsening and suicide risk, neuropsychiatric symptoms and suicide risk in smoking cessation treatment, increased risk of seizures, use in patients with a history of traumatic brain injury, potential for hepatotoxicity and hepatic impairment, increased agitation and insomnia, hypertension, altered appetite and weight, activation of psychosis or hypomanic/manic switch, potential for renal impairment, street value/abuse potential. **Pharmacogenetics:** Metabolized by 2B6. **Significant drug-drug interactions:** Inhibitor of 2D6; check all drug-drug interactions before prescribing. **Pregnancy:** Category C. **Breastfeeding:** Excreted/Use Caution. **Dosage Form:** Tablet (do not cut, crush or chew). **Generic available:** IR/SR/XL; Cost: $. **FDA label information from Drugs @FDA for Wellbutrin XL dated 7.26.11.**

Citalopram (Celexa)

DOSING INFORMATION: Week 1: Baseline weight. Consider BMP for baseline sodium in older adults and baseline QTc in all patients. **Start:** 20 mg qday. *Week 2:* Increase dose to 40 mg qday, if tolerated. **Initial, Typical Target, and Maximum Dose** of 40 mg qday (Max dose = 20 mg qday if ≥60 y/o, hepatically impaired, a CYP2C19 poor metabolizer, or taking a CYP2C19 inhibitor). **Discontinuation:** 25 percent per week to 25 percent per month depending on length of treatment in order to minimize withdrawal symptoms and relapse.

MONITORING: Weight, consider posttreatment BMP to rule out hyponatremia in older adults and posttreatment QTc in all patients.

GENERAL INFORMATION: **Mechanism of Action:** Highly selective serotonin reuptake inhibitor. **FDA Indications:** Depression. **Other Indications:** Anxiety disorders. **Pharmacokinetics:** T½ = 35 hrs. **Common Side effects (MDD):** Nausea (21 percent), dry mouth (20 percent), somnolence (18 percent), sexual side effects/ejaculatory dysfunction (6 percent). **Black-box warning:** Increased SI in patients < 25 y/o. **Contraindications:** Known hypersensitivity reaction to the product. Use of a MAOI within 14 days of stopping Celexa, concurrent use of a MAOI including drugs with significant MAOI activity (e.g., linezolid), or use of Celexa within 14 days of stopping a MAOI. **Warnings and precautions:** Clinical worsening and suicide risk, QTc prolongation and torsades de pointes, activation of hypomania/mania, serotonin syndrome, discontinuation symptoms, abnormal bleeding, hyponatremia, seizures. It is recommended that citalopram should not be used in patients with congenital long QTc syndrome, bradycardia, hypokalemia or hypomagnesemia, recent acute myocardial infarction, or uncompensated heart failure or used in combination with drugs that prolong the QTc. **Pregnancy:** Category C. **Breastfeeding:** Excreted/Use Caution. **Metabolism/Pharmacogenomics:** Primarily metabolized by 2C19 & 3A4 with 2D6 playing a less significant role. Use caution in 2C19 poor metabolizers and in patients taking 2C19 inhibitors (cimetidine). **Significant drug-drug interactions:** Weak 2D6 inhibitor; check all drug-drug interactions before prescribing. **Dosage Form:** Oral solution, Tablet. **Generic** available: Yes. Cost: ¢. FDA label information from Drugs @FDA for Celexa dated 12.3.12.

Duloxetine (Cymbalta)

DOSING INFORMATION: Week 1: Obtain blood pressure and weight. Consider BMP for baseline sodium in older adults. **Start:** 30 mg qday. *Week 2:* Increase dose to the **Initial and Typical Target Dose** of 60 mg qday or 30 mg bid, if tolerated. **Max Dose:** 120 mg qday (little evidence that higher doses are beneficial). **Discontinuation:** 25 percent per week to 25 percent per month depending on length of treatment in order to minimize withdrawal symptoms and relapse.

MONITORING: Blood pressure, weight. Consider posttreatment BMP to rule out hyponatremia in older adults.

GENERAL INFORMATION: **Mechanism of Action:** Serotonin/Norepinephrine Reuptake Inhibitor (SNRI). **FDA Indications:** MDD, GAD, diabetic peripheral neuropathic pain, fibromyalgia; chronic musculoskeletal pain. **Off-Label Indications:** Second-line ADHD, other pain, other anxiety. **Pharmacokinetics:** $T\frac{1}{2} = 12$ hrs. **Common Side effects (MDD & GAD):** nausea (25 percent), dry mouth (15 percent), diarrhea (10 percent), constipation (10 percent), fatigue (10 percent), dizziness (10 percent), somnolence (10 percent), insomnia (10 percent), decreased appetite (7 percent), hyperhidrosis (6 percent), vomiting (5 percent), agitation (5 percent). **Black-box warning:** Increased SI in patients < 25 y/o. **Contraindications:** Known hypersensitivity reaction to the product, use of a MAOI within 14 days of stopping Cymbalta, concurrent use of a MAOI including drugs with significant MAOI activity (e.g., linezolid), use of Cymbalta within 14 days of stopping a MAOI, use in patients with uncontrolled narrow angle glaucoma. **Warnings and precautions:** Suicidality, hepatotoxicity (should not be prescribed in patients with substantial alcohol use or evidence of chronic liver disease), orthostatic hypotension and syncope, serotonin syndrome, abnormal bleeding, severe skin reactions, discontinuation symptoms, manic switch, seizures, increased BP, use with 1A2 inhibitors or Thioridazine, hyponatremia, hepatic insufficiency and severe renal impairment, use caution in patient with controlled narrow-angle glaucoma and with slow gastric emptying, elevation in fasting blood glucose and HbA_{1C}, urinary hesitance and retention. **Metabolism/Pharmacogenomics:** Metabolized by 1A2 and 2D6. **Significant drug-drug interactions:** 2D6 inhibitor. Avoid coadministration with potent 1A2 inhibitors (e.g., fluvoxamine); and use cautiously with 2D6 inhibitors (e.g., Prozac). Potential for abnormal bleeding with NSAIDs or anticoagulants; Check all drug-drug interactions before prescribing. **Pregnancy:** Category C. **Breastfeeding:** Excreted/Not

Recommended. **Dosage Form:** Capsule (Do not cut, crush or chew). **Generic available:** Yes. **Cost:** $$. **FDA label information from Drugs @FDA for Cymbalta dated 10.18.2012.**

Escitalopram (Lexapro)

DOSING INFORMATION: Week 1: Baseline weight. Consider BMP for baseline sodium in older adults). **Start:** 5 mg qday. *Week 2:* Increase dose to an **Initial Target Dosage** of 10 mg qday, if tolerated. **Typical Dosage Range:** 10–20 mg qday. **Max:** 20 mg qday. **Discontinuation:** 25 percent per week to 25 percent per month depending on length of treatment in order to minimize withdrawal symptoms and relapse.

MONITORING: Weight. Consider posttreatment BMP to rule out hyponatremia in older adults.

GENERAL INFORMATION: **Mechanism of Action:** Highly selective serotonin reuptake inhibitor; S-enantiomer of the racemic derivative of citalopram. **FDA Indications:** MDD (acute and maintenance), GAD. **Off-Label Indications:** Other anxiety disorders. **Pharmacokinetics:** T½ = 27–32 hrs. **Common Side effects (MDD):** nausea (15 percent), ejaculation disorder (9 percent), insomnia (9 percent), somnolence (6 percent), fatigue (5 percent), sweating increased (5 percent). **Black-box warning:** Increased SI in patients < 25 y/o. **Contraindications:** Known hypersensitivity reaction to escitalopram or citalopram. Use of a MAOI within 14 days of stopping Lexapro, concurrent use of a MAOI including drugs with significant MAOI activity (e.g., linezolid), or use of Lexapro within 14 days of stopping a MAOI. Concomitant use with pimozide. **Warnings and precautions:** Clinical worsening and suicide risk, serotonin syndrome, discontinuation symptoms, seizures, hypomanic/manic switch, hyponatremia, abnormal bleeding. **Metabolism/Pharmacogenomics:** Primarily metabolized by 2C19 & 3A4. **Significant drug-drug interactions:** Weak 2D6 inhibitor; Use caution when coadministered with drugs metabolized by 2D6. Check all drug-drug interactions. **Pregnancy:** Category C. **Breastfeeding:** Excreted /Use Caution. **Dosage Form:** Oral solution, Tablet. **Generic available:** Yes. **Cost:** ¢. **FDA label information from Drugs @FDA for Lexapro dated 12.3.12.**

Fluoxetine (Prozac, Sarafem)

DOSING INFORMATION: **Prozac:** *Week 1:* Baseline weight. Consider BMP for baseline sodium in older adults. **Start Prozac:** 10 mg qday. *Week 2:* Increase dose to an **Initial Target Dose Prozac** of 20 mg qday (for geriatric patients, a lower initial dose or longer dosing interval is recommended and in bulimia the initial target dosage is 60 mg qday), if tolerated.

Week 4 and beyond: Consider further dose increases in 10–20 mg qday per week increments, as needed and tolerated. **Typical Dosage Range Prozac:** 20–60 mg qday. **Max Prozac:** 80 mg qday. **Discontinuation:** 25 percent per week to 25 percent per month depending on length of treatment in order to minimize withdrawal symptoms and relapse.

MONITORING: Weight. Consider posttreatment BMP to rule out hyponatremia in older adults.

GENERAL INFORMATION: **Mechanism of Action:** Selective serotonin reuptake inhibitor. **FDA Indications:** MDD (acute and maintenance), OCD, panic disorder, bulimia nervosa, premenstrual dysphonic disorder. **Off-Label Indications:** Other anxiety, fibromyalgia. **Pharmacokinetics:** T½ parent = 4–6 days, active metabolite = 4–16 days. **Common Side effects (MDD-Prozac):** nausea (21 percent), insomnia (16 percent), nervousness (14 percent), somnolence (13 percent), anxiety (12 percent), diarrhea (12 percent), anorexia (11 percent), dry mouth (10 percent), tremor (10 percent), asthenia (9 percent), sweating (8 percent). **Black-box warning:** Increased SI in patients < 25 y/o. **Contraindications:** Known hypersensitivity reaction to fluoxetine. Use of a MAOI within 5 weeks of stopping fluoxetine, concurrent use of a MAOI including drugs with significant MAOI activity (e.g., linezolid), or use of fluoxetine within 5 weeks of stopping a MAOI. Do not use pimozide or Thioridazine with fluoxetine. **Warnings and precautions:** Clinical worsening and suicide risk, increased suicidality, serotonin syndrome, allergic reactions and rash, manic switch, seizures, altered appetite and weight, abnormal bleeding, hyponatremia, anxiety and insomnia, QT prolongation, long half-life. **Metabolism/ Pharmacogenomics:** Primarily metabolized by 2D6. Use caution with 2D6 poor metabolizers. **Significant drug-drug interactions:** Potent 2D6 inhibitor; Use significant caution when coadministered with drugs metabolized by 2D6 (e.g., TCAs). Check all drug-drug interactions before prescribing. **Pregnancy:** Category C. **Breastfeeding:** Excreted/Not Recommended. **Dosage Form:** Oral solution, Capsule, Tablet. **Cost:** ¢ **Generic available:** Yes, Inexpensive. **FDA label information from Drugs @FDA for Prozac dated 7.26.2013.**

Mirtazapine (Remeron)

DOSING INFORMATION: Week 1: Baseline weight. Consider BMP for baseline sodium in older adults. **Start:** 15 mg qHS (7.5 mg qHS in older adults). *Week 2:* Increase to an **Initial Target Dose** of 30 mg qHS (15 mg qHS in older adults), if tolerated. **Typical Dosage Range:** 30–45 mg qHS (15–30 mg qHS in older adults). **Max Dose:** 45 mg qHS (30 mg qHS in older adults). **Discontinuation:** 25 percent per week to 25 percent per month depending on length of treatment in order to minimize withdrawal symptoms and relapse.

MONITORING: Weight, lipids. Consider posttreatment BMP to rule out hyponatremia in older adults.

GENERAL INFORMATION: **Mechanism of action:** Novel; central presynaptic alpha$_2$-adrenergic antagonist effects, which results in increased release of norepinephrine and serotonin. **FDA indications:** MDD. **Off-label indications:** Other anxiety, neuropathic pain, insomnia, antinausea effect (similar mechanism to odansetron). **Pharmacokinetics:** T$\frac{1}{2}$ = 26 hrs (females), 37 hrs (males). **Common side effects (MDD):** Somnolence (54 percent), dry mouth (25 percent), increased appetite (17 percent), constipation (13 percent), weight gain (12 percent), dizziness (7 percent). **Black-box warning:** Increased SI in patients < 25 y/o. **Contraindications:** Known hypersensitivity reaction to mirtazapine. Use of a MAOI within 14 days of stopping mirtazapine, concurrent use of a MAOI including drugs with significant MAOI activity (e.g., linezolid), or use of mirtazapine within 14 days of stopping a MAOI. **Warnings and precautions:** Clinical worsening and suicide risk, serotonin syndrome, hypomanic/manic switch, agranulocytosis (avoid in immunocompromised), discontinuation symptoms, akathisia/psychomotor restlessness, hyponatremia, increased cholesterol/triglycerides, dizziness, increased appetite/weight gain, transaminase elevations, seizures. **Metabolism/pharmacogenomics:** Metabolized by 1A2, 2D6, and 3A4. **Significant drug-drug interactions:** Use caution with potent 3A4 inhibitors (e.g., ketoconazole and protease inhibitors) and enzyme inducers (e.g., carbamazepine). Check all drug-drug interactions before prescribing. **Pregnancy:** Category C. **Breastfeeding:** Excreted in breast milk/Use Caution. **Dosage form:** Orally Disintegrating Tablet, Tablet. **Generic available:** Yes. **Cost:** ¢. **FDA label information from Drugs @FDA for Remeron dated 10.30.2012.**

Nortriptyline (Pamelor)

DOSING INFORMATION: **Week 1:** Baseline EKG (if any history of cardiac disease, history of arrhythmias, or over 65 y/o), pulse, HR, weight. Consider BMP for baseline sodium in older adults. **Start:** 25 mg qHS (10 mg qHS in older adults). **Week 2 and beyond:** Increase dose by 25–50 mg qHS (10 mg qHS in older adults) each week to an **Initial Target Dose** of 75 mg qHS (30 mg qHS for older adults), if tolerated. **Typical Dosage Range:** 75–100 mg qHS (30–50 mg qHS in older adults). **Max Dose:** 150 mg qHS (75 mg qHS in older adults). **Discontinuation:** 25 percent per week to 25 percent per month depending on length of treatment in order to minimize withdrawal symptoms and relapse.

MONITORING: EKG (pretreatment, initial, and annual—if any history of cardiac disease, history of arrhythmias or over 65 y/o), pulse, HR, weight. Consider posttreatment BMP to rule out hyponatremia in older adults. Blood test for serum level available with defined therapeutic range: 50–150 ng/ml; toxic >500 ng/ml. The FDA recommends testing serum levels in adults in doses above 100 mg qHS. Blood draw timed to achieve a trough level.

GENERAL INFORMATION: **Mechanism of Action:** TCA: NE > serotonin reuptake inhibitor. Generally better tolerated than other TCAs. **FDA Indications:** Depression. **Off-Label Indications:** neuropathic pain (doses up to 75 mg). **Pharmacokinetics:** T ½: highly variable 16–90+ hr. **Common side effects (MDD):** Sedation, anticholinergic side effects (blurred vision, urinary retention, dry mouth, constipation), orthostatic hypotension, weight gain, nausea, headache, sexual side effects. **Black Box:** Increased SI in patients <25 y/o. **Contraindications:** Known hypersensitivity reaction to the product, use of a MAOI within 14 days of stopping Pamelor, concurrent use of a MAOI including drugs with significant MAOI activity (e.g., linezolid), use of Pamelor within 14 days of stopping a MAOI, or use during the acute recovery period after a MI. **Warnings and precautions:** Clinical worsening and suicide risk, highly lethal in overdose, hypomanic/manic switch, serotonin syndrome, orthostatic hypotension, QTc prolongation, hepatic changes, decreased blood cell count, hyperthermia, urinary retention, SIADH, use in patients with cardiovascular disease, who have glaucoma or a history of urinary retention, with a history seizures, or with hyperthyroidism; use with quinidine. **Metabolism/Pharmacogenomics:** Metabolized by 2D6 to less active metabolites. Use caution with 2D6 poor metabolizers. **Significant drug-drug interactions:** use caution with strong 2D6 inhibitors (e.g., fluoxetine), and with medications that affect QTc; check all drug-drug interactions. **Pregnancy: Category D; associated w/increased risk of teratogenesis (need to inform women of childbearing age of this risk). Breastfeeding:** Excreted/Use Caution. **Dosage Form:** Capsules, Oral solution. **Generic available:** Yes. **Cost:** ¢. **FDA label information from Drugs @FDA for Pamelor dated 10.26.2012.**

Paroxetine (Paxil, Paxil CR, Pexeva)

DOSING INFORMATION: **Paxil (IR):** *Week 1:* Baseline weight. Consider BMP for baseline sodium in older adults. **Start IR:** 10 mg qday. *Week 2:* Increase to an **Initial Target Dose** of 20 mg qday (40 mg qday for OCD), if tolerated. *Week 4 and beyond:* Consider further increases as needed in 10 mg qday per week increments as tolerated. **Typical Dosage Range IR: 20–60 mg qday. Max Dose IR: 60 mg qday.** Paxil CR: *Week 1:* Baseline weight. Consider BMP for baseline sodium in older adults. **Start CR:** 25 mg qday (the **Initial Target Dose**). *Week 4 and beyond:* Consider further increases as needed in 12.5 mg qday per week increments. **Usual Dosage Range CR: 25–62.5 mg qday. Max Dose CR:** 62.5 mg qday. **Discontinuation:** *Often problematic.* 25 percent per week to 25 percent per month depending on length of treatment in order to minimize withdrawal symptoms and relapse.

MONITORING: Weight. Consider posttreatment BMP to rule out hyponatremia in older adults.

GENERAL INFORMATION: **Mechanism of Action:** Potent selective serotonin reuptake inhibitor, which is quite anticholinergic. **FDA Indications:** GAD, MDD, OCD, Panic Disorder, PTSD, PMDD, Social Phobia. **Pharmacokinetics:** T $\frac{1}{2}$ = 21 hrs. **Common Side effects (MDD-Paxil):** Nausea (26 percent), somnolence (23 percent), dry mouth (18 percent), asthenia (15 percent), constipation (14 percent), dizziness (13 percent), insomnia (13 percent), sexual side effects (13 percent), diarrhea (12 percent), tremor (8 percent), decreased appetite (6 percent). **Black-box warning:** Increased SI in patients < 25 y/o. **Contraindications:** Known hypersensitivity reaction to Paxil. Use of a MAOI within 4 weeks of stopping Paxil, concurrent use of a MAOI including drugs with significant MAOI activity (e.g., linezolid), or use of Paxil within 4 weeks of stopping a MAOI. Concomitant use with pimozide or thioridazine. **Warnings and precautions:** Clinical worsening and suicide risk, serotonin syndrome, hypomanic/manic switch, teratogenic effects, seizures, discontinuation syndrome, drug-drug interactions, use with tamoxifen, akathisia, abnormal bleeding, hyponatremia, bone fracture. **Metabolism/Pharmacogenomics:** Metabolized by 2D6. Use caution with 2D6 poor metabolizers. **Significant drug-drug interactions:** Strong 2D6 inhibitor. Use caution with drugs metabolized by 2D6 (e.g., TCAs); check all drug-drug interactions. **Pregnancy: Category D; associated w/ increased risk of teratogenesis (need to inform women of childbearing age of this risk). Breastfeeding:** Excreted/Use Caution. **Dosage Form:** Oral solution, Tablet, Coated Tablet (Do not cut, crush or chew). **Generic available:** IR: Yes; CR: yes, Cost: IR ¢; CR $. **FDA label information from Drugs @FDA for Paxil dated 12.18.2012.**

Sertraline (Zoloft)

DOSING INFORMATION: *Week 1:* Baseline weight. Consider BMP for baseline sodium in older adults. **Start:** 25 mg qday. *Week 2:* Increase to an **Initial Target Dose** of 50 mg qday, if tolerated. *Week 4 and beyond:* Consider further increases in dose if needed and tolerated, in 25 mg qday per week increments. **Typical Dosage Range: 50–200 mg qday. Max Dose:** 200 mg qday. **Discontinuation:** 25 percent per week to 25 percent per month depending on length of treatment in order to minimize withdrawal symptoms and relapse.

MONITORING: Weight. Consider posttreatment BMP to rule out hyponatremia in older adults. *OF NOTE:* false-positive urine immunoassay screening tests for benzodiazepines have been reported in patients taking sertraline.

GENERAL INFORMATION: Mechanism of Action: Selective serotonin reuptake inhibitor. **FDA Indications:** MDD, OCD, panic disorder, PTSD, social phobia, PMDD. **Off-Label Indications:** Other anxiety. **Pharmacokinetics:** T½ = 26 hrs. **Common Side effects (MDD):** Nausea (26 percent), diarrhea (18 percent), dry mouth (16 percent), insomnia (16 percent), somnolence (13 percent), dizziness (12 percent), tremor (11 percent), fatigue (11 percent), increased sweating, (8 percent), ejaculation failure (7 percent). **Black-box warning:** Increased SI in patients < 25 y/o. **Contraindications:** Known hypersensitivity reaction to Zoloft. Use of a MAOI within 4 weeks of stopping Zoloft, concurrent use of a MAOI including drugs with significant MAOI activity (e.g., linezolid), or use of Zoloft within 4 weeks of stopping a MAOI. Concomitant use with pimozide. **Warnings and precautions:** Clinical worsening and suicide risk, hypomanic/manic switch, serotonin symptoms, weight loss, seizure, discontinuation symptoms, abnormal bleeding, altered platelet function, hyponatremia, weak uricosuric effect, angle closure glaucoma. **Metabolism/Pharmacogenomics:** Metabolized by multiple P450 enzymes with 2C19 having the greatest pharmacogenetic and drug–drug interaction evidence. Use caution with 2C19 poor metabolizers. **Significant drug-drug interactions:** Weak 2D6 inhibitor. Use caution with drugs metabolized by 2D6 (e.g., TCAs); check all drug-drug interactions. **Pregnancy:** Category C. **Breastfeeding:** Compatible. **Dosage Form:** Oral solution, Tablet. **Generic available:** Yes. **Cost:** ¢. **FDA label information from Drugs @FDA for Zoloft dated 2.1.2013.**

Trazodone (Desyrel, Oleptro)

DOSING INFORMATION: Initiation for Depression: **Desyrel (IR)** *Week 1:* Baseline blood pressure, weight. Consider BMP for baseline sodium in older adults. **Start IR:** 25–50 mg bid-tid; increase by 25–50 mg/day per week, if tolerated, to an **Initial Target Dose IR** of 150 mg/day. *Week 4 and beyond:* Consider further increases in dose as needed and tolerated in 25–50 mg/day per week increments. **Typical Dosage Range IR:** 150–300 mg/day. **Max Dose IR:** 400 mg/day. **Oleptro (ER):** *Week 1:* Baseline blood pressure, weight. Consider BMP for baseline sodium in older adults. **Start ER:** 150 mg qHS (the **Initial Target Dose**). *Week 4 and beyond:* Can consider further increases in 75 mg/day per week increments. **Typical Dosage Range ER** of 150–300 mg qHS. **Max Dose ER:** 375 mg qHS. *Initiation for insomnia (off-label):* **Start IR:** 25–50 mg qHS (the initial target dose); increase in 25–50 mg qHS per week increments, if tolerated; **typical dose IR** 50–200 mg qHS. **Discontinuation:** 25 percent per week to 25 percent per month depending on length of treatment in order to minimize withdrawal symptoms and relapse.

MONITORING: Weight; Consider posttreatment BMP to rule out hyponatremia in older adults. Monitor for orthostatic hypotension in elderly and other vulnerable populations.

GENERAL INFORMATION: **Mechanism of Action:** Serotonin reuptake inhibitor. **FDA Indications:** Depression. **Other Indications:** Insomnia, depression augmentation. **Pharmacokinetics:** $T\frac{1}{2} = 10$ hrs. **Common Side effects (MDD-Desyrel):** Drowsiness (41 percent), dry mouth (34 percent), dizziness/lightheadedness (28 percent), headache (20 percent), blurred vision (15 percent), nausea/vomiting (13 percent), constipation (8 percent), skin condition/edema (5 percent), fatigue (6 percent), weight loss (6 percent), diarrhea (5 percent), musculoskeletal aches/pains (5 percent), tremors (5 percent), weight gain (5 percent), syncope (5 percent). **Black-box warning:** Increased SI in patients < 25 y/o. **Contraindications:** Known hypersensitivity reaction to Desyrel. Use of a MAOI within 4 weeks of stopping trazodone, concurrent use of a MAOI including drugs with significant MAOI activity (e.g., linezolid), or use of Desyrel within 4 weeks of stopping a MAOI. **Warnings and precautions:** Clinical worsening and suicide risk, serotonin syndrome, hypomanic/manic switch, QT prolongation, use in patients with heart disease (e.g., recent MI), orthostatic hypotension and syncope, abnormal bleeding, **priapism**, hyponatremia, discontinuation syndrome. **Metabolism/Pharmacogenomics:** 3A4. **Significant drug-drug interactions:** Use caution with potent 3A4 inhibitors (e.g., ketoconazole and protease inhibitors) and enzyme inducers (e.g., carbamazepine and St. John's wort). Check all drug-drug interactions. **Pregnancy:** Category C. **Breastfeeding** Excreted/Not Recommended. **Dosage Form:** Tablet (trazodone), capsule (Oleptro). **Generic available:** Desyrel: Yes; Oleptro: No. Cost: Desyrel ¢. Oleptro $$. **FDA label for Desyrel from dailymed.nlm.nih.gov, Rev. 2.2009. FDA label information from Drugs @FDA for Oleptro dated 11.13.2012.**

Venlafaxine (Effexor, Effexor XR)

DOSING INFORMATION: **Effexor (IR):** *Week 1:* Baseline blood pressure, weight. Consider BMP for baseline sodium in older adults. **Start IR:** 37.5 mg bid (37.5 qday with panic disorder). *Week 2:* Increase to the **Initial Target Dose** of 75 mg bid, if tolerated. *OF NOTE,* the initial target dose for social phobia is 37.5 mg bid qday and the initial target dose for neuropathic pain is 112.5 mg bid. *Week 3 and Beyond:* Can consider further increases in 75 mg/day increments every 2 or more weeks as needed and tolerated.

Typical Dosage Range IR: 150–300 mg/day. Max Dose IR: 375 mg/day. Effexor XR: *Week 1:* Baseline blood pressure, weight. Consider BMP for baseline sodium in older adults. Start XR: 75 mg qday (37.5 mg for panic disorder). *Week 2:* Increase to the Initial Target Dose XR of 150 mg qday, if tolerated. *OF NOTE,* the initial target dose for social phobia is 75 mg qday and the initial target dose for neuropathic pain is 225 mg qday. *Week 4 and Beyond:* Consider further increases in 75 mg/day increments every 2 or more weeks as needed and tolerated. Typical Dosage Range XR: 150–300 mg/day. Max Dose XR: 300 mg qday. Discontinuation: *Often problematic.* 25 percent per week to 25 percent per month depending on length of treatment in order to minimize withdrawal symptoms and relapse.

MONITORING: Blood pressure, weight. Consider posttreatment BMP to rule out hyponatremia in older adults

GENERAL INFORMATION: Mechanism of Action: Serotonin/ Norepinephrine Reuptake Inhibitor (SNRI). FDA Indications: GAD, MDD, Panic Disorder, Social Anxiety Disorder. Off-Label Indications: Neuropathic pain, other anxiety. Pharmacokinetics: $T \frac{1}{2} = 5$ hrs and 11 hrs (active metabolite). Common Side effects (MDD, XR): Nausea (31 percent), dizziness (20 percent), somnolence (17 percent), insomnia (17 percent), abnormal ejaculation (16 percent), sweating (14 percent), dry mouth (12 percent), nervousness (10 percent), anorexia (8 percent), constipation (8 percent), abnormal dreams (7 percent), tremor (5 percent), blurry vision (5 percent). Black-box warning: Increased SI in patients <25 y/o. Contraindications: Known hypersensitivity reaction to the product, use of a MAOI within 14 days of stopping Effexor, concurrent use of a MAOI including drugs with significant MAOI activity (e.g., linezolid), or use of Effexor within 14 days of stopping a MAOI. Warnings and precautions: Clinical worsening and suicide risk, serotonin syndrome, hypomanic/manic switch, sustained hypertension, elevations in systolic and diastolic blood pressure, seizures, mydriasis/narrow angle glaucoma, discontinuation symptoms, insomnia and nervousness, weight loss and decreased appetite, abnormal bleeding, serum cholesterol elevation, interstitial lung disease and eosinophilic pneumonia. Metabolism/Pharmacogenomics: Metabolized by 2D6. Use caution with 2D6 poor metabolizers. Significant drug-drug interactions: Limited drug-drug interactions, Low protein binding, check all drug-drug interactions before prescribing. Pregnancy: Category C. Breast-feeding: Excreted/Not Recommended. Dosage Forms: Tablet, Capsule, Coated Tablet (Do not cut, crush or chew). Generic available: IR/XR: Yes. Cost: IR ¢; XR: $. FDA label information from Drugs @FDA for Effexor XR dated 12.18.2012.

Anxiolytics & hypnotic medications

Alprazolam (Xanax; Xanax XR)

DOSING INFORMATION: **Anxiety Disorders:** Consider CBC and LFTs (see *MONITORING*); **Xanax (IR):** *Week 1:* **Start IR:** 0.25 to 0.5 mg tid; *OF NOTE:* Scheduled dosing is typically more effective than PRN dosing for control of anxiety symptoms. *Week 2 and beyond:* Increase dose as needed and tolerated in 0.5 mg–1 mg/day increments each week to the minimally effective dose. **Typical Dosage Range IR:** 0.5 to 1 mg tid. **Max Dose IR:** 4 mg/day. **Panic Disorder:** Consider CBC and LFTs (see *MONITORING*); **Xanax (IR):** *Week 1:* **Start IR:** 0.5 mg tid. *OF NOTE:* Scheduled dosing is typically more effective than PRN dosing for control of anxiety symptoms; *Week 2 and beyond:* Increase dose as needed and tolerated in 0.5–1 mg/day increments each week to the minimally effective dose. **Typical Dosage Range IR:** 4–6 mg/day. **Max Dose IR:** 9 mg/day. **Xanax XR (Panic Disorder):** *Week 1:* **Start XR:** 0.5–1mg qAM. *OF NOTE:* Scheduled dosing is typically more effective than PRN dosing for control of anxiety symptoms; *Week 2 and beyond:* Increase dose as needed and tolerated in 0.5–1 mg/day increments each week to the minimally effective dose. **Typical Dosage Range XR:** 3–6 mg/day. **Max Dose XR:** 6 mg/day. **Discontinuation:** Uniquely problematic withdrawal syndrome; Recommended taper of no more than 0.5 mg every 3 days; Doses above 4 mg/day may need slower taper of 10 percent per month. *OF NOTE:* Alprazolam concentrations may be reduced by up to 50 percent in smokers compared to nonsmokers.

MONITORING: Consider UTOX if abuse/diversion is a concern. *Per FDA:* "periodic" blood counts and liver-function tests are recommended for patients on long-term therapy.

GENERAL INFORMATION: **Mechanism of action:** enhances activity of GABA (benzodiazepine). **FDA Indications:** Panic Disorder; Anxiety disorders; Short-term use for anxiety symptoms. **Other Indications:** Insomnia. **Pharmacokinetics:** T $\frac{1}{2}$ = 11 hrs; Onset: Rapid. **Common Side effects (IR—panic disorder):** Drowsiness (77 percent), impaired coordination (40 percent), memory impairment (33 percent), increased appetite (33 percent), cognitive disorder (29 percent), weight gain (27 percent), constipation (26 percent), dysarthria (23 percent), weight loss (23 percent), decreased libido (14 percent), micturition difficulties (12 percent), increased libido (8 percent), sexual dysfunction (7 percent). **Black-box warning:** None. **Contraindications:** Known hypersensitivity reaction to the product. Use in patients with acute narrow angle glaucoma. Coadministration with ketoconazole or itraconazole. **Warnings and precautions:** Dependence and withdrawal reactions, including seizures, status epilepticus, interdose symptoms, CNS depression and impaired performance, risk of fetal harm, use with CYP 3A inhibitors, hypomanic/manic switch, weak uricosuric effect, respiratory depression, sleep apnea/COPD, physical and psychological dependence, abuse potential, use in the elderly and in patients with liver disease, paradoxical reactions. **Metabolism/Pharmacogenomics:** Metabolized by CYP3A. **Significant drug-drug interactions:** Use with a great deal of caution with potent 3A inhibitors (e.g., ketoconazole and protease inhibitors) and enzyme inducers (e.g., carbamazepine and St. John's wort)—see also under contraindications; Use with caution with other sedative/hypnotics. Check all drug-drug interactions. **Pregnancy: Category D; associated w/increased risk of teratogenesis (need to inform women of childbearing age of this risk). Breastfeeding:** Excreted/Not Recommended. **Dosage Form:** Tablet, Oral dissolving tablet, Oral solution, Coated Tablet (Do not cut, crush or chew). **Generic available:** IR/XR: Yes. Cost: IR ¢, XR $. **FDA label information from Drugs @FDA for Xanax dated 8.23.2011. FDA label information from Drugs @FDA for Xanax XR dated 8.23.2011.**

Buspirone (BuSpar)

DOSING INFORMATION: Week 1: Baseline weight. Consider BMP for baseline sodium in older adults. **Start:** 7.5 mg bid. *Week 2:* Increase to an **Initial Target Dose** of 15 mg bid, if tolerated; Consider further increases as needed and tolerated. **Typical Dose Range:** 15 mg bid to 30 mg bid mg. **Max Dose:** 30 mg bid. *OF NOTE:* Time frame for improvement similar to SSRIs and other antidepressants. **Discontinuation:** Taper slowly to minimize withdrawal symptoms.

MONITORING: Weight. Consider posttreatment BMP to rule out hyponatremia in older adults.

GENERAL INFORMATION: **Mechanism of Action:** Not specifically known; high affinity for serotonin (5-HT1A) receptors and moderate affinity for dopamine (D2) receptors; Not related to benzodiazepines and does not affect GABA binding. OF NOTE: BuSpar will not mitigate benzodiazepine withdrawal. **FDA Indications:** Anxiety. **Other Indications:** Depression augmentation. *OF NOTE:* BuSpar may be helpful for reversing SSRI/SNRI induced sexual dysfunction. **Pharmacokinetics:** T½: 2–3 hrs. **Common Side effects (Anxiety):** Dizziness (12 percent), nausea (8 percent), headache (6 percent), nervousness (5 percent). **Black-box warning:** None. **Contraindications:** Known hypersensitivity reaction to the product. **Warnings and precautions:** Use of a MAOI within 14 days of stopping BuSpar, concurrent use of a MAOI including drugs with significant MAOI activity (e.g., linezolid), or use of BuSpar within 14 days of stopping a MAOI, use in patients with severe hepatic or renal impairment, potential restlessness syndrome (e.g., akathisia). **Metabolism/Pharmacogenomics:** Metabolized by CYP3A4. **Significant drug-drug interactions:** Use with a great deal of caution with potent 3A inhibitors (e.g., ketoconazole and protease inhibitors) and enzyme inducers (e.g., carbamazepine and St. John's wort); Avoid grapefruit juice. Check all drug-drug interactions before prescribing. **Pregnancy:** Category B. **Breastfeeding:** No data/Not Recommended. **Dosage Form:** Tablet. **Generic available:** Yes. **Cost:** ¢. **FDA label information from Drugs @FDA for BuSpar dated 11.22.2010.**

Clonazepam (Klonopin)

DOSING INFORMATION: Week 1: Consider CBC and LFTs (see *MONITORING*); **Start:** 0.25 mg bid; *OF NOTE:* Scheduled dosing is typically more effective than PRN dosing for control of anxiety symptoms. *Week 2:* Increase dose as needed and tolerated to the **Typical Initial and Target Dosage** of 0.5 mg bid. Can give more of dose at qHS to target insomnia, or if causing excessive daytime sedation. *Week 3 and beyond:* Can consider further increases as needed and tolerated however most individuals experience less efficacy with more side effects at higher dosing. **Max Dose:** 4 mg/day. **Rapid Discontinuation:** 0.125 mg bid every 3 days. **Extended Discontinuation** (e.g., after months/years of use): 10 percent per month.

MONITORING: Consider UTOX if abuse/diversion is a concern. *Per FDA:* "periodic" blood counts and liver-function tests are recommended for patients on long-term therapy.

GENERAL INFORMATION: **Mechanism of action:** enhances activity of GABA (benzodiazepine). **FDA Indications:** Panic disorder. **Other Indications:** GAD, Social phobia. **Pharmacokinetics:** T½ 30–40 hrs; Onset: intermediate (1–4 hrs). **Common Side effects (Panic Disorder):** Somnolence (37 percent), dizziness (8 percent), upper respiratory tract infection (8 percent), depression (7 percent), abnormal coordination (6 percent), ataxia (5 percent). **Black-box warning:** None. **Contraindications:** Known hypersensitivity reaction to the product, patients with clinical or biochemical evidence of significant liver disease, acute narrow angle glaucoma. **Warnings and precautions:** Cognitive/motor impairment, suicidal behavior/ideation, risk of fetal harm, withdrawal symptoms, respiratory depression, sleep apnea/COPD, worsening of seizures, need for periodic blood counts and liver function tests (see above under MONITORING) physical and psychological dependence, abuse potential, use in the elderly, increased salivation, caution in renally impaired patients, paradoxical reaction. **Metabolism/Pharmacogenomics:** Metabolized by CYP3A. **Significant drug-drug interactions:** Use with a great deal of degree of caution with potent 3A4 inhibitors (e.g., ketoconazole and protease inhibitors) and enzyme inducers (e.g., carbamazepine and St. John's wort); Use caution with other sedative/hypnotics. Check all drug-drug interactions before prescribing. **Pregnancy: Category D; associated w/increased risk of teratogenesis (need to inform women of childbearing age of this risk). Breastfeeding:** Excreted/Not Recommended. **Dosage Form:** Tablet, Oral dissolving tablet. **Generic available:** Yes. Cost: ¢. **FDA label information from Drugs @FDA for Klonopin dated 10.31.2013.**

Diazepam (Valium)

DOSING INFORMATION: Week 1: Consider CBC and LFTs (see *MONITORING*); **Start:** 5 mg bid. *OF NOTE:* Scheduled dosing is typically more effective than PRN dosing for control of anxiety symptoms. *Week 2:* Increase dose as needed and tolerated by 5–10 mg/day increments per week to the minimally effective dose; Can give more of dose at qHS to target insomnia, or if causing excessive daytime sedation. **Typical Dosage Range:** 10–20 mg/day. **Max Dose:** 40 mg/d. **Rapid Discontinuation:** 10 percent of total dose every 3–4 days. **Extended Discontinuation** (e.g., after months/years of use): 10 percent per month.

MONITORING: Consider UTOX if abuse/diversion is a concern. *Per FDA:* "periodic" blood counts and liver-function tests are recommended for patients on long-term therapy.

GENERAL INFORMATION: **Mechanism of action:** Enhances activity of GABA (benzodiazepine). **FDA Indications:** Anxiety disorder, Acute alcohol withdrawal. **Pharmacokinetics:** T½ up to 48 hrs, active metabolite: up to 100 hours; Onset: immediate (1–1.5 hrs). **Common Side effects (Anxiety):** Drowsiness, fatigue, muscle weakness, ataxia. **Black-box warning:** None. **Contraindications:** Known hypersensitivity reaction to the product, myasthenia gravis, severe respiratory insufficiency, severe hepatic insufficiency, sleep apnea syndrome, acute narrow angle glaucoma. **Warnings and precautions:** Cognitive/motor impairment, suicidal behavior/ideation, risk of fetal harm, withdrawal symptoms, respiratory impairment, hepatic insufficiency, worsening of seizures, physical and psychological dependence, abuse potential, use in the elderly, paradoxical reaction, psychotic patients. **Metabolism/Pharmacogenomics:** Metabolized by CYP3A4 and 2C19 to active metabolites and largely eliminated by glucuronidation. Use caution in 2C19 poor metabolizers. **Significant drug-drug interactions:** Use with a great deal of caution with potent 3A inhibitors (e.g., ketoconazole and protease inhibitors) and enzyme inducers (e.g., carbamazepine and St. John's wort) as well as with 2C19 inhibitors; Check all drug-drug interactions before prescribing. **Pregnancy: Category D; associated w/ increased risk of teratogenesis (need to inform women of childbearing age of this** risk). **Breastfeeding:** Excreted/Not Recommended. **Significant drug-drug interactions:** Check all drug-drug interactions. Use with caution with other sedative/hypnotics. **Dosage Form:** Tablet, Oral solution. **Generic available:** Yes. Cost: ¢. **FDA label information from Drugs @FDA for Valium dated 10.22.2013.**

Hydroxyzine pamoate (Vistaril)

DOSING INFORMATION: Week 1: **Start:** 25 mg q6 hrs. *Week 2:* Increase if needed and tolerated to the **Initial Target Dose** of 50 mg q 6 hrs. *Week 3:* Can consider further increases in dose in 25 mg q6 hr increments, if needed and tolerated. *OF NOTE:* Can start at 50 mg q6 hrs and titrate up to 100 mg q 6hr more quickly, if needed. **Typical Dosage Range:** 50–100 mg q6hs. **Max Dose:** 400 mg/day. **Discontinuation:** Taper slowly to minimize withdrawal symptoms.

MONITORING: None indicated.

GENERAL INFORMATION: **Mechanism of action:** Antihistamine (H_1-receptor). **FDA Indications:** Anxiety. **Non-FDA Indications:** Insomnia. **Pharmacokinetics:** T½ 20–25 hrs. Onset within 15 to 30 minutes. **Common Side effects (Anxiety):** Drowsiness; dry mouth. **Black-box warning:** None. **Contraindications: Use in early pregnancy.** Known hypersensitivity reaction to the product. **Warnings and precautions:** Use with other CNS depressants, cognitive/motor impairment, use in elderly patients. **Metabolism/Pharmacogenomics:** Metabolized in the liver. Specific pathways are unknown. **Significant drug-drug interactions:** Check all drug-drug interactions before prescribing. **Pregnancy:** Category C (except 1st trimester). **Breastfeeding:** Excreted/Not Recommended. **Significant drug-drug interactions:** Use with caution with sedatives/hypnotics. Check all drug–drug interactions before prescribing. **Dosage Form: Generic available:** Yes. **Cost:** ¢. **FDA label for Vistaril from dailymed.nlm.nih.gov, Rev. 6.2006.**

Lorazepam (Ativan)

DOSING INFORMATION: Week 1: Consider CBC and LFTs (see *MONITORING*); **Start:** 0.5 mg bid; *OF NOTE:* Scheduled dosing is typically more effective than PRN dosing for control of anxiety symptoms. *Week 2:* Increase dose as needed and tolerated to the **Initial Target Dose** of 1 mg bid. Can give more of the dose at qHS to target insomnia or if causing excessive daytime sedation. *Week 3 and beyond:* Consider further increases as needed and tolerated to the minimally effective dose. **Typical Target Dose:** 1–3 mg bid. **Max Dose:** 10 mg/day. **Rapid discontinuation:** 10 percent every 3 days.

Extended Discontinuation (e.g., after months/years of use): 10 percent per month.

MONITORING: Consider UTOX if abuse/diversion is a concern. *Per FDA:* "periodic" blood counts and liver-function tests are recommended for patients on long-term therapy.

GENERAL INFORMATION: **Mechanism of action:** enhances activity of GABA (benzodiazepine). **FDA Indications:** Anxiety disorders; Short-term use for anxiety symptoms or anxiety associated with depressive symptoms. **Other Indications:** Insomnia (1–4 mg qHS). **Pharmacokinetics:** $T\frac{1}{2} =$ 12 hrs; Onset: intermediate (2 hrs); *OF NOTE:* no active metabolites, so safer in liver disease. **Common Side effects (Anxiety):** Sedation (15.9 percent), dizziness (6.9 percent), weakness (4.2 percent), unsteadiness (3.4 percent). **Black-box warning:** None. **Contraindications:** Known hypersensitivity reaction to the product. Acute narrow-angle glaucoma. **Warnings and precautions:** Cognitive/motor impairment, suicidal behavior/ideation, worsening of depression, risk of fetal harm, withdrawal symptoms, respiratory depression, caution in patients with sleep apnea/COPD, with hepatic insufficiency and/or encephalopathy, and in the elderly, physical and psychological dependence, abuse potential, paradoxical reaction. **Metabolism/Pharmacogenomics:** Largely eliminated by glucuronidation. **Significant drug-drug interactions:** Use with caution with other sedative/hypnotics. Check all drug-drug interactions. **Pregnancy: Category D; associated w/ increased risk of teratogenesis (need to inform women of childbearing age of this risk). Breastfeeding:** Excreted/Not Recommended. **Dosage Form:** Oral solution, Tablet, IV. **Generic available:** Yes. **Cost:** ¢. **FDA label information from Drugs @FDA for Ativan dated 4.18.2007.**

Temazepam (Restoril)

DOSING INFORMATION: Week 1: **Start:** 15 mg qHS, the **Initial Target Dose** (7.5 mg qHS in the elderly). *Week 2:* Assess for side effects, can increase as needed to 30 mg qHS (15 mg qHS in the elderly), if tolerated. **Typical Dosage Range:** 15–30 mg qHS (7.5–15 mg qHS in the elderly). *OF NOTE:* Some adult patients find the 7.5 mg qHS sufficient to improve sleep latency. **Max Dose:** 30 mg qHS (15 mg qHS in the elderly). **Discontinuation:** No taper needed, if less than 10 days use; Recommend taper 10 percent every 3 days (or longer) with long-term use.

MONITORING: Consider UTOX if abuse/diversion is a concern. *Per FDA:* "periodic" blood counts and liver-function tests are recommended for patients on long-term therapy.

GENERAL INFORMATION: **Mechanism of action:** enhances activity of GABA (benzodiazepine hypnotic). **FDA Indications:** Short-term use for insomnia (7–10 days). **Pharmacokinetics:** T$\frac{1}{2}$ = 8.8 hrs; Onset: rapid (0.5 hr). **Common Side effects (Insomnia):** Drowsiness (9 percent). **Black-box warning:** None. **Contraindications:** Known hypersensitivity reaction to the product. **Women who are or may become pregnant.** **Warnings and precautions:** Need to evaluate for comorbid diagnoses, severe anaphylactic/anaphylactoid reaction, abnormal thinking, behavioral changes and complex behaviors (e.g., "sleep driving," "sleep eating" and hallucinations), withdrawal effects, cognitive/motor impairment, use in the elderly, use in patients with hepatic impairment, impaired drug metabolism or hemodynamic responses, disinhibition, suicidal behavior/ideation, worsening of depression, physical and psychological dependence, withdrawal syndrome, abuse potential. **Metabolism/Pharmacogenomics:** Metabolized via conjugation. **Significant drug-drug interactions:** Use with caution with other sedative/hypnotics. Check all drug-drug interactions before prescribing. **Pregnancy: Category X/Established risk of congenital malformations (need to inform women of childbearing age of this risk). Breastfeeding:** Excreted/Not Recommended. **Dosage Form:** Capsule. **Generic available:** Yes. **Cost:** ¢. **FDA label information from Drugs @FDA for Restoril dated 11.8.2010.**

ADHD medications

Atomoxetine (Strattera)

DOSING INFORMATION: Week 1: Evaluate cardiovascular risk (e.g., presence of structural cardiac abnormalities or other serious heart problems) and screen for psychosis and bipolar disorder; Baseline HR, BP and consider EKG; **Start:** 40 mg qAM. *Week 2:* Increase to 80 mg qAM (or 40 mg bid, the **Initial Target and Typical Dose**), if tolerated. *Week 4–6:* Assess for side effects; can consider further increase to 100 mg/day if still symptomatic. **Max Dose:** 100 mg qAM. **Discontinuation:** Taper slowly to minimize withdrawal symptoms.

MONITORING: BP and HR at baseline, 1 month, then every 6 to 12 months; hepatic function tests if signs of liver dysfunction.

GENERAL INFORMATION: **Mechanism of action:** Selective norepinephrine reuptake inhibitor. **FDA Indication:** ADHD. **Pharmacokinetics:** T$\frac{1}{2}$ = 5.2 hrs. **Common Side effects (ADHD):** nausea (26 percent), dry mouth (20 percent), decreased appetite (16 percent), insomnia (15 percent), fatigue (10 percent), constipation (8 percent), dizziness (8 percent), somnolence (8 percent), erectile dysfunction (8 percent), abdominal pain (7 percent), urinary hesitation, (6 percent) and irritability (5 percent).

Black-box warning: Increased risk of suicidal ideation in children or adolescents, monitor closely. **Contraindications:** Known hypersensitivity reaction to the product. Use of a MAOI within 14 days of stopping Strattera, concurrent use of a MAOI including drugs with significant MAOI activity (e.g., linezolid), use of Strattera within 14 days of stopping a MAOI, narrow angle glaucoma, pheochromocytoma, severe cardiovascular disorders. **Warnings and precautions:** Suicidal ideation, severe liver injury, serious cardiovascular events, emergent cardiovascular symptoms, effects on blood pressure and heart rate including hypertension, tachycardia, orthostatis and syncope, emergent psychotic or manic symptoms—screening for bipolar disorder is recommended, aggressive behavior/hostility, possible severe allergic reactions including anaphylaxis, urinary hesitancy and retention, **priapism**, use in patients receiving potent 2D6 inhibitors (e.g., fluoxetine or paroxetine) or who are know to be 2D6 poor metabolizers as dosage adjustments may be necessary. **Metabolism/Pharmacogenomics:** Metabolized by 2D6. Use with great caution and consider alternatives to Strattera in 2D6 poor metabolizers. **Significant drug-drug interactions:** Use with great caution and consider alternatives to Strattera when considering use with 2D6 inhibitors (e.g., fluoxetine or paroxetine); Check all drug-drug interactions and *CONSIDER CONSULTATION WITH A PHARMACIST BEFORE PRE-SCRIBING THIS MEDICATION.* **Pregnancy:** Category C. **Breastfeeding:** Limited data/Not recommended. **Dosage Form:** Capsule. **Generic available:** No. **Cost:** $$$. **FDA label information from Drugs @FDA for Strattera dated 2.20.14.**

D-amphetamine and L-amphetamine salts (Adderall, Adderall XR)

DOSING INFORMATION: **Adderall (IR):** *Week 1:* Evaluate cardiovascular risk (e.g., presence of structural cardiac abnormalities or other serious heart problems); Baseline HR, BP and consider EKG; Screen for bipolar disorder; **Start IR:** 5 mg qAM and 5 mg qPM (use intervals of 4–6 hours between doses—can take earlier in the afternoon if insomnia results). *Week 2:* Increase to 10 mg qAM and 5 mg qPM, if needed and tolerated. *Week 3 and beyond:* Consider further increases in 5 mg qday per week increments, if tolerated, until treatment of symptoms or max dose is reached. **Adderall XR:** *Week 1:* Evaluate cardiovascular risk (e.g., presence of structural cardiac abnormalities or other serious heart problems); Baseline HR, BP and consider EKG; Screen for bipolar disorder. **Start XR:** 10 mg qAM. *Week 2:* Consider increase to 20 mg qAM, if needed and tolerated. *Week 3 and beyond:* Consider further increases in 10 mg qAM increments per week, if tolerated, until treatment of symptoms, or max dose is reached. **Typical Target Dose**

(IR/XR): Lowest effective individualized dose. **Usual Max Dose (IR/XR):** 40 mg/day.

MONITORING: BP and HR at baseline, 1 month, then every 6 to 12 months; Signs of aggressive behavior or hostility; Consider UTOX if abuse/diversion is a concern.

GENERAL INFORMATION: **Mechanism of action:** CNS stimulant. **FDA Indication: IR:** ADHD in children, narcolepsy. **XR:** ADHD in children and adults. **Pharmacokinetics:** $T\frac{1}{2} = 10\text{-}13$ hrs. **Common Side effects (ADHD-XR):** Dry mouth (35 percent), loss of appetite (33 percent), insomnia (27 percent), headache (26 percent), weight loss (10 percent), nausea (8 percent), anxiety, (8 percent), dizziness (7 percent), tachycardia (6 percent), diarrhea (6 percent), urinary tract infections (5 percent). **Black-box warnings:** High potential for abuse/dependence; Misuse may cause sudden death and serious cardiovascular adverse events. **Contraindications:** Known hypersensitivity reaction to the product. Advanced arteriosclerosis, symptomatic cardiovascular disease, moderate to severe hypertension, hyperthyroidism, known hypersensitivity or idiosyncrasy to the sympathomimetic amines, glaucoma, agitated states, history of drug abuse, concurrent use of a MAOI including drugs with significant MAOI activity (e.g., linezolid), use of Adderall within 14 days of stopping a MAOI. **Warnings and precautions:** Serious cardiovascular events (death, stroke, and myocardial infarction)—**stimulant drugs should not be used in patients with known structural cardiac abnormalities, cardiomyopathy, serious heart rhythm abnormalities, coronary artery disease, or other serious heart problems,** increased blood pressure, adverse psychiatric events (may worsen preexisting psychosis or bipolar disorder or trigger the emergence of new psychotic or manic symptoms—screening for bipolar disorder is recommended), monitor for aggressive behavior, seizures, peripheral vasculopathy including Raynaud's phenomenon, visual disturbance, may worsen tics, potential for abuse of dependence. **Metabolism/Pharmacogenomics:** Metabolized by 2D6. **Significant drug-drug interactions:** Check all drug-drug interactions before prescribing. **Pregnancy:** Category C. **Breastfeeding:** No data/Not recommended. **Dosage Form:** Tablet (IR), Capsule (XR). **Generic available: IR/XR:** Yes. **Cost: $. FDA label information from Drugs @FDA for Adderall XR dated 2.7.2007. FDA label information from Drugs @FDA for Adderall XR dated 12.3.2013.**

Lisdexamfetamine (Vyvance)

DOSING INFORMATION: Week 1: Evaluate cardiovascular risk (e.g., presence of structural cardiac abnormalities or other serious heart problems); Baseline HR, BP and consider EKG; **Start:** 30 mg qAM. *Week 2:* Increase dose in weekly increments of 10 mg–20 mg, if tolerated, until treatment of symptoms or max dose is reached. **Typical Target Dose:** Lowest effective individualized dose. **Usual max dose:** 70 mg/day.

MONITORING: BP and HR at baseline, 1 month, then every 6 to 12 months; Signs of aggressive behavior or hostility; Consider UTOX if abuse/diversion is a concern.

GENERAL INFORMATION: **Mechanism of action:** CNS stimulant. **FDA Indication:** ADHD in children and adults. **Pharmacokinetics:** $T\frac{1}{2} = < 1$ hour (prodrug for dextroamphetamine $T\frac{1}{2} = 10$ hrs). **Common Side effects (ADHD):** Decreased appetite (27 percent), insomnia (27 percent), dry mouth (26 percent), diarrhea (7 percent), nausea (7 percent), anxiety (6 percent) and anorexia (5 percent). **Black-box warnings:** CNS stimulants have a high potential for abuse/dependence; Assess for risk of abuse prior to and after prescribing. **Contraindications:** Known hypersensitivity reaction to the product. Concurrent use of a MAOI including drugs with significant MAOI activity (e.g., linezolid), use of Vyvanse within 14 days of stopping a MAOI. **Warnings and precautions:** Serious cardiovascular events (death, stroke, and myocardial infarction)—**stimulant drugs should not be used in patients with known structural cardiac abnormalities, cardiomyopathy, serious heart rhythm abnormalities, coronary artery disease, or other serious heart problems,** blood pressure and heart rate increases, adverse psychiatric events (may worsen preexisting psychosis or bipolar disorder or trigger the emergence of new psychotic or manic symptoms—screening for bipolar disorder is recommended), monitor for aggressive behavior, peripheral vasculopathy including Raynaud's phenomenon, potential for abuse of dependence. **Metabolism/Pharmacogenomics:** Converted to dextroamphetamine in the blood. Dextroamphetamine metabolized by 2D6. **Significant drug-drug interactions:** Check all drug-drug interactions before prescribing. **Pregnancy:** Category C. **Breastfeeding:** No data/Not recommended. **Dosage Form:** Capsule. **Generic available:** No. **Cost: $$.** **FDA label information from Drugs @FDA for Vyvanse dated 12.6.13.**

Methylphenidate (Ritalin, Metadate ER, Methylin ER, Ritalin SR; Metadate CD, Ritalin LA, Concerta, Daytrana-patch, Quillivant XR)

DOSING INFORMATION: **Ritalin (IR):** *Week 1:* Evaluate cardiovascular risk (e.g., presence of structural cardiac abnormalities or other serious heart problems); Baseline HR, BP and consider EKG; **Start IR:** 5 mg qAM and 5 mg qPM (preferably before meals; use intervals of 4–6 hours between doses; can take earlier in the afternoon if insomnia results). *Week 2:* Increase dose to 10 mg qAM and 5 mg qPM, if needed and tolerated. *Week 3 and beyond:* Consider further increase in dose in 5 mg/day per week increments, if tolerated, until treatment of or max dosage is reached. **Ritalin SR:** *Week 1:* Evaluate cardiovascular risk (e.g., presence of structural cardiac abnormalities or other serious heart problems); Baseline HR, BP and consider EKG; **Start SR:** 10 mg qAM (preferably before meals). *Week 2:* Consider increase to 20 mg qAM, if needed and tolerated. *Week 3 and beyond:* Consider further increase in dose in 10 mg increments qday per week, if tolerated until treatment of symptoms or max dose is reached. **Concerta:** *Week 1:* Evaluate cardiovascular risk (e.g., presence of structural cardiac abnormalities or other serious heart problems); Baseline HR, BP and consider EKG; **Start Concerta:** 18 mg qAM. *Week 2:* Increase dose to 36 mg qAM if needed and tolerated; *Week 3 and beyond:* Consider further increases in 18 mg qday per week increments, if tolerated, until treatment of symptoms or max dose is reached. **Daytrana:** Patch; Special dosing (see FDA guidelines). **Typical Target Dose (IR/SR/Concerta):** Lowest effective individualized dose. **Usual Max Dose (IR/SR):** 60 mg/day (**Concerta** 72 mg/day).

MONITORING: BP and HR at baseline, 1 month, then every 6 to 12 months; Signs of aggressive behavior or hostility; Consider UTOX if abuse/diversion is a concern. Per FDA: "Periodic CBC, differential, and platelet counts are advised during prolonged therapy."

GENERAL INFORMATION: **Mechanism of action:** CNS stimulant. **FDA Indication:** ADHD; Narcolepsy. **Pharmacokinetics:** T½ for Concerta: 3.5 hrs (others vary). **Common side effects (ADHD-Concerta):** Decreased appetite (25 percent), headache (22 percent), dry mouth (14 percent), nausea (13 percent), insomnia (12 percent), anxiety (8 percent), weight decreased (7 percent), irritability (6 percent), and hyperhidrosis (5 percent), tachycardia (5 percent). **Black-box warnings:** Caution in use in patients with history of drug or alcohol dependence. Chronic abusive use can lead to tolerance and psychological dependence including abnormal behavior. **Contraindications:** Known hypersensitivity reaction to the product, marked anxiety, tension, and agitation, glaucoma, tics or a family history or diagnosis of Tourette's syndrome, concurrent use of a MAOI including drugs with significant MAOI activity (e.g., linezolid), use of methylphenidate within 14 days of stopping a MAOI. **Warnings and precautions:** Serious cardiovascular events (death, stroke, and myocardial infarction)—**stimulant drugs should not be used in patients with known structural cardiac abnormalities, cardiomyopathy, serious heart rhythm abnormalities, coronary artery disease, or other serious heart problems,** blood pressure and heart rate increases, adverse psychiatric events (may worsen preexisting psychosis or bipolar disorder or trigger the emergence of new psychotic or manic symptoms—screening for bipolar disorder is recommended), monitor for aggressive behavior, seizures, **priapism,** visual disturbance, tics, peripheral vasculopathy including Raynaud's syndrome, GI obstruction with preexisting GI narrowing, hematologic monitoring advised (see above under MONITORING). **Metabolism/Pharmacogenomics:** Primarily metabolized by de-esterification. **Significant drug-drug interactions:** May inhibit the metabolism of Coumadin, anticonvulsants and some antidepressant, e.g., TCAs and SSRIs. Check all drug-drug interactions before prescribing. **Pregnancy:** Category C. **Breastfeeding:** No data/Not recommended. **Significant drug-drug interactions: Dosage Form:** Tablet, Capsule Extended Release, Patch, Solution, Suspension, Tablet Chewable. **Generic available: IR/ER. Cost: IR $, ER $$. FDA label information from Drugs @FDA for Concerta dated 12.12.13.**

Miscellaneous medications

Prazosin (Minipress)
DOSING INFORMATION: Week 1: **Start:** 1 mg qHS increase to 2 mg qHS after 3–4 days. *Week 2:* Continue titration in 1 mg qHS increments every 3–4 days, if tolerated, until symptom remission, or max dose reached. **Typical Dosage Range:** 3–5 mg qHS. **Max Dose:** 10 mg qHS (in severe PTSD).

MONITORING: Blood pressure.

GENERAL INFORMATION: **Mechanism of action:** Antihypertensive (alpha-1 blocker). **Non-FDA Indication:** PTSD-related nightmares/night sweats. **Pharmacokinetics:** T ½ = 2–3 hrs. **Common Side effects (Hypertension):** Dizziness (10 percent), headache (8 percent), drowsiness (8 percent), lack of energy (7 percent), weakness (6 percent), palpitations (5 percent), nausea (5 percent). **Black-box warnings:** None listed. **Contraindications:** Known hypersensitivity reaction to the product or quinazolines. **Warnings and precautions:** Syncope with loss of consciousness (occasionally associated with severe tachycardia), orthostatic hypotension, cataract surgery, dizziness or drowsiness may occur after first dose. **Metabolism/Pharmacogenomics:** Metabolized primarily by demethylation and conjugation. **Significant drug-drug interactions:** Taking with trazodone or Viagra may increase risk of **priapism.** Check all drug-drug interactions. **Pregnancy:** Category C. **Breastfeeding:** No data/Not recommended. Check all drug-drug interactions before prescribing. **Dosage Form:** Capsules. **Generic available:** Yes. **Cost: ¢. FDA label information from Drugs @FDA for Minipress dated 11.4.13.**

Mood stabilizers

Carbamazepine extended release (Equetro)

DOSING INFORMATION: Week 1: Check baseline labs (urine pregnancy test, CBC with differential, CMP—see below for guidelines regarding Asian patients). Discuss birth control method with women of childbearing age due to severe risk to fetus. **Avoid in pregnancy. Start:** 200 mg bid. *Week 2–8:* Check trough carbamazepine plasma level before the morning dose. If level is subtherapeutic, increase dosage by 200 mg/day, if tolerated. This process is repeated weekly over 8 weeks due to autoinduction of metabolism. **Target Plasma Level:** Therapeutic levels: 4–12 mcg/ml (**Typical Dosage Range:** 600–1200 mg/day; **Max Dose:** 1600 mg/day). **Toxic concentration:** >15 mcg/ml. **Discontinuation:** Taper slowly to minimize withdrawal symptoms.

ONGOING MONITORING: Baseline labs: urine pregnancy test, CBC with differential, CMP. Monitoring of blood levels is recommended with the usual adult therapeutic drug levels between 4 and 12 mcg/ml. This medication induces autoinduction of metabolism, which is usually complete 3–5 weeks after initiation of a fixed carbamazepine regimen. Monitoring frequency (blood level & CBC with differential): *Qweekly* X 8 weeks, *Q2 months* X 2, and then *q6 months.* LFTs: *q6 months.*

GENERAL INFORMATION: **Mechanism of action:** Antiepileptic drug with mood stabilizer efficacy chemically related to tricyclic antidepressants. **FDA Indications:** Bipolar I, acute manic and mixed episodes. **Pharmacokinetics:** T½ variable due to autoinduction; Initial: 35–40 hours Steady state: 12–17 hours. **Common Side effects Equetro (Mania):** Dizziness (44 percent), somnolence (32 percent), nausea (29 percent), vomiting (18 percent), ataxia (15 percent), constipation (10 percent), pruritis (8 percent), dry mouth (8 percent), asthenia (8 percent), rash (7 percent), blurred vision (6 percent), speech disorder (6 percent). **Black-box warnings:** (1) Serious and sometimes fatal dermatologic reactions, including toxic epidermal necrolysis (TEN) and Stevens-Johnson syndrome (SJS). Estimated occurrence: 1 to 6 per 10,000 new users in countries w/ mainly Caucasian populations, but the risk in some Asian countries is estimated 10X higher and are associated with the presence of HLA-B*1502. **Asian patients and other high-risk patients should be screened for the presence of HLA-B*1502 prior to starting Equetro.** Discontinue, if these reactions occur. (2) Aplastic anemia and agranulocytosis. Obtain pretreatment hematological testing (SEE ABOVE). Discontinue if significant bone marrow depression develops. **Contraindications:** Hypersensitivity to carbamazepine, tricyclic antidepressants, or any component of the formulation; bone marrow depression; concurrent use of a MAOI including drugs with significant MAOI activity (e.g., linezolid), use of Equetro within 14 days of stopping a MAOI; concomitant use with nefazodone; concomitant use with delavirdine or other nonnucleoside reverse transcriptase inhibitors. **Warnings and precautions:** Serious dermatologic reactions (SJS/TEN associated with HLA-B*1502 allele—as noted above, and hypersensitivity reactions associated with HLA-A*3101 allele—consider testing prior to treatment to reduce risk), aplastic anemia and agranulocytosis, drug reaction with eosinophilia and systemic symptoms, suicidal behavior and ideation, embryofetal toxicity, abrupt discontinuation and risk of seizure, hyponatremia, cognitive and motor impairment, hepatic porphyria, decreased antiviral effect of nonnucleoside reverse transcriptase inhibitors. **Metabolism/Pharmacogenomics:** Metabolized by 3A4. **Significant drug-drug interactions:** Equetro is a strong 3A4 inducer and is inhibited by many drugs include fluoxetine. Examples of interactions include with Warfarin (resulting in decreased Warfarin levels) and hormone contraceptives (resulting in reduced efficacy). Check all drug-drug interactions as they are common with this medication and *CONSIDER CONSULTATION WITH A PHARMACIST BEFORE PRESCRIBING THIS MEDICATION.* **Pregnancy: Category D; associated w/ increased risk of teratogenesis (need to inform women of childbearing age of this risk) and should be avoided in pregnancy. Breastfeeding:** Excreted/Not recommended. Would recommend checking blood levels in the infant/toddler to confirm minimal maternal transfer of this medication given the variability in excretion between mothers. **Dosage Form:** Capsule, Tablet. **Generic Available:** Yes; **Cost:** $. **FDA label information from Drugs @FDA for Equetro dated 11.13.12.**

Divalproex sodium (Depakote, Depakote ER)

DOSING INFORMATION: **Depakote ER:** *Week 1:* Check baseline labs (urine pregnancy test, CBC for thrombocytopenia, coagulation tests, and liver function tests). Discuss birth control method with women of childbearing age due to severe risk to fetus. **Avoid in pregnancy. Start ER:** 500 mg qHS. *Week 2:* Check trough ER plasma level before, but as close to the dosing time as possible. If level is subtherapeutic, add 250–500 mg to qHS dose, if tolerated. Repeat weekly as need to reach therapeutic dosage. **Target plasma level ER:** 85 to 125 mcg/ml. **Usual Max Dose ER:** 60 mg/kg/day. **Formulation:** Depakote (DR) is a less preferable delayed release formulation due to increased side effect profile. If used, Depakote DR typically requires lower doses divided bid or TID and a trough plasma level of 50 to 125 mcg/ml. **Discontinuation:** Taper slowly to minimize withdrawal symptoms.

ONGOING MONITORING: Weight, CBC, coagulation tests, and liver function tests are recommended before initiating therapy and at least q6 months.

GENERAL INFORMATION: **Mechanism of action:** Antiepileptic drug with mood stabilizer efficacy. **FDA Indications:** Bipolar I disorder, mania or mixed. **Off-Label Indications:** Bipolar I disorder, rapid cycling. **Pharmacokinetics:** $T\frac{1}{2}$ = 9–16 hrs. **Common side effects (Depakote ER):** Somnolence (26 percent), dyspepsia (23 percent), nausea (19 percent), vomiting (13 percent), diarrhea (12 percent), dizziness (12 percent), abdominal pain (10 percent). **Black-box warnings:** (1) Hepatotoxicity (usually during the first 6 months), (2) pancreatitis and (3) fetal risk particularly including neural tube defects, other major malformations, and decreased IQ. **Contraindications:** Known hypersensitivity reaction to the product. Hepatic disease or significant hepatic dysfunction, known mitochondrial disorders caused by mutations to DNA polymerase gamma, urea cycle disorders, pregnant patients treated for prophylaxis of migraine headaches. **Warnings and precautions:** Hepatotoxicity, patients with known or suspected mitochondrial disease, birth defects, decreased IQ following in utero exposure, use in women of child bearing potential, pancreatitis, suicidal behavior or ideation, urea cycle disorders, thrombocytopenia, hyperammonemia, hyperammonemia and encephalopathy associated with concomitant topiramate use, hypothermia, multiorgan hypersensitivity reactions, interaction with carbapenem antibiotics, somnolence in the elderly, periodic drug plasma concentration monitoring, effect on ketone and thyroid function tests, effect of HIV and CMV replication, medication in the stool, Stevens-Johnson syndrome (~1:5000). **Metabolism/Pharmacogenomics:** Major metabolic pathways involve glucuronidation and beta-oxidation. **Significant drug-drug interactions:** Check all drug-drug interactions as they are common with this medication and *CONSIDER CONSULTATION WITH A PHARMACIST BEFORE PRESCRIBING THIS MEDICATION.* OF NOTE: aspirin at antipyretic dosages can increase free valproic acid level up to 4X and both carbapenem antibiotics and carbamazepine can significantly increase the clearance of valproic acid. Also, hyperammonemia and encephalopathy are associated with concomitant topiramate use. **Pregnancy: Category X (migraine prophylaxis/D (other indication); associated w/ increased risk of teratogenesis/fetal risk, particularly neural tube defects, other major malformations, and decreased IQ (need to inform women of childbearing age of this risk and recommend birth control) and should be avoided in pregnancy.** **Breastfeeding:** Excreted/Use caution. Recommend checking valproic acid blood levels in the infant/toddler to confirm minimal maternal transfer of this medication given the variability in excretion between mothers as well monitoring for excessive bleeding or bruising in the infant/toddler. Also consider periodically checking (e.g., q 6 months) the infant/toddler's platelets, LFTs, and coagulation tests. **Dosage Form:** Capsule, Coated Tablet (Do not cut, crush or chew), Solution. **Generic Available:** Yes (DR, ER). **Cost:** DR: $; Divalproex ER $$. **FDA label information from Drugs @FDA for Depakote ER dated 7.31.2013.**

Lamotrigine (Lamictal)

DOSING INFORMATION: Week 1 and 2: **Start:** 25 mg qday. *Week 3 and 4:* 50 mg qday, if tolerated. *Week 5:* 100 mg qday, if tolerated. *Week 6:* 200 mg qday, if tolerated (the **Initial Target and Typical Dose** as there is no compelling evidence of increased mood stabilization benefit at higher doses). Dosage will need to be adjusted for patients taking carbamazepine, phenytoin, phenobarbital, primidone, or valproate (see FDA guidelines). *OF NOTE:* Estrogen containing oral contraceptives increase metabolism of Lamictal such that target dose may need to be increased. Starter packs are available. **Restarting therapy after discontinuation:** If lamotrigine has been withheld for 3 days, restart according to initial dosing recommendations. **Nonurgent discontinuation:** Decrease by 50 percent per week (over at least 2 weeks).

ONGOING MONITORING: Drug levels are not typically measured.

GENERAL INFORMATION: **Mechanism of action:** Antiepileptic drug with mood stabilizer efficacy. **FDA Indications:** Bipolar Disorder, maintenance. **Off-Label Indications:** Bipolar depression. **Pharmacokinetics:** $T\frac{1}{2} = 25$ hrs. **Common side effects:** Nausea (14 percent), insomnia (10 percent), fatigue (8 percent), rhinitis (7 percent), abdominal pain (6 percent), constipation (5 percent), vomiting (5 percent). **Black-box warning:** For serious, life-threatening rashes requiring hospitalization and discontinuation of treatment (Stevens-Johnson syndrome @ approx. 1: 1000). Nearly all cases of life-threatening rashes associated with lamotrigine have occurred within 2 to 8 weeks of treatment initiation. The risk of rash may also be increased by coadministration of lamotrigine with Depakote (valproic acid) exceeding the recommended initial dose of lamotrigine, or exceeding the recommended dose escalation for lamotrigine. Lamotrigine should ordinarily be discontinued at the first sign of rash, unless the rash is clearly not drug related. **Contraindications:** Known hypersensitivity reaction to the product. **Warnings and precautions:** Serious skin rashes, multiorgan hypersensitivity reactions and organ failure, blood dyscrasias, suicidal behavior and ideation, increased aseptic meningitis risk, dosage adjustments needed for oral contraceptives, withdrawal seizures, increased risk of status epilepticus, sudden unexplained death in epilepsy. **Metabolism/Pharmacogenomics:**

Metabolized primarily by glucuronidation. **Significant drug-drug interactions:** Notable interactions decreasing lamotrigine levels include estrogen containing oral contraceptives (~50 percent), and carbamazepine (~40 percent). Valproate increases lamotrigine concentrations slightly more than two-fold. Check all drug-drug interactions before prescribing. **Pregnancy:** Category C; North American Antiepileptic Drug Pregnancy Registry (NAAED) suggest an increased incidence of cleft lip and/or cleft palate following first trimester exposure. **Breastfeeding:** Excreted in breast milk/Not Recommended. **Dosage Form:** Tablet, Chewable, Oral Dissolving Tablet. **Generic Available:** Yes. Cost: ¢. **FDA label information from Drugs @FDA for Lamictal dated 12.20.2013.**

Lithium carbonate (Lithobid)

DOSING INFORMATION: Week 1: Check baseline labs (urine pregnancy, basic metabolic panel (baseline Cr), Ca^{2+}, CBC (for baseline WBC) TSH, EKG (for patients over 40 y/o). **Start lithium carbonate (IR)/Lithobid (ER) 300 mg bid or 600 mg qHS** (may start with 300 mg/qHS, if the patient is less acute or sensitive to side effects, to increase tolerability). *Week 2 and Beyond:* Check lithium level weekly (ideally 12 hours after the last dose) and as indicated and tolerated increase dose in 300 mg/day increments to target plasma level of 0.8–1.0 meq/L. **Typical Target Plasma Level and Dose IR/ER:** Plasma level 0.8–1.0 meq/L which usually equates with daily dose of 1200–1800 mg. *OF NOTE:* For less severe conditions and for maintenance, a target plasma level between 0.6 and 0.8 may be desirable. **Dosing Schedule** should be determined by tolerability and compliance; Typically bid or qHS. **Formulation:** There are both immediate release and sustained release formulations. Nausea is more common with IR formulations and diarrhea with ER formulations. **Discontinuation:** Taper slowly (e.g., 25 percent per week) to minimize withdrawal symptoms and/or relapse.

ONGOING MONITORING: Check lithium levels 5–7 days after dose change (ideally 12 hours after last dose) and Q6 months when stable. Other labs: Baseline labs as above, Repeat at Q3 months X2 and Q6 months *GENERAL INFORMATION:* **Mechanism of action:** Natural salt with mood stabilizer efficacy. **FDA Indications:** Bipolar disorder, mania; bipolar disorder, maintenance. **Off-Label Indications:** Bipolar disorder, depression; depression augmentation; antisuicide effect. **Pharmacokinetics:** T½ = ~24 hrs. **Common Side Effects:** Nausea, tremor, polyuria (related to nephrogenic diabetes insipidus) and thirst, weight gain, loose stools, cognitive impairment (sedation, including changes in memory, concentration, apathy, and decreased creativity). **Black-box warning:** Toxicity can occur at levels close to therapeutic dosing: Mild symptoms occur at 1.5–2.5 meq/L (increase tremor, slurred speech, and increased lethargy), Moderate 2.5–3.5 meq/L (clonus, coarse tremors, worsening lethargy), and Severe above 3.5 meq/L which can be lethal. **Contraindications:** Known hypersensitivity reaction to the product. Significant renal impairment, significant cardiovascular disease, psoriasis, sodium depletion, dehydration, or debilitation. **Warnings and precautions:** Lithium toxicity, unmasking of Brugada syndrome (disorder characterized by abnormal EKG findings and a risk of sudden death), renal effects (including long-term diminution of concentrating ability, morphologic changes), encephalopathic syndrome when coadministered with an antipsychotic, concomitant use with neuromuscular blocking agents, increased risk of hypothyroidism and hyperparathyroidism with long term use, drug–drug interactions (see below). **Metabolism/Pharmacogenetics:** Excreted renally. **Significant drug-drug interactions:** Use with a great deal of caution with drugs that increase lithium levels including thiazide diuretics, NSAIDS (except aspirin), ACE-inhibitors, tetracyclines, metronidazole, potassium-sparing diuretics, and loop diuretics. Avoid or use alternatives with most calcium channel blockers. Increased risk of EPS and neurotoxicity with 1st generation antipsychotics. Check all drug-drug interactions before prescribing. **Pregnancy: Category D; associated w/ increased risk of teratogenesis (need to inform women of childbearing age of this risk).** Cardiac malformations, including Ebstein's anomaly (background rate of this defect is 1/20,000 births compared to the ~1/1000 rate among infants exposed to lithium in utero), are the primary risk of using lithium during the first trimester. **Breastfeeding:** Contraindicated. **Dosage Form:** Capsule, Tablet, Coated Tablet (Do not cut, crush or chew). **Generic Available:** IR/ER: Yes. **Cost: $. FDA label information from Drugs @FDA for Lithobid and lithium carbonate dated 10.20.2011.**

Antipsychotics

Aripiprazole (Abilify)
ANTIPSYCHOTIC RISK PROFILE: EPS: Mild; TD Risk: Mild; Sedation: Mild; Metabolic Effects: Mild.

DOSING INFORMATION: Week 1: Assess baseline weight, waist circumference, blood pressure, fasting plasma glucose, fasting lipid profile, CBC (for baseline WBC), EKG (to assess QTc) and AIMS test. **Initiation for Schizophrenia: Start:** 7.5 mg qday. *Week 2:* increase dose to an **Initial Target Dose** of 15 mg qday, if tolerated. **Typical Dosage Range:** 15–30 mg qday. **Max Dose:** 30 mg qday, although there is little compelling evidence for benefit of doses above 15 mg qday. **Initiation for Bipolar Manic/Mixed Episode: Start:** 7.5–15 mg qday depending on episode severity.

Week 2: Increase dose to an **Initial Target Dosage** between 15–30 mg qday depending on tolerability and response to Abilify. **Typical Dosage Range:** 15–30 mg qday. **Max Dose:** 30 mg qday. **Initiation for Major Depressive Disorder, Adjunctive: Start:** 2 mg qday (the **Initial Target Dose**). Continue for at least 2 weeks. *Week 3:* Consider further increase to 5 mg qday, if tolerated, and if still severely symptomatic. **Typical Dosage Range:** 2–5 mg qday. **Max Dose:** 10 mg qday. **Discontinuation:** Taper slowly to minimize withdrawal symptoms.

ONGOING MONITORING: EKG at target dose (at least once to assess QTc). *At 4 weeks:* weight. *At 8 weeks:* weight. *At 12 weeks:* weight, blood pressure, fasting plasma glucose, fasting lipid profile. *Quarterly thereafter:* weight. *Annually ongoing:* waist circumference, weight, blood pressure, fasting plasma glucose, fasting lipid profile, and AIMS test. Repeat CBC in patients with previous low WBC.

GENERAL INFORMATION: Atypical antipsychotic/partial dopamine agonist. **FDA Indications:** Schizophrenia; Bipolar mania and mixed episode (also as adjunctive to lithium and valproate); Major depressive disorder, adjunctive; Irritability associated with autism (pediatrics). **Off-Label Indications:** PTSD/OCD augmentation. **Pharmacokinetics:** $T\frac{1}{2} = 75$ h. **Common side effects (MDD, adjunctive):** Akathisia (25 percent), restlessness (12 percent), insomnia (8 percent), fatigue (8 percent), blurred vision (6 percent), constipation (5 percent). **Common side effects (Mania):** Akathisia (13 percent), sedation (8 percent), restlessness (6 percent), tremor (6 percent), extrapyramidal symptoms (5 percent). **Black-box warnings:** (1) Increased mortality in elderly patients with dementia related psychosis. (2) Increased risk of suicidal thinking and behavior in children, adolescents and young adults. **Contraindications:** Known hypersensitivity reaction to the product. **Warnings and precautions:** Use in elderly patients with dementia-related psychosis, clinical worsening of depression and suicide risk, NMS, TD, metabolic changes including hyperglycemia and diabetes mellitus, dyslipidemia and weight gain, orthostatic hypotension, increased risk of leukopenia, neutropenia and agranulocytosis, seizures/convulsions, potential for cognitive and motor impairment, body temperature dysregulation, dysphagia, QTc prolongation, sudden cardiac death, cerebrovascular accident. **Metabolism/Pharmacogenomics:** Metabolized by 3A4 and 2D6. **Significant drug–drug interactions:** Caution with 3A4 inducers (e.g., carbamazepine)—Abilify dosage should be doubled when coadministered with carbamazepine. Caution when coadministered with strong 3A4 inhibitors (e.g., ketoconazole and protease inhibitors) and strong 2D6 inhibitors (e.g., fluoxetine and paroxetine). In both cases the Abilify dosage should be cut in half. Potential to enhance the effect of certain antihypertensives due to its α1-adrenergic receptor antagonism; Check all drug-drug interactions before prescribing. **Pregnancy:** Category C. Developmental toxicity and teratogenic effects in animal studies. **Breastfeeding:** Excreted/Not Recommended. **Dosage Form:** Tablet, Soluble, Oral Dissolving Tablet. **Generic Available:** yes, **Cost: $$$**. **FDA label information from Drugs @FDA for Abilify dated 7.20.13.**

Asenapine (Saphris)

ANTIPSYCHOTIC RISK PROFILE: EPS: Mild to moderate; TD Risk: Unknown; Sedation: Mild to moderate Metabolic Effects: Mild

DOSING INFORMATION: Week 1: Assess baseline weight, waist circumference, blood pressure, fasting plasma glucose, fasting lipid profile, EKG (to assess QTc) and AIMS test. **Initiation for Schizophrenia: Start:** 5 mg bid (the **Initial Target and Typical Dose**). *OF NOTE:* This is a sublingual medication and the patient should not eat or drink for 10 min after administration. **Max Dose:** 10 mg bid, although there is little compelling evidence in schizophrenia for additional efficacy of 10 mg bid. **Initiation for Bipolar Manic/Mixed Episode: Start:** 5–10 mg bid (the **Initial Target and Typical Dose**) depending on episode severity. **Typical Dosage Range:** 5–10 mg bid. **Max Dose:** 10 mg bid. **Discontinuation:** Taper slowly to minimize withdrawal symptoms.

ONGOING MONITORING: EKG at target dose (at least once to assess QTc). *At 4 weeks:* Weight. *At 8 weeks:* Weight. *At 12 weeks:* Weight, blood pressure, fasting plasma glucose, fasting lipid profile. *Quarterly thereafter:* Weight. *Annually ongoing:* Waist circumference, weight, blood pressure, fasting plasma glucose, fasting lipid profile, AIMS test. Repeat CBC in patients with previous low WBC.

GENERAL INFORMATION: Atypical antipsychotic. **FDA Indications:** Acute schizophrenia; Acute bipolar mania or mixed (monotherapy or as adjunctive). **Off-Label Indications:** None. **Pharmacokinetics:** T½ = 24 hrs. **Common side effects (Schizophrenia):** Somnolence (13 percent), EPS excluding akathisia (10 percent), akathisia (6 percent), oral hypoesthesia (5 percent). **Black-box warnings:** Increased mortality in elderly patients with dementia related psychosis. **Contraindications:** Known hypersensitivity reaction to the product. **Warnings and precautions:** Increased mortality and risk of cerebrovascular adverse events including stroke in elderly patients with dementia-related psychosis, NMS, TD, hyperglycemia and diabetes mellitus, weight gain, hypersensitivity reactions, orthostatic hypotension and syncope, increased risk of leukopenia, neutropenia and agranulocytosis, QT prolongation, sudden cardiac death, hyperprolactinemia, seizures, potential for cognitive and motor impairment, body temperature regulation, dysphagia. **Metabolism/Pharmacogenomics:** Cleared primarily by glucuronidation and metabolism by 1A2. **Significant drug-drug interactions:** Saphris is a weak 2D6 inhibitor. Use caution when coadministered with drugs metabolized by 2D6 (e.g., venlafaxine). Caution when coadministered with potent 1A2 inhibitors (e.g., fluvoxamine); Check all drug-drug interactions before prescribing. **Pregnancy:** Category C. **Breastfeeding:** No data/Not recommended. **Dosage Form:** Sublingual tablet. **Generic Available:** No. **Cost: $$$. FDA label information from Drugs @FDA for Saphris dated 3.21.13.**

Haloperidol (Haldol)

ANTIPSYCHOTIC RISK PROFILE: EPS: High; TD Risk: High; Sedation: Mild; Metabolic Effects: Mild.

DOSING INFORMATION: Week 1: Assess baseline weight, waist circumference, blood pressure, fasting plasma glucose, fasting lipid profile, EKG (to assess QTc) and AIMS test. **Start:** 1 mg bid (0.5 mg bid in the elderly)*. *Week 2:* Increase to an **Initial Target Dose** of 2 mg bid (1 mg bid in the elderly), if tolerated. *Week 3 and beyond:* Assess for side effects and consider further increases to 1 mg bid increments, if tolerated, until symptom remission or max dose is reached. If qAM dosage is excessively sedating consider consolidating more of the dose to qHS. **Typical Dosage Range:** 4–10 mg (2–5 mg in the elderly). **Max Dose:** 20 mg (10 mg in the elderly). *OF NOTE:* It is frequently necessary to prescribe an anticholinergic medication with Haldol to treat Parkinsonian side effects (Benadryl 25 mg or Cogentin 1–2 mg PRN or scheduled). **Discontinuation:** Taper slowly to minimize withdrawal symptoms.

ONGOING MONITORING: EKG at target dose (at least once to assess QTc). *At 4 weeks:* weight. *At 8 weeks:* weight. *At 12 weeks:* weight, blood pressure, fasting plasma glucose, fasting lipid profile. *Quarterly thereafter:* weight. *Annually ongoing:* waist circumference, weight, blood pressure, fasting plasma glucose, fasting lipid profile, and AIMS test.

GENERAL INFORMATION: Typical antipsychotic. **FDA Indications:** "Management of manifestation of psychotic disorders." **Pharmacokinetics:** T½ = up to 3 weeks. **Common side effects (Psychosis):** Extrapyramidal symptoms (Parkinsonism, akathisia), orthostatic hypotension, sedation/fatigue, weight gain, dry mouth, nausea, insomnia, dizziness, anxiety. **Black-box warning:** Increased mortality in elderly patients with dementia related psychosis. **Contraindications:** Known hypersensitivity reaction to the product. Severe toxic central nervous system depression or comatose states. Parkinson's disease. **Warnings and precautions:** Increased risks in elderly patients with dementia-related psychosis, cardiovascular effects (sudden death, QT-prolongation, and torsades de pointes), TD, NMS, usage in pregnancy, combined use with lithium, increased risk of bronchopneumonia, potential for cognitive and motor impairment, use with alcohol, increased risk of leukopenia, neutropenia and agranulocytosis, hypotension, caution in patient with severe cardiovascular disease, seizures, hyperprolactinemia, potential for severe neurotoxicity in patients with thyrotoxicosis, dysphagia, body temperature regulation. **Metabolism/Pharmacogenomics:** Metabolized by glucuronidation and 3A4 and 2D6. **Significant drug–drug interactions:** Caution with 3A4 inducers (e.g., carbamazepine and St. John's wort) and inhibitors of 3A4 (ketoconazole and protease inhibitors) and 2D6 (e.g., fluoxetine and paroxetine); Check all drug-drug interactions before prescribing. **Pregnancy:** Category C. **Breastfeeding:** Excreted /Use caution. Would recommend checking blood levels in the infant/toddler to confirm minimal maternal transfer of this medication given the variability in excretion between mothers. **Dosage Form:** Tablet, Concentrate. **Generic Available:** Yes. **Cost:** ¢. **FDA label for Haldol from dailymed.nlm.nih.gov, Rev. dated 10.2011.**

Iloperidone (Fanapt)

ANTIPSYCHOTIC RISK PROFILE: EPS: Very low; TD Risk: Mild; Sedation: Unknown, likely low; Metabolic Effects: Moderate

DOSING INFORMATION: Week 1: Assess baseline weight, waist circumference, blood pressure, fasting plasma glucose, fasting lipid profile, EKG (to assess QTc) and AIMS test. **Titration schedule:** *Day 1:* 1 mg bid. *Day 3:* 2 mg bid. *Day 8:* 4 mg bid. *Day 15:* 6 mg bid (the **Initial Target Dose**). Titration can be slowed for orthostatic hypotension or other side effects. *Week 3:* Consider further titration to max dosing as needed and tolerated. **Typical Dosage Range:** 6–12 mg bid. **Max Dose:** 24 mg/day. **Restarting therapy after discontinuation:** if medication has been stopped for greater than 3 days, the initial titration schedule should be followed. **Discontinuation:** Taper slowly to minimize withdrawal symptoms.

ONGOING MONITORING: EKG at target dose (at least once to assess QTc). *At 4 weeks:* Weight. *At 8 weeks:* Weight. *At 12 weeks:* Weight, blood pressure, fasting plasma glucose, fasting lipid profile. *Quarterly thereafter:* Weight. *Annually ongoing:* Waist circumference, weight, blood pressure, fasting plasma glucose, fasting lipid profile, AIMS test. Repeat CBC in patients with previous low WBC.

GENERAL INFORMATION: Atypical antipsychotic. **FDA Indications:** Schizophrenia. **Off-Label Indications:** None. **Pharmacokinetics:** T½ = 18 hrs, active metabolite = 26 hrs. **Common side effects:** Dizziness (10 percent), somnolence (9 percent), dry mouth 8 percent), nasal congestion (5 percent). **Black-box warnings:** Increased mortality in elderly patients with dementia related psychosis. **Contraindications:** Known hypersensitivity reaction to the product. **Warnings and precautions:** Increased risks in elderly patients with dementia-related psychosis, QTc prolongation, NMS, TD, metabolic changes including hyperglycemia and diabetes, dyslipidemia and weight gain, seizures, orthostatic hypotension and syncope, increased risk of leukopenia, neutropenia and agranulocytosis, hyperprolactinemia, body temperature regulation, dysphasia, **priapism**, potential for cognitive and motor impairment, sudden cardiac death, cardiovascular accident. **Metabolism/Pharmacogenomics:** Metabolized by 3A4 and 2D6. Caution with 2D6 poor metabolizers. **Significant drug-drug interactions:** Caution when coadministered with strong 3A4 inhibitors (e.g., ketoconazole) and strong 2D6 inhibitors (e.g., fluoxetine and paroxetine). In both cases the Fanapt dosage should be cut in half. Caution with centrally acting antihypertensives (due to its α1-adrenergic receptor antagonism). Should not be used with any other drugs that prolong the QT interval; Check all drug-drug interactions before prescribing. **Pregnancy:** Category C. **Breastfeeding:** No data/Not recommended. **Dosage Form:** Tablet. **Generic Available:** No. **Cost: $$$. FDA label information from Drugs @FDA for Fanapt dated 4.21.2014.**

Lurasidone (Latuda)

ANTIPSYCHOTIC RISK PROFILE: EPS: Mild to Moderate; TD Risk: Unknown; Sedation: Moderate; Metabolic Effects: Mild.

DOSING INFORMATION: Week 1: Assess baseline weight, waist circumference, blood pressure, fasting plasma glucose, fasting lipid profile, CBC (for baseline WBC), EKG (to assess QTc) and AIMS test. *OF NOTE:* It is critical to take Latuda with food (at least 350 calories) for optimal absorption (increased by up to three fold). Also, grapefruit juice should be avoided. **Initiation for Schizophrenia: Start:** 40 mg qday (the **Initial Target Dosage**). *Week 2:* Assess for side effects. **Typical Dosage Range:** 40–160 mg qday. **Max Dose:** 160 mg/day. **Initiation for Bipolar Depression: Start:** 20 mg qday (**the Initial Target Dose**). *Week 2:* Assess for side effects. **Typical Dosage Range:** 20–60 mg/day. **Max Dose:** 120 mg/day. **Discontinuation:** Taper slowly to minimize withdrawal symptoms.

ONGOING MONITORING: EKG at target dose (at least once to assess QTc). *At 4 weeks:* Weight. *At 8 weeks:* Weight. *At 12 weeks:* Weight, blood pressure, fasting plasma glucose, fasting lipid profile. *Quarterly thereafter:* Weight. *Annually ongoing:* Waist circumference, weight, blood pressure, fasting plasma glucose, fasting lipid profile, AIMS test. Repeat CBC in patients with previous low WBC.

GENERAL INFORMATION: Atypical antipsychotic. **FDA Indications:** Schizophrenia; Bipolar I, depression as monotherapy or adjunct to lithium or valproate. **Off-Label Indications:** No data yet. **Pharmacokinetics:** T $\frac{1}{2}$ = 18 hrs. **Common Side Effects (Schizophrenia):** Somnolence (17 percent), EPS (14 percent), akathisia (13 percent), nausea (10 percent). **Common Side Effects (Bipolar Depression):** Nausea (14 percent), somnolence (11 percent), akathisia (9 percent), EPS (7 percent). **Black-box warnings:** (1) Increased mortality in elderly patients with dementia related psychosis. (2) Increased risk of suicidal thinking and behavior in children, adolescents, and young adults taking antidepressants. (3) Monitor for worsening and emergence of suicidal thoughts and behaviors. **Contraindications:** Known hypersensitivity reaction to the product. Coadministration with strong CYP3A4 inhibitors (e.g., ketoconazole and protease inhibitors) and inducers (e.g., carbamazepine and St. John's wort). **Warnings and precautions:** Increased mortality and risk of cerebrovascular adverse events including stroke in elderly patients with dementia-related psychosis, suicidal thoughts and behaviors in adolescents and young adults, NMS, TD, metabolic changes including hyperglycemia and diabetes, hyperprolactinemia, increased risk of leukopenia, neutropenia and agranulocytosis, orthostatic hypotension and syncope, seizures, potential for cognitive and motor impairment, body temperature dysregulation, hypomanic/manic switch, dysphagia, neurological adverse reactions in patient with Parkinson's disease or dementia with Lewy Bodies. **Metabolism/Pharmacogenomics:** Metabolized by 3A4. **Significant drug-drug interactions: Do not use Latuda in combination with strong 3A4 inhibitors (e.g., ketoconazole or protease inhibitors) or inducers (e.g., carbamazepine or St. John's wort).** Latuda dosage should be cut in half with moderate 3A4 inhibitors (e.g., diltiazem). Dosage adjustment may be necessary with coadministered with moderate 3A4 inducers. Grapefruit juice should be avoided. Check all drug-drug interactions and *CONSIDER CONSULTATION WITH A PHARMACIST BEFORE PRESCRIBING THIS MEDICATION.* **Pregnancy:** Category B. **Breastfeeding:** No data/Not recommended. **Dosage Form:** Tablet. **Generic Available:** No. **Cost: $$$.** **FDA label information from Drugs @FDA for Latuda dated 7.12.2013.**

Olanzapine (Zyprexa)

ANTIPSYCHOTIC RISK PROFILE: EPS: Mild; TD Risk: Mild; Sedation: Moderate to high; Metabolic Effects: Severe.

DOSING INFORMATION: Week 1: Assess baseline weight, waist circumference, blood pressure, fasting plasma glucose, fasting lipid profile, CBC (for baseline WBC), EKG (to assess QTc) and AIMS test. **Initiation for**

Schizophrenia: Start: 5 mg qHS. *Week 2:* Increase dose to the **Initial Target Dose** of 10 mg qHS, if tolerated. *Week 3 and beyond:* If still symptomatic, consider further increases, if tolerated, to 15–20 mg qHS. **Typical Dosage Range:** 10–20 mg qHS. **Max Dose:** 20 mg qHS. **Initiation for Bipolar Manic/Mixed Episode: Start:** 10 mg qHS (the **Initial Target Dose**). *Week 2 and beyond:* Increase dose to 15 mg qHS as needed and tolerated. **Typical Dosage Range:** 10–20 mg qHS mg. *OF NOTE:* Maintenance dosage is usually lower than dose used in acute episodes. **Max Dose:** 20 mg qHS. **Discontinuation:** Taper slowly to minimize withdrawal symptoms.

ONGOING MONITORING: EKG at target dose (at least once to assess QTc). *At 4 weeks:* Weight, Fasting lipid profile. *At 8 weeks:* Weight. *At 12 weeks:* Weight, blood pressure, fasting plasma glucose, fasting lipid profile. *Quarterly thereafter:* Weight. *Annually ongoing:* Waist circumference, weight, blood pressure, fasting plasma glucose, fasting lipid profile, and AIMS test.

GENERAL INFORMATION: Atypical antipsychotic. **FDA Indications:** Schizophrenia, Bipolar I disorder (manic or mixed episodes) with and without lithium or valproate. **Off-Label Indications:** PTSD/OCD augmentation, Depression augmentation. **Pharmacokinetics:** $T\frac{1}{2}$ = 30 hr. **Common Side Effects:** Weight gain/increased appetite (~17 percent >11 lb. gain at six weeks; ~40 percent >11 lb. gain at 6 months), somnolence (29 percent), dizziness (11 percent), dry mouth (9 percent), constipation (9 percent). **Black-box warnings:** Increased mortality in elderly patients with dementia related psychosis. **Contraindications:** Known hypersensitivity reaction to the product. **Warnings and precautions:** Elderly patients with dementia-related psychosis, NMS, hyperglycemia, hyperlipidemia, weight gain, TD, orthostatic hypotension, leukopenia, neutropenia, and agranulocytosis, dysphagia, seizures, potential for cognitive and motor impairment, body temperature dysregulation, hyperprolactinemia, QT prolongation, sudden cardiac death, cerebrovascular accident. **Metabolism/ Pharmacogenomics:** Primarily metabolized by direct glucuronidation and 1A2. **Significant drug-drug interactions:** Caution when coadministered with 1A2 inducers (e.g., carbamazepine) and potent 1A2 inhibitors (e.g., fluvoxamine—consider dosage adjustment); *OF NOTE:* tobacco induces the metabolism of Zyprexa—consider dosage adjustment when starting or stopping tobacco; Check all drug-drug interactions before prescribing. **Pregnancy:** Category C. **Breastfeeding:** Excreted /Not recommended. **Dosage Form:** Tablet, Tablet Dispersible. **Generic Available:** Yes. **Cost:** ¢. **FDA label information from Drugs @FDA for Zyprexa dated 7.12.2013.**

Olanzapine and fluoxetine (Symbyax)

ANTIPSYCHOTIC RISK PROFILE: EPS: Mild TD Risk: Mild Sedation: Moderate to high Metabolic Effects: Severe

DOSING INFORMATION: **Initiation for Bipolar Depression and Treatment Resistant Depression:** *Week 1:* Assess baseline weight, waist circumference, blood pressure, fasting plasma glucose, fasting lipid profile, EKG (to assess QTc) and AIMS test. Consider BMP for baseline sodium in older adults. **Start:** olanzapine 6 mg/fluoxetine 25 mg qHS (the **Initial Target Dose**). In patients with risk for orthostasis, start olanzapine 3 mg/fluoxetine 25 mg qHS. *Week 4 and beyond:* Consider increase in dose if needed and tolerated. **Typical Dosage Range:** olanzapine 6 mg/fluoxetine 25 mg-olanzapine 12 mg/fluoxetine 50 mg qHS. **Max Dose:** olanzapine 12 mg /fluoxetine 50 mg qHS. **Discontinuation:** Taper slowly to minimize withdrawal symptoms.

ONGOING MONITORING: EKG at target dose (at least once to assess QTc). *At 4 weeks:* Weight, Fasting lipid profile. *At 8 weeks:* Weight. *At 12 weeks:* Weight, blood pressure, fasting plasma glucose, fasting lipid profile. *Quarterly thereafter:* Weight. *Annually ongoing:* Waist circumference, weight, blood pressure, fasting plasma glucose, fasting lipid profile, AIMS test. Repeat CBC in patients with previous low WBC. Consider posttreatment BMP to rule out hyponatremia in older adults.

GENERAL INFORMATION: Atypical antipsychotic combined with SSRI. **FDA Indications:** Depressive Episodes Associated with Bipolar I disorder and Treatment Resistant Depression. **Off-Label Indications:** None. **Pharmacokinetics:** T½ (olanzapine) = 30 hr; T½ (fluoxetine) = 4–6 days. **Common Side Effects:** Somnolence (27 percent), Weight gain (25 percent), increased appetite (20 percent), dry mouth (15 percent), edema (15 percent), fatigue (12 percent), tremor (9 percent), vision blurred (5 percent), disturbance in attention (5 percent). **Black-box warnings:** (1) Increased risk of suicidal thinking and behavior in children, adolescents, and young adults taking antidepressants, (2) Monitor for worsening and emergence of suicidal thoughts and behaviors, (3) Increased mortality in elderly patients with dementia related psychosis. **Contraindications:** Known hypersensitivity reaction to fluoxetine or olanzapine. Use of a MAOI within 5 weeks of stopping Symbyax, concurrent use of a MAOI including drugs with significant MAOI activity (e.g., linezolid), or use of Symbyax within 5 weeks of stopping a MAOI. Do not use pimozide or thioridazine with Symbyax because of QT prolongation risk. **Warnings and precautions:** Clinical worsening and suicide risk, elderly patients with dementia-related psychosis, NMS, hyperglycemia, hyperlipidemia, weight gain, serotonin syndrome, allergic reactions and rash, hypomanic/manic switch, TD, orthostatic hypotension, leukopenia, neutropenia, and agranulocytosis, dysphagia, seizures, abnormal bleeding, hyponatremia, potential for cognitive and motor impairment, body temperature dysregulation, QT prolongation, hyperprolactinemia, long elimination half-life of fluoxetine, discontinuation reactions, sudden cardiac death, cerebrovascular accident. **Metabolism/Pharmacogenomics:** *Fluoxetine:* primarily metabolized by 2D6. Use caution with 2D6 poor metabolizers. *Olanzapine:* primarily metabolized by direct glucuronidation and 1A2. **Significant drug-drug interactions:** *Fluoxetine:* potent 2D6 inhibitor; Use significant caution when coadministered with drugs metabolized by 2D6 (e.g., TCAs). *Olanzapine:* caution when coadministered with 1A2 inducers (e.g., carbamazepine) and potent 1A2 inhibitors (e.g., fluvoxamine—consider dosage adjustment). *OF NOTE:* tobacco induces the metabolism of olanzapine—consider dosage adjustment when starting or stopping tobacco. Check all drug-drug interactions before prescribing. **Pregnancy:** Category C. **Breastfeeding:** Excreted/Not recommended. **Dosage Form:** Capsule. **Significant drug-drug interactions:** Check all drug-drug interactions. **Generic Available:** Yes. **Cost: $$ (if components purchased separately, $). FDA label information from Drugs @FDA for Symbyax dated 8.7.2013.**

Paliperidone (Invega)

ANTIPSYCHOTIC RISK PROFILE: EPS: Moderate; TD Risk: Moderate; Sedation: Moderate; Metabolic Effects: Moderate.

DOSING INFORMATION: **Initiation for Schizophrenia and Schizoaffective Disorder:** *Week 1:* Assess baseline weight, waist circumference, blood pressure, fasting plasma glucose, fasting lipid profile, and EKG (to assess QTc) and AIMS test. **Start:** 3 mg qAM. *Week 2:* Increase to an **Initial Target Dose** of 6 mg qAM, if tolerated. *Week 3 and beyond:* Consider further increases in 3 mg increments up to a maximum of 12 mg/day, if tolerated. **Typical Dosage Range:** 3–12 mg qday. **Max Dose:** 12 mg/day. **Discontinuation:** Taper slowly to minimize withdrawal symptoms.

ONGOING MONITORING: EKG at target dose (at least once to assess QTc). *At 4 weeks:* Weight. *At 8 weeks:* Weight. *At 12 weeks:* Weight, blood pressure, fasting plasma glucose, fasting lipid profile. *Quarterly thereafter:* Weight. Annually ongoing: Waist circumference, weight, blood pressure, fasting plasma glucose, fasting lipid profile, AIMS test. Repeat CBC in patients with previous low WBC.

GENERAL INFORMATION: Atypical antipsychotic. **FDA Indications:** Schizophrenia; Schizoaffective disorder (monotherapy or as adjunctive). **Off-Label Indications:** Bipolar, mixed or manic. **Pharmacokinetics:**

T ½ =23 hrs. **Common Side Effects (Schizophrenia):** Somnolence (20 percent), extrapyramidal symptoms (18 percent), akathisia (11 percent), tachycardia (9 percent). **Black-box warnings:** Increased mortality in elderly patients with dementia related psychosis. **Contraindications:** Known hypersensitivity reaction to the product or risperidone, or to any components in the formulation. **Warnings and precautions:** Increased mortality and risk of cerebrovascular adverse events including stroke in elderly patients with dementia-related psychosis, NMS, QT prolongation, sudden cardiac death, cerebrovascular accidents, TD, metabolic changes including hyperglycemia and diabetes, dyslipidemia and weight gain, hyperprolactinemia, potential for gastrointestinal obstruction, orthostatic hypotension and syncope, increased risk of leukopenia, neutropenia and agranulocytosis, potential for cognitive and motor impairment, seizures, dysphagia, **priapism**, potential increased risk for thrombotic thrombocytopenic purpura, body temperature dysregulation, antiemetic effect. **Metabolism/Pharmacogenomics:** Majority of absorbed dose is renally excreted unchanged. Multiple minor hepatic metabolic pathways. **Significant drug-drug interactions:** Caution with use of other drug that can cause orthostatic hypotension; Carbamazepine increases the renal clearance of Invega by ~40 percent whereas valproate increases the effective dosage of Invega by ~50 percent. Check all drug-drug interactions before prescribing. **Pregnancy:** Category C. **Breastfeeding:** Excreted/Not recommended. **Dosage Form:** Tablet, Suspension. **Generic Available:** No. **Cost:** $$$. **FDA label information from Drugs @FDA for INVEGA dated 4.6.2011.**

Perphenazine (Trilafon)

ANTIPSYCHOTIC RISK PROFILE: EPS: Moderate; TD Risk: High; Sedation: Moderate; Metabolic Effects: Mild.

DOSING INFORMATION: Week 1: Assess baseline Weight, waist circumference, blood pressure, fasting plasma glucose, fasting lipid profile, CBC (for baseline WBC) and EKG (to assess QTc) and AIMS test. **Start:** 4 mg bid. *Week 2:* Increase to an **Initial Target Dose** of 8 mg bid, if tolerated. *Week 3 and beyond:* Assess for side effects and consider further increases to 12 mg bid if still symptomatic. If qAM dosage is excessively sedating consider consolidating more of the dose to qHS. **Typical Dosage Range:** 8–24 mg/day. **Max Dose:** 24 mg/day in an outpatient setting. *OF NOTE:* Consider lower overall dosing in the elderly. **Discontinuation:** Taper slowly to minimize withdrawal symptoms.

ONGOING MONITORING: EKG at target dose (at least once to assess QTc). *At 4 weeks:* Weight. *At 8 weeks:* Weight. *At 12 weeks:* Weight, blood pressure, fasting plasma glucose, fasting lipid profile. *Quarterly thereafter:* Weight.

Annually ongoing: Waist circumference, weight, blood pressure, fasting plasma glucose, fasting lipid profile and AIMS test.

GENERAL INFORMATION: Typical antipsychotic. **FDA Indications:** Schizophrenia. **Pharmacokinetics:** T½ = 9–12 hrs. **Common Side Effects:** Extrapyramidal symptoms (seen at higher doses; Parkinsonism, akathisia), orthostatic hypotension, sedation/fatigue and anticholinergic side effects (blurred vision, urinary retention, xerostomia, constipation). **Black-box warnings:** Increased mortality in elderly patients with dementia related psychosis. **Contraindications:** Known hypersensitivity reaction to the product. Use in comatose or greatly obtunded patients and in patients receiving large doses of CNS depressants, in patients with suspected or established subcortical brain damage, with or without hypothalamic damage, in the presence of existing blood dyscrasias, bone marrow depression, or liver damage. **Warnings and precautions:** Increased mortality and risk of cerebrovascular adverse events including stroke in elderly patients with dementia-related psychosis, tardive dyskinesia, NMS, suicidality, seizures, caution in patient with depression, potential for cognitive and motor impairment, orthostatic hypotension, QTc prolongation, hyperprolactinemia, sudden cardiac death, cerebrovascular accident, body temperature dysregulation, increased risk of leukopenia, neutropenia and agranulocytosis long term use associated with potential liver damage, corneal and lenticular deposits. **Metabolism/Pharmacogenomics:** Metabolized by 2D6. Use caution with 2D6 poor metabolizers. **Significant drug-drug interactions:** Use caution with potent 2D6 inhibitors (e.g., fluoxetine and paroxetine). Check all drug-drug interactions before prescribing. **Pregnancy:** Category C. **Breastfeeding:** Excreted/Not recommended. **Dosage Form:** Tablet. **Generic Available:** Yes. **Cost:** $. **FDA label information from Drugs @FDA for Trilafon dated 5.2.2002. FDA label for perphenazine from dailymed.nlm.nih.gov, Rev. dated 12.2013.**

Quetiapine (Seroquel, Seroquel XR)

ANTIPSYCHOTIC RISK PROFILE: EPS: Mild; TD Risk: Mild; Sedation: Moderate; Metabolic Effects: Moderate to severe.

DOSING INFORMATION: Week 1: Assess baseline weight, waist circumference, blood pressure, fasting plasma glucose, fasting lipid profile, CBC (for baseline WBC), EKG (to assess QTc) and AIMS test. **Initiation for Schizophrenia or Bipolar Manic/Mixed Episode: Start Seroquel (IR):** Day 1, 25 mg bid; Day 2, 50 mg bid; Day 3, 100 mg bid; Day 4, 150 mg bid and Day 5, 200 mg bid (**Initial Target Dose IR**). This titration schedule can be slowed down because of side effects. At higher daily dosages consider scheduling a greater proportion of dose qHS to limit daytime sedation.

Start Seroquel XR: Day 1, 50 mg qHS; Day 2, 100 mg qHS; Day 3, 200 mg qHS; Day 4, 300 mg qHS and Day 5, 400 mg qHS (**Initial Target Dose XR**). This titration schedule can be slowed down because of side effects. *Week 2:* Can consider further increases in 100 mg increments, if tolerated, up to **Max Dose (IR/XR)** of 800 mg/day. **Typical Dosage Range (IR/XR):** 400–800 mg/day. **Initiation for Bipolar Depression: Start Seroquel IR/XR:** Day 1, 50 mg qHS; Day 2, 100 mg qHS; Day 3, 200 mg qHS; and Day 4, 300 mg qHS (**Initial Target Dose IR/XR**). **Typical Dosage Range (IR/XR):** 300–600 mg/day. **Max Dose (IR/XR):** 600 mg/day. **Initiation for Adjunctive Treatment for Major Depression: Start Seroquel XR:** Day 1, 50 mg qHS; Day 2, 100 mg qHS; Day 3, 150 mg qHS (**Initial Target Dosage XR**). **Typical Dosage Range (XR):** 150–300 mg qHS. **Maximum Dose (XR):** 300 mg qHS. *OF NOTE:* for the elderly consider a slower rate of dose titration and a lower target dose for all indications. **Discontinuation:** Stopping medication abruptly may cause discontinuation syndrome (insomnia, nausea, headache, diarrhea, vomiting, irritability).

ONGOING MONITORING: EKG at target dose (at least once to assess QTc). *At 4 weeks:* Weight, Fasting lipid profile. *At 8 weeks:* weight. *At 12 weeks:* weight, blood pressure, fasting plasma glucose, fasting lipid profile. *Quarterly thereafter:* weight. *Annually /ongoing:* Waist circumference, weight, blood pressure, fasting plasma glucose, fasting lipid profile and AIMS test. Consider checking for cataracts.

GENERAL INFORMATION: Atypical antipsychotic. **FDA Indications:** Schizophrenia (IR, XR), Bipolar I – manic (IR, XR), Bipolar I – mixed (XR), Bipolar disorder – depressive episode (IR, XR), Bipolar maintenance as adjunctive to lithium or divalproex (IR, XR), Adjunctive treatment of MDD (XR). **Off-Label Indications:** Anxiety disorders augmentation. **Pharmacokinetics:** T $\frac{1}{2}$ = 6 hr (IR); 7 hrs (XR). **Common Side Effects (Schizophrenia and Bipolar Mania—Seroquel IR):** Headache (21 percent), somnolence (18 percent), dizziness (11 percent), dry mouth (9 percent), constipation (8 percent), weight gain (5 percent), dyspepsia (5 percent), ALT increased (5 percent). **Common Side Effects (Bipolar Depression—Seroquel XR):** Somnolence (52 percent), dry mouth (37 percent), Increased appetite (12 percent), dyspepsia (7 percent), weight gain (7 percent), fatigue (6 percent). **Black-box warnings:** (1) Increased mortality in elderly patients with dementia related psychosis. (2) Increased risk of suicidal thinking and behavior in children, adolescents, and young adults taking antidepressants. (3) Monitor for worsening and emergence of suicidal thoughts and behaviors. **Contraindications:** Known hypersensitivity reaction to the product. **Warnings and precautions:** Increased mortality and risk of cerebrovascular adverse events including stroke in elderly patients with dementia-related psychosis, suicidal thoughts and behaviors in adolescents and young adults, NMS, metabolic changes including hyperglycemia and diabetes, dyslipidemia and weight gain, TD, hypotension, increased risk of leukopenia, neutropenia and agranulocytosis, cataracts, QT prolongation, seizures, hypothyroidism, hyperprolactinemia, potential for cognitive and motor impairment, body temperature dysregulation, dysphagia, discontinuation syndrome, seizures, dysphagia QTc prolongation, sudden cardiac death, cerebrovascular accident. **Metabolism/Pharmacogenomics:** Metabolized by 3A4. **Significant drug-drug interactions:** Dosage adjustment is required when quetiapine is coadministered with strong 3A4 inhibitors (e.g., reduce the dosage to one sixth with ketoconazole and ritonavir) or with chronic treatment (>7–14 days) with potent 3A4 inducers (e.g., increase the dosage by 5 fold with phenytoin, rifampin, St. John's wort). Caution with medications that cause QTc prolongation. Check all drug-drug interactions and *CONSIDER CONSULTATION WITH A PHARMACIST BEFORE PRESCRIBING THIS MEDICATION.* **Pregnancy:** Category C. **Breastfeeding:** Excreted/Not recommended. **Dosage Form:** Tablet, Tablet-24-hour. **Generic Available:** IR: yes; XR: No. **Cost:** IR: $, XR: $$$. **FDA label information from Drugs @FDA for Seroquel IR dated 10.29.14. FDA label information from Drugs @FDA for Seroquel XR dated 4.30.2013.**

Risperidone (Risperdal)

ANTIPSYCHOTIC RISK PROFILE: EPS: Moderate; TD Risk: Moderate; Sedation: Moderate; Metabolic Effects: Moderate.

DOSING INFORMATION: Week 1: Assess baseline weight, waist circumference, blood pressure, fasting plasma glucose, fasting lipid profile, CBC (for baseline WBC), EKG (to assess QTc) and AIMS test. **Initiation for Schizophrenia: Start:** 1 mg qHS. *Week 2:* Increase to 1 mg bid, if tolerated. *Week 3:* Increase to an **Initial Target Dose** of 1 mg qAM and 2 mg qHS, if tolerated. If qAM dosage is excessively sedating consider consolidating more of the dose to qHS. *Week 4 and beyond:* Assess side effects and consider further increases in 1 mg increments, if tolerated until symptom remission or **Max Dose** of 6 mg reached. **Typical Dosage Range:** 3–4 mg/day. *OF NOTE:* dosages above 4 mg/day are much more likely to be associated with EPS and it may be necessary to prescribe an anticholinergic medication to deal with Parkinsonian side effects (Benadryl 25 mg or Cogentin 1–2 mg PRN or scheduled). **Initiation for Bipolar Mania and Mixed Episodes: Start:** 1–2 mg/day (bid or qHS) depending on episode severity. *Week 2:* Increase to an **Initial Target Dose** of 2–3 mg/day (with more at HS), if tolerated and depending on episode severity. *Week 3 and beyond:* Assess for side effects and consider further increases in 1 mg increments until symptom remission or **Max Dose** of 6 mg reached. If qAM dosage is excessively sedating consider consolidating more of the dose to qHS. In severe cases of mania consider accelerating this titration schedule. **Typical Dosage Range:** 1–4 mg/day. *OF NOTE:* dosages above 4 mg/day are much more likely to be associated with EPS and it may be necessary to prescribe an anticholinergic medication to deal with Parkinsonian side effects (Benadryl 25 mg or Cogentin 1–2 mg PRN or scheduled). **Discontinuation:** Taper slowly to minimize withdrawal symptoms.

ONGOING MONITORING: EKG at target dose (at least once to assess QTc). *At 4 weeks:* Weight. *At 8 weeks:* Weight. *At 12 weeks:* Weight, blood pressure, fasting plasma glucose, fasting lipid profile. *Quarterly thereafter:* Weight. *Annually ongoing:* Waist circumference, weight, blood pressure, fasting plasma glucose, fasting lipid profile, and AIMS test.

GENERAL INFORMATION: Atypical antipsychotic. **FDA Indications:** Bipolar mania and mixed episode; Schizophrenia. **Off-Label Indications:** Depression augmentation, anxiety disorders augmentation. **Pharmacokinetics:** $T\frac{1}{2} = 3$ hrs for risperidone and 21 hours the active metabolite. **Common side effects (mania):** Parkinsonism (25 percent), sedation (11 percent), akathisia (9 percent), tremor (6 percent), dystonia (5 percent), nausea (5 percent). **Black-box warnings:** Increased mortality in elderly patients with dementia related psychosis. **Contraindications:** Known hypersensitivity reaction to the product. **Warnings and precautions:** Increased mortality and risk of cerebrovascular adverse events including stroke in elderly patients with dementia-related psychosis, NMS, TD, metabolic changes including hyperglycemia and diabetes, dyslipidemia and weight gain, hyperprolactinemia, orthostatic hypotension, increased risk of leukopenia, neutropenia and agranulocytosis, cataracts, potential for cognitive and motor impairment, seizures, dysphagia, **priapism,** body temperature dysregulation, patients with phenylketonuria, QTc prolongation, sudden cardiac death, cerebrovascular accident. **Metabolism/Pharmacogenomics:** Metabolized by 2D6 and 3A4 (minor). Use caution with 2D6 poor metabolizers. **Significant drug–drug interactions:** The dosage of Risperdal should be adjusted with 2D6 inhibitors (e.g., fluoxetine, and paroxetine) and enzyme 3A4 inducers (e.g., carbamazepine and St. John's wort). See the FDA label for specific recommendations. Check all drug-drug interactions before prescribing. **Pregnancy:** Category C. **Breastfeeding:** Excreted/Not recommended. **Dosage Form:** Solution, Tablet, Dispersible Tablet. **Generic available:** Yes. **Cost: ¢. FDA label information from Drugs @FDA for Risperdal 4.18.2014.**

Ziprasidone (Geodon)

ANTIPSYCHOTIC RISK PROFILE: EPS: Moderate; TD Risk: Mild; Sedation: Moderate; Metabolic Effects: Mild.

DOSING INFORMATION: Week 1: Assess baseline weight, waist circumference, blood pressure, fasting plasma glucose, fasting lipid profile, CBC (for baseline WBC), CMP for patients at risk of significant electrolyte disturbances should have baseline serum potassium and magnesium measurements and EKG (to assess QTc) and AIMS test. **Initiation for Schizophrenia: Start:** 20 mg twice daily (with food). *Week 2 and beyond:* Consider increasing dose by 20 mg bid per week as needed and tolerated. **Typical Dosage Range:** 20–80 mg bid. **Initiation for Bipolar Mania and Mixed Episodes: Start:** 40 mg bid (with food). *Week 2 and beyond:* Increase dose in 20 mg bid per week increments as needed and tolerated. In severe cases of mania consider accelerating this titration schedule (can increase to 60–80 mg bid on day 2 of treatment if needed). **Typical Dosage Range:** 40–80 mg bid (Mean ~60 mg bid). **Max Dose:** 100 mg bid. **Discontinuation:** Taper slowly to minimize withdrawal symptoms.

ONGOING MONITORING: EKG at target dose (at least once to assess QTc). Geodon should be discontinued in patients who are found to have persistent QTc measurements >500 msec. At *4 weeks:* Weight. *At 8 weeks:* Weight. *At 12 weeks:* Weight, blood pressure, fasting plasma glucose, fasting lipid profile. *Quarterly thereafter:* Weight. *Annually ongoing:* Waist circumference, weight, blood pressure, fasting plasma glucose, fasting lipid profile, and AIMS test.

GENERAL INFORMATION: Atypical antipsychotic. **FDA Indications:** Treatment of schizophrenia. Acute treatment of a mixed or manic episode in bipolar I disorder. Bipolar I disorder maintenance therapy as an adjunct to lithium or valproate. **Off-Label Indications:** Schizoaffective disorder. **Pharmacokinetics:** T½ = 7 hrs. **Common Side Effects (Schizophrenia):** Somnolence (14 percent), extrapyramidal symptoms (14 percent), nausea (10 percent), respiratory track infection (8 percent), dizziness (8 percent). **Black-box warnings:** Increased mortality in elderly patients with dementia related psychosis. **Contraindications:** Known hypersensitivity reaction to the product. Do not use in patients with (1) a known history of QT prolongation, (2) a recent acute myocardial infarction, (3) with uncompensated heart failure. Do not use in combination with other drugs that have demonstrated QT prolongation. **Warnings and precautions:** Increased mortality in elderly patient with dementia-related psychosis, QT prolongation and risk of sudden death, NMS, TD, metabolic changes including hyperglycemia and diabetes, rash, orthostatic hypotension, increased risk of leukopenia, neutropenia and agranulocytosis, seizures, dysphagia, hyperprolactinemia, potential for cognitive and motor impairment, **priapism**, body temperature dysregulation, cerebrovascular accident. **Metabolism/Pharmacogenomics:** Primarily metabolized by aldehyde oxidase. Some metabolism via 3A4. **Significant drug-drug interactions: methadone, and any medications that prolong the QT interval are contraindicated.** Potent 3A4 inhibitors (e.g., ketoconazole) and inducers (e.g., carbamazepine) increase and decrease Geodon levels by approximately 35–40 percent respectively. Check all drug-drug interactions before prescribing. **Pregnancy:** Category C. **Breastfeeding:** No data/Not recommended. **Dosage Form:** Capsule. **Generic available:** Yes. **Cost: $$. FDA label information from Drugs @FDA for Geodon 12.17.2013.**

References
Online resources
- Drugs@FDA http://www.accessdata.fda.gov/scripts/cder/drugsatfda/. Accessed April 30, 2014
- DailyMed http://dailymed.nlm.nih.gov/dailymed/about.cfm
- DrugBank http://www.drugbank.ca/
- PharmGKb https://www.pharmgkb.org/index.jsp
- LactMed http://toxnet.nlm.nih.gov/cgi-bin/sis/htmlgen?LACT Accessed April 30, 2014.

Article

Kroon, L. A. (2007). Drug interactions with smoking. *American Journal of Health-System Pharmacy, 64*(18), 1917–21.

Textbook

Thomas, W. (2012). *Medications and Mother's Milk 2012: A Manual of Lactational Pharmacology, 15th edition.* Hale Publisher.

Appendix: Resources

Screeners

Adult ADHD Self-Report Scale V1.1 (ASRS v1.1)
ADHD
http://www.hcp.med.harvard.edu/ncs/asrs.php

Alcohol Use Disorders Identification Test (AUDIT-C)
Substance use, alcohol, stimulants, opioids
http://www.integration.samhsa.gov/images/res/tool&uscore;auditc.pdf

Child Behavior Check List (CBCL)
ADHD
http://www.aseba.org/forms/schoolagecbcl.pdf (purchase required)

Clinical Institute Withdrawal Assessment of Alcohol Scale (revised) (CIWA-Ar)
Substance use, alcohol, stimulants, opioids
http://www.chce.research.va.gov/apps/PAWS/pdfs/ciwa-ar.pdf

Composite International Diagnostic Interview (CIDI-3)
Mood disorders, bipolar; Mood disorders, depression
http://medicine.yale.edu/intmed/vacs/instruments/3299&uscore;CIDI&
    uscore;Lifetime&uscore;Paper&uscore;Version&uscore;WHO-1.pdf

Confusion Assessment Method (CAM)
Mood disorders, depression; Psychotic disorders
https://www.healthcare.uiowa.edu/igec/tools/cognitive/CAM.pdf

Integrated Care: Creating Effective Mental and Primary Health Care Teams, First Edition.
Anna Ratzliff, Jürgen Unützer, Wayne Katon, and Kari A. Stephens.
© 2016 John Wiley & Sons, Inc. Published 2016 by John Wiley & Sons, Inc.

Conjoint Questionnaire for Alcohol and Other Drug Abuse (CAGE-AID)
Substance use, alcohol, stimulants, opioids
http://www.agencymeddirectors.wa.gov/Files/cageover.pdf

Drug Abuse Screening Test (DAST)
Substance use, alcohol, stimulants, opioids
http://www.integration.samhsa.gov/clinical-practice/screening-tools#drugs

Generalized Anxiety Disorder (GAD-7)
Anxiety disorders
http://www.phqscreeners.com/

Mini-Mental State Examination (MMSE)
Psychotic disorders
http://www4.parinc.com/Products/Product.aspx?ProductID=MMSE-2
   (purchase required)

Montreal Cognitive Assessment (MoCA)
Psychotic disorders
http://www.mocatest.org/

Pain Intensity and Opioid Interference Risk, Three-item scale assessment tool (PEG three-item scale)
Chronic pain
http://www.ncbi.nlm.nih.gov/pmc/articles/PMC2686775/pdf/11606_2009
   _Article_9 81.pdf

Patient Health Questionnaire (PHQ-2, PHQ-9, PHQ-15)
Mood disorders, depression
http://www.phqscreeners.com/

PTSD Checklist - civilian version (PCL-C)
Trauma disorders
http://www.mirecc.va.gov/docs/visn6/3&uscore;PTSD&uscore;CheckList&
   uscore;and&uscore;Scoring.pdf

UCLA PTSD Index Trauma Screen (UCLA PTSD Index)
Trauma disorders
http://www.ptsd.va.gov/professional/assessment/child/ucla-ptsd-dsm-iv
   .asp **(purchase required)**

Social Communication Questionnaire (SCQ)
Autism Spectrum Disorders
http://www.wpspublish.com/store/p/2954/social-communication-questionnaire-scq **(purchase required)**

Yale Obsessive Compulsive Checklist (Y-BOC)
Anxiety disorders
http://www.adaa.org/screening-obsessive-compulsive-disorder-ocd

Online Content Available

1. Collaborative Care Toolkit Inventory: Are you ready for Collaborative Care?
2. Building a Registry
   a. Sample Excel-based
   b. Registry Example
3. Collaborative Care Tools
   a. Initial Care Manager Assessment & Care Plan - Template
   b. Initial Care Manager Assessment & Care Plan Example
   c. Follow-up Care Manager Note - Template
   d. Follow-up Care Manager Note - Example
   e. Relapse Prevention Plan - Template
   f. Relapse Prevention Plan – Example
   g. Initial Psychiatric Consultant Case Review – Template
   h. Initial Psychiatric Consultant Case Review – Example
   i. Follow-up Psychiatric Case Review - Template
   j. Follow-up Psychiatric Case Review - Example
   k. Developing Primary Care Protocols for Psychiatric Emergencies - Guide
   l. Sample Safety Protocol and Credible Plan Questions
4. Care Manager, Job Description and Summary of Responsibilities
5. Psychiatric Consultant, Job Description and Summary of Responsibilities
6. Screeners (Quick Reference Links)
7. Brief Medication Prescribing Protocols

About the Authors and Contributors

Patricia Areán, PhD, is a Professor, clinical psychologist and expert in behavioral interventions for mood disorders in the Department of Psychiatry and Behavioral Sciences at the University of Washington.

Amy Bauer, MD, MS, Assistant Professor of Psychiatry and Behavioral Sciences at the University of Washington, is a consulting psychiatrist for primary care settings and conducts research to improve mental health services in primary care settings for underserved populations. She also co-leads a career development pathway for Psychiatry residents to foster workforce development in Integrated Care.

Carolyn Brenner, MD, is an Assistant Professor and Associate Residency Director in the University of Washington Psychiatry and Behavioral Sciences Department and the Medical Director of Harborview Mental Health & Addictions Services, where her clinical work focuses on people with severe mental illness and psychosis.

Joseph Cerimele, MD, MPH, is a psychiatrist at the University of Washington currently practicing Collaborative Care in primary care clinics. His Collaborative Care research focuses on improving quality of care for patients with bipolar disorder seen in primary care settings.

Lydia Chwastiak, MD, MPH, is an Associate Professor in the UW Department of Psychiatry and Behavioral Sciences and assists with education and training efforts at the AIMS Center. Her current clinical work includes psychiatric consultation to two care managers in a large urban safety net primary care clinic through the WA State Mental Health Integration Program.

Integrated Care: Creating Effective Mental and Primary Health Care Teams, First Edition.
Anna Ratzliff, Jürgen Unützer, Wayne Katon, and Kari A. Stephens.
© 2016 John Wiley & Sons, Inc. Published 2016 by John Wiley & Sons, Inc.

Susan E. Collins, PhD, is a licensed clinical psychologist and Associate Professor in the Department of Psychiatry and Behavioral Sciences at the University of Washington. She codirects the Harm Reduction Research and Treatment lab at Harborview Medical Center where she works with substance users and their communities to co-develop, evaluate and disseminate community-driven and patient-centered substance use programming.

Kyl Dinsio, MD, is an adult and geriatric psychiatrist providing psychiatric consultation in the Collaborative Care model and also direct consultation to primary care in the Swedish medical system in Seattle, Washington.

Mark H. Duncan, MD, is board certified in family medicine, adult psychiatry, and addiction psychiatry, and is an Acting Assistant Professor at the University of Washington providing psychiatric consultation in the Collaborative Care model for both rural and urban primary care clinics.

William French, MD, is board certified in child and adolescent and general psychiatry and is an Assistant Professor at the University of Washington and Seattle Children's Hospital. He provides pediatric Collaborative Care psychiatric consultation at local primary care clinics, school-based health centers, and through a statewide telephone program, which connects pediatric primary care providers with child psychiatrists.

David A. Harrison, MD, PhD, is an Assistant Professor in the Department of Psychiatry and Behavioral Sciences at the University of Washington School of Medicine and specializes in both inpatient hospital-based consult-liaison psychiatry as well as team-based integrative mental health care in the primary care setting.

Catherine Q. Howe, MD, PhD, is an Assistant Professor in the Department of Psychiatry and Behavioral Sciences at the University of Washington, where she provides psychiatric consultation in the integrated care model for both primary care and specialty care medical clinics.

Wayne Katon, MD, was a professor of Psychiatry, Director of the Division of Health Services and Epidemiology, and Vice Chair of the Department of Psychiatry and Behavioral Sciences at the University of Washington Medical School. He passed away March 1, 2015. Dr. Katon's original 1995 *JAMA* publication paved the way for the Collaborative Care model that is widely implemented in clinics today. The effectiveness of the model has since been tested in over 80 randomized controlled trials and has helped countless people receive better care.

Kim Kensington, PsyD, is a clinical psychologist who works with, and presents internationally about, adults with Attention-Deficit/Hyperactivity Disorder.

Ryan Kimmel, MD, is an Associate Professor in the University of Washington's Department of Psychiatry and Behavioral Sciences. He is the Medical Director of Hospital Psychiatry at the University of Washington Medical Center and teaches a psychopharmacology series for the Psychiatry Residency Training Program.

Evette Ludman, PhD, is a clinical psychologist and research scientist who has been studying innovative models of Collaborative Care for over 20 years.

Joseph O. Merrill, MD, MPH, is an Associate Professor of Medicine at the University of Washington who has broad clinical, research and teaching experience in primary care internal medicine and addiction medicine, including Collaborative Care treatment models.

Anna Ratzliff, MD, PhD, is an Associate Professor and serves as the Director for the Integrated Care Training Program in the Department of Psychiatry and Behavioral Sciences at the University of Washington. She works as a psychiatric consultant in safety-net primary care settings and develops strategies to educate members of integrated care teams.

Richard K. Ries, MD, is Professor of Psychiatry and Director of the Addictions Division in the University of Washington School of Medicine, Seattle, WA.

Andrew J. Saxon, MD, is Professor of Psychiatry in the Department of Psychiatry and Behavioral Sciences at the University of Washington. He is board certified with additional qualifications in addiction psychiatry by the American Board of Psychiatry and Neurology. Dr. Saxon's current research work is supported by the VA, the Department of Defense, and the National institute on Drug Abuse. His work involves pharmacotherapies and psychotherapies for alcohol, cocaine, tobacco, and opioid use disorders, as well as work in the co-occurrence of substance use disorders and posttraumatic stress disorder and on reducing homelessness.

Jennifer Sexton, MD, previously worked within the Collaborative Care model as a clinician teacher at the University of Washington; she now resides in Minneapolis, MN and works at Park Nicollet Mental Health Clinic.

Stacy Shaw Welch, PhD, is a practicing clinical psychologist specializing in anxiety disorders and a clinical researcher studying practical applications of evidence based treatments in community settings. She is the Clinical Director of the Evidence Based Treatment Centers of Seattle and on the adjunct faculty at the University of Washington.

Kari A. Stephens, PhD, is a practicing clinical psychologist specializing in working within integrated care teams and a clinical researcher studying dissemination of evidenced based behavioral practices in medical settings.

Jürgen Unützer, MD, MPH, is an internationally recognized psychiatrist and health services researcher. He is a Professor and Chair of Psychiatry and Behavioral Sciences at the University of Washington, where he also directs the AIMS Center, dedicated to "advancing integrated mental health solutions."

Index

abdominal pain, 159–160
Abilify. *See* aripiprazole
abstinence, motivation for, 144–145
acamprosate, 138–139
accountable practice, 7, 237
acetaminophen, 165, 167
action, 229
acute depression, 63, 66–67
acute mania, 63, 66–67
Adderall. *See* dextroam-
    phetamine/amphetamine
Adderall XR. *See* dextroam-
    phetamine/amphetamine
    ER
ADHD. *See* attention-deficit hyperactivity
    disorder
adjustment disorder, 35, 84
adolescents
    ADHD in, 181–183, 185, 188, 192–197,
      200
    depression in, 53
Advil. *See* ibuprofen
AEDs. *See* antiepileptic drugs
agonists, 140
alcohol use
    disorders, 35, 124–128, 132–133, 135,
      137–139, 144
    harm reduction ideas for, 144
    history, 8

suicide and, 128
withdrawal from, 137
alcohol-induced depressive disorder,
    35
Aleve. *See* naproxen sodium
alprazolam (Xanax, Xanax XR), 90
    prescribing protocols, 258–259
    quick reference, 242
Ambien. *See* zolpidem
amitriptyline (Elavil), 42, 242
amphetamines, 141
antagonists, 140–141
antianxiety medications
    black-box warnings for, 258–264
    dosing information for, 242–243,
      258–264
    in evidence-based
      psychopharmacology, 242–243,
      258–264
    monitoring of, 258–264
    prescribing protocols for, 258–264
    quick reference for, 242–243
    side effects of, 258–264
anticonvulsants, 67
antidepressants, 38–41, 45–50, 65–66,
    141
    anxiety treatment and, 95
    black-box warnings for, 247–257
    chronic pain and, 165, 167, 169

Integrated Care: Creating Effective Mental and Primary Health Care Teams, First Edition.
Anna Ratzliff, Jürgen Unützer, Wayne Katon, and Kari A. Stephens.
© 2016 John Wiley & Sons, Inc. Published 2016 by John Wiley & Sons, Inc.

chronic pain (*continued*)
  mental health and, 153, 159–160,
    170–171, 178
  nonpharmacological approaches to,
    165, 169–170
  pathophysiology of, 155
  patient and, 157–158, 161–162, 166,
    170, 172–173, 177–179
  PC and, 157, 162, 172–173, 177,
    179
  PCP and, 157–158, 162, 165–170,
    172–175, 177–179
  physical functioning and, 154
  provisional diagnosis of, 161–163
  psychosocial functioning and,
    154–155
  psychosocial interventions for, 166
  PTSD and, 160, 169
  questionnaire, 156
  referrals for, 174
  relapse prevention of, 178–179
  resources for, 179
  safety and, 155, 167
  substance-use disorders and, 153,
    159–161, 175
  suicide and, 155
  syndrome, 160
  therapeutic alliance for, 166
  treatment of, 89, 153, 159, 163–179,
    165
  types of, 159–160
  unspecified, 160
CIDI. *See* Composite International
    Diagnostic Interview
citalopram (Celexa), 88, 169
  prescribing protocols, 248–249
  quick reference, 241
clinical flowchart, 3–4
clinical impact
  of ADHD, 181
  of anxiety and trauma disorders,
    78
  of bipolar disorder, 55
  of challenging clinical situations,
    207–208
  of chronic pain, 153
  of major depression, 27–28

  of psychotic disorders, 101–102
  of substance-use disorders, 124–125
clonazepam (Klonopin), 90, 116
  prescribing protocols, 260–261
  quick reference, 242
clonidine (Catapres), 139, 195
clonidine ER (Kapvay), 195
CM. *See* care manager
cognitive behavioral therapy (CBT)
  for ADHD, 191, 196–197
  for anxiety and trauma disorders, 87,
    90–91
  for bipolar disorder, 69
  for chronic pain, 166, 169–170
  for depression, 39, 44
  for psychotic disorders, 119, 121
cognitive deficits, 103, 113
Collaborative Care team. *See also*
    challenging clinical situations;
    evidence-based behavioral
    interventions, for Collaborative
    Care team; evidence-based
    psychopharmacology, for
    Collaborative Care team; team
    goals
  assessment by, 8–15
  BHP on, 2–5, 7, 9–10, 15, 17–23
  blame among, 209
  bond, 229–230
  case example of, 10, 15, 18–21, 23
  functioning, 6
  introduction of, 3–6, 37
  overview of, 1
  partners, 3
  patient on, 1, 3–10, 14–23
  PC on, 2, 4–6, 9, 15, 18–22
  PCP on, 2–6, 8–11, 14–15, 17–23
  principles of, 19
  problematic behaviors of, 212–218
  roles, 1–3, 6
  skills, 3–8
  structure, 4
  support for, 224–225
  tasks, 5, 229–230
  tools, 3–8
  treatment by, 5, 15–23
  workflow, 3–4, 6